PROGRESS IN INFLAMMATION RESEARCH

PROGRESS IN INFLAMMATION RESEARCH

JAMES A. PITZER
EDITOR

Nova Biomedical Books
New York

For permission to use material from this book please contact us:
Telephone 631-231-7269; Fax 631-231-8175
Web Site: http://www.novapublishers.com

Library of Congress Cataloging-in-Publication Data
Progress in inflammation research / James A. Pitzer, editor.
p. ; cm.
Includes bibliographical references and index.
ISBN 1-59454-277-5 (hardcover)
1. Inflammation.
[DNLM: 1. Inflammation--physiopathology.] I. Pitzer, James A.
RB131.P745 2004
616'.0473--dc22 2004031123

Published by Nova Science Publishers, Inc. ✢New York

Contents

Preface

The process of inflammation, which causes the swelling and redness around a wound, is a vital part of the body's system for fighting off infections. When the body is hurt, the immune system produces chemical signals telling cells to multiply without dying, allowing skin to close over a gash, for example. Other chemicals spur the growth of new blood vessels to feed the recovering tissue. Scientists have linked inflammation to cancer and recently to heart disease in several ways. Doctors suspect that long-term inflammation or infection is involved in up to 20% of cancers, including those of the esophagus, colon, skin, stomach, liver, bladder, breast and some kinds of lymphoma.

C-reactive protein (CRP) is one of the acute phase proteins that increase during systemic inflammation. It's been suggested that testing CRP levels in the blood may be a new way to assess cardiovascular disease risk. A high sensitivity assay for CRP test (hs-CRP) is now widely available. This new book presents recent leading edge research from around the world.

As reported in chapter I, retroperitoneal fibrosis (RPF) is an uncommon collagen vascular or connective tissue disease known since 1905. Although difficult to establish, the incidence of RPF is certainly less than 1 per 10,000 patients. The disease is more frequent in man with a peak between 40 and 60 years of age. Retroperitoneal fibrosis may be divided into primary idiopathic (or chronic periaortitis) or secondary disease. The primary cases are associated with atherosclerotic inflammatory abdominal aortic aneurysms. Secondary cases may be related to various etiologies including medications, infections, connective tissue diseases or surgery, and malignancies. Irrespective of its cause, RPF should be regarded as a generalized inflammatory disease with different pathophysiological entities, which have at their end result, fibrosis involving the structures within the retroperitoneal space. Beside fibrosis, histology confirms the presence of a variable chronic inflammatory cell infiltrate. The majority of lymphocytes and macrophages as well as most vascular endothelial cells are HLA-DR positive. B and T cells are present with the majority of T cells of the T helper phenotype. In perianeurysmal RPF, the suggested mechanism, which has been confirmed by immunohistochemical studies, is a local immuno-allergic reaction to components of atherosclerotic plaques. The allergen may be a component of ceroid, which is elaborated within the atheroma. Once ruptured, atheroma liberates ceroids in peri-aortic tissue inducing a chronic fibrosing inflammatory reaction. Cytokines gene expression analysis shows the presence of IL-1α, IL-2, IL-4, IFNγ and IL-2 receptors. Adhesion molecules such as E selectin, ICAM and VCAM were also found in aortic inflammatory aneurysm, and may play a significant role in RPF pathogenesis. The clinical course is insidious with nonspecific symptoms and signs including at the early phase of the disease abdominal, back or flank pain, and weight loss accompanied with anemia and an erythrocyte sedimentation rate. In time, if ureteral obstruction increases progressively, features of renal failure predominate. Treatment of RPF should be adapted to the etiology and the clinical manifestations. The most commonly used approach is the association of long-term corticosteroids or immunosuppressive treatment with laparotomy or more recently laparoscopic ureterolysis and ureteral stenting. Accumulating data suggest that alternative treatment strategies such as tamoxifen or mycophenolate mofetil may be of interest in some cases. When diagnosed early and treated adequately, RPF does not affect survival. However, long-term follow-up is mandatory since late recurrences are not uncommon.

As reported in chapter II, Neuropathic pain is a serious clinical concern, arising from various diseases as well as physical damage of the central and peripheral nervous systems. Neuropathic pain is usually manifested as spontaneous pain, hyperalgesia and allodynia. Due to unclear mechanisms, the treatment is largely unsatisfactory. Therefore, it adversely affects the life quality of the patients. Damage of a nerve is inevitably followed by infiltration of blood-borne inflammatory cells into degenerating axons, of which macrophages are the principal effecter cells. Macrophages not only clean myelin debris, but also produce pro-inflammatory cytokines, growth factors and pain inducing mediators including prostaglandins (PGs). The role of this inflammatory event in the pathogenesis of neuropathic pain is yet to be determined. The purpose of the book chapter is to address morphological and pharmacological evidence that invading macrophage derived PGs are involved in the pathogenesis of neuropathic pain following nerve injury. In this chapter, it was demonstrated that PG synthesizing enzyme cyclooxygenase 2 (COX2) is dramatically up-regulated in invading macrophages in injured nerve of rats following partial sciatic nerve ligation (PSNL), chronic constriction injury of sciatic nerve (CCI) and spinal nerve ligation (SNL). COX2-IR cells appear as early as 3 days postlesion, reach a peak by 2 to 4 weeks, then gradually decrease and completely disappear by 7 month postlesion. PGE2 released from injured nerve explants is significantly increased compared to that from intact nerve explants. Both non-selective and selective COX inhibitors suppress the release of PGE2 from injured nerve explants. Perineural and intraplantar injection of a non-selective COX inhibitor ketorolac effectively relieves mechanical allodynia in rats treated with PSNL, CCI and SNL. Local ketorolac achieved maximum anti-allodynia during 2-4 weeks postlesion. Seven months after lesion, the anti-allodynia induced by local ketorolac completely disappears. Two and 4 weeks following PSNL, cell profiles expressing EP1, EP2, EP3, and EP4 receptors are dramatically increased in injured nerve. EP4 up-regulation in these cells is the most prominent and widespread among other EP receptors. About half of macrophages express EP1 and EP4, only small fraction of macrophages express EP2 and EP3. Local ketorolac significantly suppress the phosphorylation of cAMP responsive element binding protein and the expression of pain-related neuropeptide substance P, calcitonin gene-related peptide and dynorphin in the dorsal horn. The hypothesis that macrophage derived PGE2 is involved in the up-regulation of pro-inflammatory cytokine interleukin-6 (IL-6) in injured nerve was tested. PSNL increased IL-6 IR cell profiles in injured nerves and most of them were identified as invading macrophages. PGE2 and IL-6 releases from cultured cells derived from injured nerves are significantly increased and suppressed by both non-selective and selective COX2 inhibitors. Treatment with PGE2 further enhanced IL-6 release in a concentration- and time-dependent manner. A selective EP4 receptor antagonist and a protein kinase C inhibitor suppressed IL-6 release, suggesting that IL-6 induction by PGE2 is mediated through EP4 receptor and PKC signaling pathway. All above data suggest that PG over-production in invading macrophages in injured nerve is a common event following peripheral nerve injury, which contributes to the plasticity in signal transduction events and neuropeptide expression in primary sensory neurons and dorsal horn neurons and to the development of neuropathic pain during initial several months. Up-regulation of EP receptors in invading macrophages suggests that, through autocrine or paracrine pathways, over-produced PGE2 may influence macrophage functions, including pro-inflammatory cytokine production, which indirectly contributes to the development of neuropathic pain.

Chapter III focuses on, that stroke is among the most common diseases of advanced age becoming a steadily increasing financial healthcare problem in the industrialized world with the increasing longevity and aging of the population. To-date there are not effective therapeutics. However, during the last years promising findings suggest that systemic inflammation and neuroinflammation are central features in cerebrovascular disease. Atherosclerosis, the pathologic process underlying most coronary artery disease and the majority of ischemic stroke (IS) in humans, is an inflammatory process. Complex interactions occur between the classic risk factors for atherosclerosis and its clinical consequences. These interactions appear to involve inflammatory mechanisms both in the periphery and in the central nervous system (CNS). Inflammation in the CNS or in the periphery may be a risk factor for the initial development of cerebral ischemia. Peripheral infection and inflammatory processes are likely to be important in this respect. CNS inflammation is important in the pathophysiologic processes occurring in IS, subarachnoid hemorrhage and following hemorrhagic stroke. Stroke elicits an inflammatory response in the injured brain that is mediated by various factors, leading to the accumulation of inflammatory cells. The inflammatory reaction, which has a rapid onset and continues after the stroke, is thought to acutely contribute to the evolution of tissue injury. It appears that inflammation may be important both before, in predisposing to a stroke, and afterwards, where it is important in the mechanisms of cerebral injury and repair. Many compounds have been identified in stroke, which are known to promote and sustain inflammatory responses at local and systemic level, producing a neuroinflammatory response and a systemic acute phase response. The acute phase inflammatory response after stroke is a reflection of an unspecific Systemic Inflammatory Response Syndrome. Classic acute-phase reactants and body temperature are also modified in stroke, and may be useful in the prediction of events, outcome, and as therapeutic targets. The pentraxin C-reactive protein is found as a stronger and independent predictor of stroke risk and of prognosis in stroke patients when compared to other prothrombotic and inflammatory markers. Its synthesis is markedly upregulated in stroke. Since it as known to activate the complement cascade in an antibody-independent fashion and chronic activation can cause destruction of host tissue, this pentraxin may be important initiators of an autodestructive process influencing short-term and long-term prognosis of stroke patients. Considerable opportunities therefore exist for the development of novel therapies. Whether these targets will be useful in the development of therapies for the treatment of stroke in humans is far from clear, they provide fertile ground for scientific investigation. At the moment, beyond the traditional anti-thrombotic agents, statins and angiotensin-converting enzyme inhibitors may prove to be important additions to our armamentarium for stroke prevention and treatment acting partly via anti-inflammatory mechanisms.

Chapter IV presents endotoxemia and septic shock occurs with an exacerbated inflammatory response that damages tissue mitochondria. Skeletal muscle appears as one of the main target organs in septic shock, showing an increased nitric oxide (NO) production and an early oxidative stress. Heart and diaphragm mitochondria produced, in normal conditions, 67 and 24% of maximal total cellular NO production, and endotoxemic rats showed 30-90% increased mtNOS activity. Heart and diaphragm mitochondrial $O_2^{\bullet -}$ and H_2O_2 production were 2-3 increased during endotoxemia and Mn-SOD activity showed a 2 fold increase in treated animals. One of the current hypotheses for the molecular mechanisms underlying the complex condition of septic shock is that the enhanced NO production by mtNOS and cytosolic iNOS leads to excessive peroxynitrite production and protein nitration in the mitochondrial matrix, causing mitochondrial dysfunction and contractile failure. The available data suggest that impairment of mitochondrial function based on the pathological alteration of NO metabolism and on the production of toxic oxidative and nitrosative species, constitutes the basis of the molecular mechanism of organ dysfunction in endotoxic and septic shock. The high NO production by mtNOS and mitochondrial dysfunction, which are characteristics of the septic shock syndrome, open new avenues for experimentation and for the analisis of clinical data.

The gut has long been suspected of being involved in the pathology of shock. It seems to contribute in a significant way to the development of SIRS and sepsis. In the past, the proposed mechanisms of action were typically based on one of two hypotheses. The first hypothesis is that bacterial and endotoxin translocation in the intestine contribute to the morbidity and mortality seen in shock. The second hypothesis is that a major part of the pathophysiology seen in patients with sepsis is due to a production of secondarily induced inflammatory mediators. Chapter V's investigations have served to demonstrate that *pancreatic enzymes* appear to be directly involved in the production of the inflammatory mediators which have been observed in the blood of animals during experimental shock.

In: Progress in Inflammation Research
Editor: James A. Pitzer, pp. 1-38
ISBN 1-59454-277-5

Chapter I

Retroperitoneal Fibrosis, a True Inflammatory Disease: New Insights in an Old Entity

Pascal Meier[1,2*]***, Samuel Rotman***[3]***, Edouard Blanc***[1] ***and Michel Burnier***[2]

[1]Division of Nephrology, Department of Medicine, Hôpital de Sion; [2]Division of Nephrology, Department of Medicine; [3]Institute of Pathology, Centre Hospitalier Universitaire Vaudois/Switzerland

Abstract

Retroperitoneal fibrosis (RPF) is an uncommon collagen vascular or connective tissue disease known since 1905. Although difficult to establish, the incidence of RPF is certainly less than 1 per 10,000 patients. The disease is more frequent in man with a peak between 40 and 60 years of age. Retroperitoneal fibrosis may be divided into primary idiopathic (or chronic periaortitis) or secondary disease. The primary cases are associated with atherosclerotic inflammatory abdominal aortic aneurysms. Secondary cases may be related to various etiologies including medications, infections, connective tissue diseases or surgery, and malignancies. Irrespective of its cause, RPF should be regarded as a generalized inflammatory disease with different pathophysiological entities, which have at their end result, fibrosis involving the structures within the retroperitoneal space. Beside fibrosis, histology confirms the presence of a variable chronic inflammatory cell infiltrate. The majority of lymphocytes and macrophages as well as most vascular endothelial cells are HLA-DR positive. B and T cells are present with the majority of T cells of the T helper phenotype. In perianeurysmal RPF, the suggested mechanism, which has been confirmed by immunohistochemical studies, is a local immuno-allergic reaction to components of atherosclerotic plaques. The allergen may be a component of ceroid,

* Corresponding Author :Pascal Meier, MD,Division de Néphrologie,Centre Hospitalier Universitaire Vaudois (CHUV), 17, Ouest Bugnon, 1011 Lausanne, Suisse, Tel : +41/21.314.11.14, Fax : +41/21.314.11.39, E-mail : Pascal.Meier@chuv.hospvd.ch

which is elaborated within the atheroma. Once ruptured, atheroma liberates ceroids in peri-aortic tissue inducing a chronic fibrosing inflammatory reaction. Cytokines gene expression analysis shows the presence of IL-1α, IL-2, IL-4, IFNγ and IL-2 receptors. Adhesion molecules such as E selectin, ICAM and VCAM were also found in aortic inflammatory aneurysm, and may play a significant role in RPF pathogenesis. The clinical course is insidious with nonspecific symptoms and signs including at the early phase of the disease abdominal, back or flank pain, and weight loss accompanied with anemia and an erythrocyte sedimentation rate. In time, if ureteral obstruction increases progressively, features of renal failure predominate. Treatment of RPF should be adapted to the etiology and the clinical manifestations. The most commonly used approach is the association of long-term corticosteroids or immunosuppressive treatment with laparotomy or more recently laparoscopic ureterolysis and ureteral stenting. Accumulating data suggest that alternative treatment strategies such as tamoxifen or mycophenolate mofetil may be of interest in some cases. When diagnosed early and treated adequately, RPF does not affect survival. However, long-term follow-up is mandatory since late recurrences are not uncommon.

Key words: Retroperitoneal fibrosis, Aortic aneurysm, Renal failure, Immunosuppression, Atherosclerosis, Inflammation, Systemic disease

Introduction

Retroperitoneal fibrosis (RPF) is an uncommon disease first described in 1905 by Alberan [1] and further documented by Ormond in 1948 [2]. Retroperitoneal fibrosis is a descriptive term for a heterogeneous group of disease processes that can lead to urinary tract obstruction and renal failure (Table 1). The term “fibrosis” is a misnomer because RPF is an inflammatory process that may lead to fibrosis [3]. Macroscopically it is characterized by fibrosis of the retroperitoneum along the great vessels. The fibrosis spreads down to the pelvis or up to involve the mediastinum; it may also infiltrate the base of the mesenterium (Table 2) [1-5]. The hallmark of the disease and its main complication is ureteral entrapment, which is often silent and progressive. Retroperitoneal fibrosis is an unusual cause of renal insufficiency that presents as an insidious process. Typically, patients, who present with renal failure (75% of cases), have already progressed to bilateral urinary tract obstruction by the time of diagnosis. Clinically, they may present with flank pain, or urinary tract infection or may remain asymptomatic, with RPF detected during follow-up of their primary disease [6, 7]. Initially believed to represent an idiopathic, non-malignant, inflammatory process of unknown etiology [8-12], it later was proven that about one third of all cases are related to specific predisposing factors. The etiology of RPF is postulated to be secondary to either a local or systemic inflammation process. Indeed, it may be discovered in coexistence with other systemic inflammatory process such as mediastinitis, Riedel’s thyroiditis, sclerosing cholangitis, and orbital pseudotumor [13-16]. Some studies have shown an association of RPF with a local inflammation involving retroperitoneal structures, including the aorta, bowel, and lymph nodes [17]. The etiology, clinical presentation, and radiologic features of this condition are variable, and RPF is often misdiagnosed at presentation. Although surgery may relieve the ureteral obstruction, the etiology or the pathophysiological process remains present with the risk of local recurrence and the possibility of systemic effects including compression of other retroperitoneal structures. Additional medical treatment of RPF may be warranted including corticosteroids, immunosuppressive drugs and more recently tamoxifen.

Table 1. Classification of Retroperitoneal Fibrosis

Idiopathic		70%
Secondary		30%
Neoplasia		
	retroperitoneal metastasis	
	retroperitoneal tumor (urinary tract, lymphoma)	
	carcinoid tumor	
Retroperitoneal trauma		
	hemorrhage	
	enteritis	
	complicated diverticulitis	
	appendiceal abscess	
	urinary extravasation	
	irradiation	
	surgical intervention	
	iatrogenic	
Infectious agents		
	urogenital tract infection	
	tuberculosis	
	histoplasmosis	
	syphilis	
Medication[1]		
	methysergide, ergotamine, bromocryptine, pergolide, hydralazine, methyldopa, hydrochlorothiazide, reserpine, paracetamol, aspirin, phenacetin, codeine, beta-adrenergic blocking agents, haloperidol, sulpha-derivatives, anticonvulsivants, antihistamines, ampicilin, glibenclamide	
Others		
	vasculitis	
	Weber-Christian syndrome (paniculitis)	
	mesenteric paniculitis	
	fibrosclerosis	
	Crohn's disease	
	familial	

[1]firm data only exist for methysergide-induced RPF with more than 40 reported cases in the literature

Table 2. Localisations of Fibrosing Process

Retroperitoneum
Kidneys
Adrenals
Peridural space
Psoas
Pelvis
Bladder
Prostate
Genitalia (scrotum)
Uterus and adnexa
Intra-abdominal
Extra-hepatic biliary tree
Liver
Spleen
Pancreas
Small intestine, caecum, colon and rectum
Intra-peritoneal vessels
Thoracic
Mediastinum
Diaphragm
Lungs
Heart and pericardium
Aorta and pulmonary vessels

Epidemiology

The incidence of RPF is difficult to establish [9, 18, 19]. Based on recent systematic literature reviewing and on the annual number of new patients with RPF seen at the Centre Hospitalier Universitaire Vaudois (4 patients/year over the last 10 years) and at the Mayo Clinic, it is less than 1 per 10'000 patients [10, 11, 13, 20]. It is likely, however, that the pathologic entity of periaortic fibrosis occurs more frequently than it is clinically evident or diagnosed. Available histopathologic evidence suggests that asymptomatic periaortic fibrosis is present in 4.5% of patients undergoing surgery for abdominal aortic aneurysms [21, 22]. Retroperitoneal fibrosis is primarily a disease of middle-aged adults. However, RPF can occur in children and older adults (range 5-85 years old) [9, 12, 21, 23, 24]. The disease is more common in males than in females in most series (2:1 ratio). This is probably due to the higher incidence of symptomatic atherosclerotic disease of the aorta in men. There does not appear to be an ethnic predisposition for RPF, but there seems to be some genetic predispositions [16].

Clinical Features

The diversity of symptoms, most of which are not directly referable to the urinary tract, makes this condition a diagnostic problem to the non-specialist. Because of the non-specific nature of the presenting symptoms and the paucity of physical findings, there is often a significant delay from onset of symptoms to diagnosis. Retroperitoneal fibrosis should always be considered in the differential diagnosis of chronic renal failure [9, 10, 18-20].

During the inflammatory phase that represents the active and often the initial phase of the disease, symptoms are non-specific and source of diagnostic delay [9, 25-27]. Considering all the clinical signs related to RPF, it is worth mentioning the symptomatology of pain (Table 3) [25, 28] associated with general signs and non-specific digestive manifestations [29, 9]. The pain is often described as aching and dull in nature with no specific pattern of radiation or intensity. The pain is usually constant and not exacerbated by movement or palpation. Despite the frequent occurrence or ureteral obstruction, renal colic is rare. The pain may spread to the lower abdomen or to the thighs. Lumbar, groin or testicular pain has also been described [8, 25, 30]. Other unusual presenting symptoms include claudication, hematuria, Raynaud's phenomena, spinal stiffness, polyuria, and oliguria [12, 21, 31-35]. Less commonly, patients may present with fever or anorexia [36].

In a retrospective study, Baker *et al.* reviewed 60 patients presenting with an idiopathic RPF [30]. The commonest presenting symptoms were flank and abdominal pain, weight loss, nausea and polyuria.

In advanced cases, hypertension, uremia, vena cava obstruction, duodenal obstruction, or rectal obstruction can occur [6]. The physical examination in patient with RPF is usually unrevealing [12, 21, 25, 31-34, 37]. Sometimes, a painless abdominal mass around the umbilic or in the lower abdomen may be palpable (26%) [9, 12]. In this context, the presence of abdominal pain associated with signs of ureteral obstruction (i.e. urinary dysfunction, renal failure) and biological inflammatory syndrome should evoke an inflammatory aortic aneurysm [21, 38]. Swellings of the lower limbs and even of the scrotum are possible [9]. Although the median time from symptom onset to diagnosis is 3 to 4 months, this interval may be 1 year or longer in some patients [9, 12, 24]. In a more advanced stage, clinical signs are the consequence of the extension of fibrosis to various retroperitoneal, abdominal, pelvic and thoracic structures [38-42].

Table 3. Clinical Presentation

Usual	Occasional	Rare
Initial		
Back pain	Nausea and vomiting	Swelling of the lower limbs
Flank pain	Testicular pain	Intermittent claudication
Abdominal pain	Nycturia	Livedo reticularis
Gastrointestinal transit alteration	Oliguria - anuria	Raynaud's phenomenon
General signs and symptoms	General signs and symptoms	Polyuria
Fever	Discomfort	Hematuria
		Nephrogenic diabetes insipidus
Lack of appetite	Weight loss	Nephrotic syndrome
	Weakness	
Advanced		
Lower abdomen and groin pain	Abdominal mass	Inferior vena caval thrombosis
Anuria	Groin mass	Varices of the lower limbs
Arterial hypertension	Ischemia of the lower limbs	Testicular mass
Anorexia - nausea - vomiting	Swelling of the lower limbs	Testicular ischemia
Wasting		Hydrocele - varicocele
General state alteration		Impotence
		Jaundice
		Portal hypertension
		Rectal bleeding
		Superior vena caval syndrome
		Irritative cough
		Hemoptysis
		Pleural or pericardial effusion

The renal impairment due to urinary tract compression is found in almost 50% of the patients. The urinary output may be either preserved [38, 43], or significantly reduced [44]. Anuria is rarely found but is highly suggestive for RPF [45]. Nycturia that represents a classical symptom is somewhat uncommon and is found in only 13% of the patients with RPF. One can find along to high blood pressure, digestive symptoms such as anorexia, nausea and vomiting, all due to the severity of the renal impairment. Retroperitoneal extension of the fibrosis leads to extrinsic compression of the great vessels with concomitant risk of iliocaval thrombosis (2%) [40].

In summary, the clinical manifestations of RPF are polymorphous. However, the association of dorsal or lumbar pains and alteration of the general status to renal failure and inflammatory syndrome should suggest the diagnosis of RPF.

Laboratory findings are often non-specific. However, mild normochromic normocytic anemia and significantly elevated erythrocyte sedimentation rate (ESR) or C-reactive protein (CRP) are expected findings in more than 70% of the patients [9, 44]. Leukocytosis, thrombocytosis, hypergammaglobulinemia, antinuclear antibodies and rheumatoid factor are seen less commonly. Immune thrombocytopenia, anti-smooth muscle cells antibodies; c- or p-anti-neutrophil cytoplasmic antibodies, anti-cardiolipin antibodies or anti-beta 2 glycoprotein 1 antibodies have been described [18, 45-50]. The results of serum complement, immunoglobulin profile and lymphocyte subpopulations showed the typical features observed in any chronic systemic inflammatory disease. The variability of lymphocyte subpopulation abnormalities could be due to characteristic variations related to a particular phase of the disease. In chronic phase, azotemia occurs in almost 50% of the patients and may be associated with hematuria [9, 12, 20]. Although, some 30% of the patients with RPF have proteinuria, possibly as an expression of segmental glomerulosclerosis due to ureteral obstruction, the nephrotic syndrome is quite rare. Significant bacteriuria is uncommon [25, 51].

Imaging

Morphological investigations are essential to establish the diagnosis of RPF. The choice of the imaging technique depends on the clinical signs and the renal function (Table 4). In first intent, it might be an intravenous urography (IU), an abdominal CT scanner or an arteriography. In every case, a CT scanner or a magnetic resonance imaging (MRI) should be done at the initial phase or during the follow-up. Although MRI may have several theoretical advantages to CT scanner, its superiority has not yet been shown [52, 53]. Additional measures, such as nuclear medicine may provide useful information regarding the stage of disease, thus indicating a potential response to medical treatment.

The urographic appearance of RPF reflects the variable course of the disease. The scout film may demonstrate obscuration of the psoas margin, although this is an inconsistent finding [53]. The classic triad of urographic findings in RPF includes: delayed excretion of contrast material with unilateral (20%) or bilateral (68%) hydronephrosis [12]; medial deviation of the middle one third of the ureters (74-91%); and tapered narrowing of the ureters at the L4/L5 level [25]. Medial deviation of the ureters was at one time considered almost pathognomonic of RPF. However, it was found not to be a consistent finding in all patients as further investigation revealed that approximately 20% of normal patients demonstrate similar medial deviation of the ureters [12]. A review of 21 patients with RPF and 60 without RPF revealed no significant difference in the position of the ureters between the two groups [36]. Interestingly, the obstruction in RPF often appears minimal despite profound clinical renal failure [54]. This suggests that the obstruction in RPF relates to interference of the normal peristaltic activity of the ureter rather than mechanical obstruction.

This is supported by histological examination of the ureters, which often demonstrates the presence of edema and inflammation, but rarely shows fibrosis within the ureter [55]. Of note, unilateral stenosis of the ureter is uncommon [56, 57]. Though the complete spectrum of obstructive uropathy may be seen, acute obstruction is extremely rare in patients with RPF. In these cases, the nephrogram is increasingly dense with only marginal dilatation of the pelvicalyceal system. When the obstruction has been present for more than 5 days and up to 5 weeks, the nephrogram is no longer increasingly dense [55]. This is the post-acute phase of obstruction. As the disease progresses further, the typical changes of chronic ureteral obstruction have time to develop and the pelvicalyceal system then shows obvious dilatation. In some cases there may be no pelvivalyceal opacification in the presence of a persistent nephrogram and there are cases where a nephrogram faded without subsequent pelvicalyceal opacification. This is generally because the obstruction is complete. In case of anuria, IU showed either minimal dilatation of the pelvicalyceal system or no pelvicalyceal opacification. Analysis of follow-up urograms indicates that kidneys, which show minimal dilatation of the pelvicalyceal system often return to normal. Absence of a nephrogram may be associated with post-obstructive atrophy.

Retrograde pyelography is used to establish the diagnosis of RPF in patients with significantly impaired renal function in whom intravascular contrast material is contraindicated, or to further characterize the extent of the disease in patients in whom the diagnosis has already been made. The findings are generally the same as on IU with the added finding of nondistensibility of the ureters. Interestingly, small catheters can usually be passed retrograde up the ureters despite the extensive extrinsic fibrosis [58].

Lymphography has been used as a complimentary study to IU in making the diagnosis of RPF. The retroperitoneal lymphatics, due to their delicate structure, should be more easily compressible by RPF than the adjacent ureters. Thus, obstruction of the lymphatics should occur before compression of the ureters or major retroperitoneal blood vessels, and the changes of RPF should be detectable by lymphangiography before the change become apparent in the urinary tract [59]. Normal lymphangiograms, however, have been reported, even in patients with extensive RPF and severe ureteral compression [59]. The appearance of RPF on lymphangiography includes delay in passage of contrast through the iliac and para-aortic lymphatics, obstruction of lymphatic flow at the L3-4 level resulting in nonvisualization of the lymphatics above the fourth lumbar vertebra, filling of collateral lymphatic channels with reflux into lymphatic channels not normally visualized, and small irregular filling defects within the mesenteric and para-aortic lymph nodes [60]. In addition, the absence of lymph node metastases helps to exclude malignancy.

Venography of the inferior vena cava shows pathological findings in more than 50% and can be coupled to a renal phase, which can realize a veno-urography [8, 43]. Usually forward shifted, inferior vena cava shows more or less regular contours' narrowing and is accompanied with collateral circulation [33, 40].

Table 4. Imaging Procedures in Retroperitoneal Fibrosis Evaluation

Radiological Procedure	Typical findings	Comment
Intravenous urography / retrograde pyelography	Extrinsic ureteric compression at the level of L4/L5; hydroureteronephrosis; during retrograde studies, a 5F or 6F catheter can be usually be passed easily through the strictured area	Medial deviation of the ureter, long considered a classic sign of RPF, has been shown to be a normal variant
Ultrasound	Hypo/anechoic, well-demarcated and irregularly contoured retroperitoneal mass; hydronephrosis	Examination of the retroperitoneum may be precluded by abdominal bowel gas orobesity; RPF may be missed unless its presence is sought along the entire length of the prevertebral and paravetrebral areas
CT scanner	Paraspinal, well-demarcated retroperitoneal mass, isodense with the surrounding muscles; no displacement of psoas muscles or great vessels; degree of contrast enhancement correlates with activity of disease	May demonstrate possible causes of RPF; differenciating RPF from lymphoma, sarcoma or retroperitoneal adenopathy may occasionally be difficult
Magnetic resonance imaging	Low or medium intensity retroperitoneal mass similar to adjacent psoas muscle on T1-weighted images; vascular structure and patency well defined; high signal intensity or inhomogeneity of the plaqueon T2-weighted images may suggest malignancy	Avoids the risk of contrast medium related nephrotoxicity; benign RPF may also exhibit high signal intensity on T2-weighted images; multiplanar capabilities
^{67}Gallium scintigraphy	Avid uptake of ^{67}gallium in early, cellular stage of RPF; no uptake in late, fibrotic stage	May suggest potential beneficial effect of steroids; no information about actual fibrosis; limited experience
Fludeoxyglucose F 18 positron emission tomography	RPF exhibited low fludeoxyglucose F 18 uptake, whereas malignant lymphoma exhibited high fludeoxyglucose F 18 uptake. The fibrosis of postoperative scar tissue has low fludeoxyglucose F 18 uptake	Recent data suggest that increased thoracic or abdominal vascular fludeoxyglucose F 18 uptake is highly specific with a high positive predictive value for the diagnosis of periaortitis and FRP active phase; PET is an expensive imaging modality

Other procedures providing additional information, include colour doppler ultrasound, venography of the inferior vena cava and 123I-MIBG scintigraphy
RPF: retroperitoneal fibrosis. CT: computed tomography. PET: positron emission tomography

Ultrasound has been used as a less invasive means of diagnosing and following RPF. The ultrasound appearance of RPF is that of an extensive, well-defined, smooth-margined, retroperitoneal mass centered over the sacral promontory, enveloping the aorta and inferior vena cava circumferentially and extending laterally to involve the ureters with obliteration of the adjacent tissue planes [61]. The mass is generally hypoechogenic due to the homogeneity of the tissue [62]. There may be variable degrees of hydronephrosis and hydroureter. An attempt has been made to use doppler sonography to differentiate malignant from non-malignant RPF. However, there appear to be no distinguishing features [63]. Color doppler is useful in defining the tubular retroperitoneal structures. To distinguish between RPF and retroperitoneal mass, which could invade inferior vena cava, Kikumori *et al.* investigated the diagnostic value of intracaval endovascular ultrasonography (ICEUS) for invasion of the inferior vena cava by retroperitoneal tumors [64]. The sensitivity, specificity, and positive predictive values of ICEUS for the diagnosis of the inferior vena cava invasion were 100% for each statistical test. However, these values for computed tomography were 100%, 14%, and 25%, respectively. The authors conclude that ICEUS provides confirmatory information regarding tumor invasion of the inferior vena cava compared to RPF. This modality also can assist in formulating an operative strategy for retroperitoneal tumors.

The CT scanner is the modality of choice for the diagnosis and follow-up of patients with RPF. The appearance is quite variable. In typical cases, the attenuation value is similar to that of muscle and resemble to a well-marginated soft tissue mass with obstruction of the aorta and inferior vena cava. The mass tends not to displace the aorta anteriorly [65]. There is obliteration of the fat plane between the mass and the adjacent psoas musculature. The degree of intravenous contrast enhancement depends on the histological type and the stage of the disease (active vascular *vs* late avascular). The early, active inflammatory and vascular stage shows significant enhancement, whereas the avascular fibrotic late stage enhances very little. The distinction between early and late stage by CT scanner may allow disease progression or regression to be followed during medical management. In rare cases, RPF presents as a single or multiple soft tissue irregular masses and the differential diagnosis from primary retroperitoneal tumor or malignant lymphadenopathy is difficult [66]. Malignant causes cannot be differentiated from non-malignant causes only on CT findings [61]. However, CT scanner allows not only evaluation of the extent of the mass beyond the urinary tract, but also can show significant disease before the urinary tract is involved. Primary differential diagnosis for the CT scanner appearance of RPF includes retroperitoneal hemorrhage, primary retroperitoneal sarcoma, and metastases to the retroperitoneum. In addition, retroperitoneal amyloidosis has mimicked the appearance of RPF in at least one case [67]. Morphology is somewhat useful in the differentiation. Unlike RPF, most retroperitoneal neoplasms displace the ureters laterally and significant displacement of the aorta from the spine is suggestive of a malignancy, although a small amount of anterior displacement may occur in RPF [58, 68]. Retroperitoneal fibrosis, unlike malignant tumors, does not produce local bone destruction. Attenuation values and contrast enhancement have been less useful and are not believed to distinguish fibrosis from malignant tumor [69].

More recently, spiral computed tomography has been used to evaluate the postoperative response of RPF in patients with inflammatory abdominal aortic aneurysm (AAA) [70]. In this condition, spiral CT angiography may be an accurate and reliable method for evaluating inflammatory AAAs. These aneurysms are characterized by the presence of distinct concentric layers with patent endoluminal space surrounded by thrombus, which shows no contrast enhancement. The wall itself is enhanced with calcified plaques on the inner aspect. Beyond this is a layer of low-density fibrous tissue, which generally surrounds only the anterior and the lateral aspects of the aorta. Enhancement of the fibrotic mantle depends on the amount of contrast medium used, as well as the injection rate. Thus, spiral CT angiography can be used to evaluate the preoperative inflammation process and its extension, and to monitor the postoperative evolution of the fibrotic process.

The multiplanar capabilities of MRI, in addition to the advantages of not requiring iodinated contrast material and of providing better vascular definition, have made MRI an attractive option in the evaluation of RPF. Indeed, MRI has an excellent soft tissue contrast and great value in distinguishing benign from malignant fibrosis [71, 72]. Benign RPF has a homogeneous low signal intensity on both T1- and T2-weighted images. The presence of acute inflammatory process sometimes leads to areas of high signal intensity. If ill-defined margin heterogeneity and increased signal intensity on T2-predominant images are shown, histological study must be done to exclude malignancy [72, 73]. Retroperitoneal fibrosis is generally of low signal intensity on T1-weighted images and variable signal intensity on T2-weighted images depending on the stage of the disease. In the early active inflammatory phase of RPF, there is a high signal intensity on T2-weighted images as a result of local capillaries with leaky epithelial junctions and a high fluid content within the tissues. In the late fibrous phase of the disease, there is a characteristic low signal intensity on T2-weighted images consistent with the avascular, acellular fibrosis with low fluid content. Similarly, a decrease in the tissue edema in the early stage of the disease following corticosteroid therapy may be reflected as lower signal intensity on T2-weighted imaging. Thus, MRI may be able to assess response to therapy. Retroperitoneal fibrosis cannot be differentiated with certainty even intraoperatively from lymph node metastases or retroperitoneal sarcoma. It has also been described that progression of abnormal tissue and the extensive perirenal involvement are strongly indicative of malignancy [74]. The main conditions that must also be ruled out in cases of perirenal involvement are non-Hodgkin's lymphoma, histiocytosis, amyloidosis, and extramedullary hematopoiesis [75, 76]. T2-weighted images in these entities usually revealed moderate to high signal intensity masses. But as mentioned previously, this finding is not specific. Rapidly growing benign plaque or early stage of RPF may also exhibit heterogeneity with high signal intensities due to the increased water content caused by acute inflammation. Therefore, multiple tissue samples are necessary as very few malignant cells may be mixed with inflammatory ones [72]. Most authors agree that, although ultrasound and renal scintigraphy may contribute to the evaluation of patients with extensive RPF, CT is the preferred imaging method. The multiplanar imaging capability of MRI appears to facilitate assessment of disease extent.

Today, nuclear medicine has no definite role in the diagnosis or follow-up of RPF. Yet it may be promising in the differentiation of malignant from non-malignant RPF. Indeed, gallium 67 imaging has been used in selected patients with RPF but has not been adopted to any great extent [77, 78]. The rational for using gallium 67 is that this isotope binds to lymphocytes localized in the region of inflammation. Thus, a gallium 67 uptake may reflect the early inflammatory stage of the disease. Identification of somatostatin receptor sst2A on epithelioid cells, multinucleated giant cells, and a subset of $CD68^+$ macrophages in patients with periaortitis also suggests a potential role for indium 111–labeled octreotide in the noninvasive imaging of this condition [79]. Positron emission tomography (PET) is a nuclear imaging modality based on the differential uptake of 2-deoxy-2-(F-18)fluoro-D-glucose (fludeoxyglucose F 18), a glucose analogue, by actively metabolizing cells. Intravenously injected fludeoxyglucose F 18 is actively transported into cells in proportion to their rate of glycolysis. Because of its deoxy substitution, fludeoxyglucose F 18, unlike glucose, is unable to be further metabolized, and thus accumulates. This feature has been particularly well exploited in tumor imaging [80]. Because of the markedly increased glycolytic rate of malignant cells, high concentrations of fludeoxyglucose F 18 are achieved relative to surrounding normal tissues, representing areas of focal hypermetabolism that appear as "hot spots" on the resulting scintigram. The noninvasive PET scan has the advantage of being able to provide a visual representation of the whole body in a single image that can be displayed in axial, coronal, and sagittal orthogonal tomographic planes, as well as in a volume-rendered 3-dimensional rotational display. It can therefore demonstrate easily the overall extent, distribution, and metabolic activity of the vasculitic process. Positron emission tomography has an advantage over other imaging modalities in that the severity of metabolic abnormalities can be quantitated, with standardized uptake values providing an objective measure of disease activity, a useful parameter when evaluating response to therapy and disease recurrence. Recent data suggest that increased thoracic or abdominal vascular fludeoxyglucose F 18 uptake is highly specific with a high positive predictive value for the diagnosis of periaortitis and FRP active phase [81-84]. Presently, PET is an expensive imaging modality not readily available in most hospitals and is approved for use principally in oncologic conditions. Other uses may include vasculitis such as giant cell arteritis, extracranial vasculitis, periaortitis, true aortitis and potentially RPF. In a limited study of fludeoxyglucose F 18 PET, Kubota *et al.* observed that RPF exhibited low fludeoxyglucose F 18 uptake, whereas malignant lymphoma exhibited high fludeoxyglucose F 18 uptake [84]. The fibrosis of postoperative scar tissue has been demonstrated to have low fludeoxyglucose F 18 uptake.

Etiology

A wide variety of factors may incite fibrosis in the retroperitoneum. The list of associations appears to be growing since the introduction of this disease by Ormond (Table 5a,b). This includes hemorrhage; extravasation of urine; irradiation; surgery; non-specific gastrointestinal inflammation including Crohn's disease, appendicitis and diverticulitis; and numerous infections including tuberculosis, histoplasmosis, syphilis, and actinomycosis [9]. These etiologies result in fibrosis that has a variety of distributions and presentations, which are quite distinct, however, from the well-characterized periaortic fibrosis present in the RPF [12]. Although, the majority of cases of true RPF (± 70%) are considered idiopathic, it may be part of a systemic fibrosing disease such as fibrous pseudotumor of the orbit [85, 86], Riedel's thyroiditis [87, 88], sclerosing cholangitis [89], and mediastinal fibrosis (Table 1) [14, 41, 42]. Of all patients with RPF, 8% to 15% have additional fibrosis outside the peritoneum [35].

Case reports and clinical series have provided a lot of various medical conditions and pharmacological agents related to RPF [90-102]. While each of these factors may be associated with RPF, the pathophysiological mechanism responsible for the development of the fibrosis remains unclear.

Table 5a. Related Findings in 481 Patients with Retroperitoneal Fibrosis

Findings	Percentage
Idiopathic	67.8
Methysergide	12.4
All malignancies	7.9
Mediastinal fibrosis	3.3
Periaortic inflammation - arteritis	2.4
Mesenteric fibrosis	2
Sclerosing cholangitis	1.6
Abdominal aortic aneurysm	1.8
Crohn's disease	1.2
Thrombophlebitis	1
Riedel's thyroiditis	0.8
Other	5.3

From reference [12].

Much attention has focused on drug-related RPF but convincing evidence exists only for the long-term use of methysergide, an ergot-alkaloid used as prophylaxis for migrainous headache. Several case reports have also linked the long-term use of other ergot-alkaloids, notably bromocryptine, to RPF [48, 102-109]. Several beta-blocking agents have been implicated as a possible cause of RPF [109]. However, there is doubt whether beta-adrenergic blocking agents or other antihypertensive drugs cause RPF. It seems more likely that they were used to treat hypertension caused by unrecognized RPF [110]. Only anecdotal data are available for other drugs and the association is probably coincidental rather than causal.

In rare situation, RPF may be related to the so-called multifocal fibrosclerosis (less than twenty cases reported in the literature) [111]. This condition is characterized by fibrous lesions occurring in various sites, and presenting in the form of orbital pseudotumor, RPF, Riedel's thyroiditis, sclerosing cholangitis, mediastinal and pulmonary fibrosis, fibrosis of the parotid and lacrimal glands.

The incidence of co-existing RPF and aortic aneurysm (perianeurysmal fibrosis), which is certainly underestimated, ranges from 4% to 12% [21, 23, 39, 112-114].

The occurrence of RPF in patients with connective tissue diseases or autoimmune phenomena is frequently mentioned (Table 5b) [46, 99, 115-117]. The concomitant presence of generalized vasculitis with RPF, the similarity between idiopathic RPF and other sclerosing diseases and the beneficial effect of corticoids in some cases suggest that fibrosis may be a local manifestation of a systemic connective tissue disease [22, 98-100]. Using the vasculitis' histological criteria (vessel wall infiltration by acute or chronic inflammatory cells, fibrinoid wall necrosis), Littlejohn *et al.* found 37 cases of vasculitis and RPF in a review of

Table 5b. Pathological Findings Related to Retroperitoneal Fibrosis

Fibrosing pathologies
Orbital pseudotumor
Riedel's thyroiditis
Sclerosing cholangitis
Pulmonary fibrosis
Pancreas pseudotumor
Collagen diseases, vasculitides and systemic autoimmune diseases
Periarteritis nodosa
Giant cell arteritis
Henoch-Scönlein purpura
Takayasu's arteritis
Systemic sclerosis
Systemic lupus erythematosus
Sjogren's syndrome
Ankylosing spondylitis
Recurrent polychondritis
Rheumatoid arthritis
Granulomatous diseases
Sarcoidosis
Primary biliary cirrhosis
Wegener's granulomatosis
Autoimmune phrnomena[1]
Positive direct Coombs
Anti-nuclear antibody positivity
Hypocomplementemia C3, C4
ANCA positivity
Others
Uveitis
Membranous glomerulonephritis
Hypereosinophilic syndrome
Immune thrombocytopenia
Sickle cell anemia
Marfan's syndrome
Cryoglobulinemia

[1]autoimmune phenomena detectable but not definite systemic disease.
ANCA: anti-neutrophil cytoplasmic antibody

500 cases, giving a prevalence of 7% [16]. As the authors mentioned, this prevalence represents the tip of the iceberg as many cases were inadequately reported. Most vasculitic changes occurred in vessels situated within the inflammatory tissue of the retroperitoneum. If the mediastinum or thyroid are involved in a similar process, vasculitis could also be seen in these areas (multifocal fibrosclerosis). Involvement of vessels outside these tissues constituted systemic vasculitis and could include almost any organ system such as the kidneys, the heart, the mesentery, the liver, the gall bladder, the testes, the prostate, the spleen and the adrenals. A review of these reports indicates that systemic vasculitis occurred in about 33% of all patients with RPF, and suggests that vasculitis in the retroperitoneal tissues may not simply be secondary to local inflammation, but resulted from a primary vasculitic process.

Some studies investigated a possible genetic predisposition by testing for the HLA-B27 immunophenotype, which might be positive in 30% to 50% of cases of RPF. The absence of familial cases suggests a polygenic hereditary mechanism, based on multiple genetic factors [8, 16]. However, the relationship between sacroiliitis, the major histocompatibility complex antigen HLA-B27 and RPF remains unclear, and needs further studies.

Approximately 8% is associated with malignancy, mostly metastatic disease from lung, breast, prostate, or digestive tract, and malignant lymphoma or sarcoma [9, 12]. Retroperitoneal fibrosis has been associated with both benign and malignant carcinoid [9, 12, 112] and in rare cases with cervix carcinoma [118] and tumors of the urinary system [119]. The fibrosis in these cases is the result of the intense desmoplasia following the tumor infiltration of the retroperitoneum.

Pathological Findings

Imaging alone can never provide absolute proof of the diagnosis, which depends upon histology. CT-guided biopsy may be feasible and appropriate in some patients but in others open biopsy will be necessary to confirm the diagnosis beyond doubt. The histological appearance of RPF is of a non-specific inflammatory process and varies according to stage and activity of the disease [120, 121]. The common denominator in all of the cases of RPF is the exuberant formation of fibrous tissue, which compresses nearby hollow organs and vessels [10, 122]. Idiopathic RPF belong to a family of inflammatory diseases of similar morphological appearance (including inflammatory aneurysm, idiopathic mediastinal fibrosis and perianeurysmal fibrosis) now called chronic periaortitis [115, 123-125]. A common characteristic is represented by marked adventitial infiltration by lymphocytes, plasma cells and fibrosis around advanced aortic atherosclerotic plaques.

Gross Pathology

Retroperitoneal fibrosis represents a white, dense and fibrous plaque that is usually found at the level of the aortic bifurcation, near the sacra promontory. As it progresses, RPF engulfs the aorta and inferior vena cava, and spreads through the retroperitoneum along the great vessels within the pelvis. Less frequently, the plaque extends anteriorly along the celiac trunk. The fibrosis often extends laterally to the ureters and the psoas muscles, and is responsible for the hydronephrosis, which represents the hallmark of the disease. One or both ureters may be involved at any point along their course, though usually in the middle one third. Although RPF is usually localized between the renal hila and the pelvic brim, it may be contiguous across the diaphragm with mediastinal fibrosis [25, 26, 126, 127]. No specific macroscopic feature exists to distinguish RPF secondary to malignancy (malignant RPF) from non malignant or idiopathic RPF.

Histology

Microscopically, the disease appears as a subacute, non-specific inflammatory reaction in fibrous tissue (Figure 1a-d). Early in the disease, there are collagen bundles interspersed with lymphocytes, pleomorphic cells, polynuclear leucocytes, eosinophils, and macrophages [126]. Giant cells, granulomas and histiocytes can also be seen in the earlier inflammatory stage of the disease [122, 128]. Later stages of the disease manifest as an acellular fibrosis [18, 129]. Malignant RPF is histologically indistinguishable from idiopathic RPF. Only the demonstration of the small islands of tumor cells within the fibrotic mass can indicate malignancy as the probable cause of RPF. Furthermore, the differential diagnosis to distinguish between RPF and a sclerosing lymphoma may be sometimes challenging. Retroperitoneal fibrosis characteristically discloses areas of dense, homogeneous, eosinophilic, and hypocellular connective tissue interlaced with areas where the fibrous tissue is of the immature type containing numerous lymphocytes, plasma cells, and fewer eosinophils, with normal widely spaced germinal centers. Sclerosing lymphomas involving the retroperitoneum are usually B-cell lymphomas of follicular center cell origin, disclosing a monotonous population of small-cleaved cells or large cleaved and noncleaved cells. These lymphomas may have a follicular or diffuse pattern [130]. In these cases, the immunostains for kappa and lambda light chains may help to establish the diagnosis. To exclude the possibility of Hodgkin's disease and sclerosing retroperitoneal lymphoma, other immunostains such as c-Kit, Leu-M1, Ki-1 and LCA may be helpful [130, 131].

Chronic periaortitis is usually considered to be a result of atherosclerosis. Its location is not limited to the abdominal aorta, and has been described in its thoracic portion [132]. The pathology described in chronic periaortitis shows ulcerated fibrolipid plaques with thinning of the media [132, 133]. The adventitia contains chronic inflammatory cells consisting of lymphocytes, plasma cells, giant cells and granulomas with varying degrees of fibrosis (Figure 2a-e). Similar inflammation and fibrosis may be seen in the coronary arteries. This inflammation may range from a minimal inflammatory response in a non inflammatory aneurysm to an exaggerated exudative reaction seen in inflammatory lesions. It is uncertain as to the cause of this exaggerated response in certain individuals. Predisposing environmental or constitutive factors have not been evaluated.

Pathogenesis

Apart from direct causes such as retroperitoneal hemorrhage or metastases, the pathogenesis of RPF may be presented as a chronic inflammatory response to a number of possible inciting factors, including medication, infection, and systemic processes such as vasculitis and systemic lupus erythematosus (Tables 1 and 5a,b). An immune phenomenon may play a role in the pathogenesis of malignant RPF, involving both tumor antigens and antigens associated with tumor growth but unrelated to tumor cells. The mechanism by which drugs cause RPF remains unknown. Methysergide acts as a strong serotonin-antagonist. By analogy to the carcinoid tumor, rebound release of serotonin following a prolonged intake of this drug might be possible. However, this does not explain the association of RPF with other drugs, which seemed to serve as haptens, thereby inducing a hypersensitivity or autoimmune reaction.

Reported familial occurrence of RPF and presence of HLA-B27 in some patients with idiopathic RPF suggest that the liability to develop this disorder may sometimes be governed by genetic factors [16, 134-136]. However, no abnormal loci have been demonstrated.

However, in a subset of patients with so-called idiopathic RPF, it may be a local complication of advanced systemic atherosclerosis [14, 51, 123, 132, 137]. In this respect, the term "idiopathic RPF" should probably be abandoned in favour of "chronic periaortitis" or "auto-allergic periaortitis" as much more is now known of the etiology of the condition thanks in particular to the work of Mitchinson and Parums. In 1970, Mitchinson [14] suggested that the condition may represent an auto-allergic reaction to several components of atheromatous plaques confirmed by immunohistochemical studies [132, 138]. Chronic periaortitis is present to a variable degree in association with atherosclerotic abdominal aortic aneurysms. In contrast with atherosclerotic plaques where the intimal layer is mainly affected, abdominal aortic aneurysms are characterized by the formation of inflammatory infiltrates, predominantly in the media and adventitia. In contrast with primary atherosclerosis, where T lymphocytes are exclusively present, the adventitial infiltrates in abdominal aortic aneurysms contain a large number of both B cells and T cells. Many of the lymphocytes are activated and proliferating, and germinal centers are common. The majority of lymphocytes and macrophages and most vascular endothelial cells are HLA-DR positive. Ki67 and BerH2 staining is found in B cells and T helper cells, indicating that these cells were proliferating and activated. These findings compare with the characterization of inflammatory cells associated with "inflammatory aneurysms" and with the inflammatory cells present in the spectrum of inflammation seen as a complication of advanced atherosclerosis. Except for the degree of aortic dilatation, the histopathological findings appear similar between RPF and inflammatory aortic abdominal aneurysms. This could indicate that mechanisms involved in aneurysm formation link atherosclerosis to retroperitoneal fibrosis.

The concept that atherosclerosis is a specific form of chronic inflammatory process resulting from interactions between plasma lipoproteins, cellular components (monocyte/macrophages, T lymphocytes, endothelial cells and smooth muscle cells) and the extracellular matrix of the arterial wall is now well accepted (Figure 3). Histologically, atherosclerotic lesions from the early-stage (fatty streak) to more complicated lesions possess all the features of chronic inflammation. It has been demonstrated that atherogenic lipoproteins such as oxidized LDL, remnant lipoprotein (beta-VLDL) and lipoprotein-a play a critical role in the pro-inflammatory reaction, whereas high density lipoprotein, anti-atherogenic lipoproteins, exert anti-inflammatory functions. In cholesterol-fed animals, the earliest events in the arterial wall during atherogenesis are the adhesion of monocytes and lymphocytes to endothelial cells followed by the migration of these cells into the intima. It has been shown that these early events in atherosclerosis are triggered by the presence of high levels of atherogenic lipoproteins in the plasma and are mediated by inflammatory factors such as adhesion molecules and cytokines in the arterial wall. The development of genetically modified laboratory animals has provided a powerful approach for dissecting individual candidate genes and studying their cause-and-effect relationships in lesion formation and progression. It appears then that chronic periaortitis is caused by an auto-allergic reaction to oxidized LDL formed in the developing atheromatous plaque and which is normally sequestered unless the media is breached. In 1990, Parums *et al.* reported the presence of serum antibodies (mostly IgG) to oxidized LDL or ceroid (usually both) [139, 140]. These antibodies would be produced when the aortic media surrounding the atherosclerotic plaques is breached so that the antigen can be recognized by lymphocytes [139]. This proposed cause explains much. For instance, the occasional association of chronic periaortitis with mediastinal fibrosis is explicable on the basis that the latter condition is simply a similar periaortitis involving the thoracic aorta [140, 141]. It is probably no coincidence that a drug such as methysergide, which has ergot like activity and hence causes arterial spasm, has been associated with the condition in a few cases. Beside the presence in the inflammatory mass of predominantly B cells, T cells and especially T-helper ($CD4^+$) cells were commonly observed [115, 124, 125, 142, 143]. Other inflammatory leucocytes such as plasma cells, polynuclear cells and macrophages were also present. Once entrapped in the atherosclerotic plaque, the macrophages become lipid-laden foam cells and secrete interleukines (ILs) and chemokines that cause cell proliferation (e.g. lymphoctes and fibroblasts). Studies with appropriate antibodies to IgG and IgM locate these immunoglobulins to areas within the atheromatous plaques where the oil-red O technique shows the presence of ceroid. The dominant immunoglobulin is IgG. Ceroid laden macrophages have been identified in the adventitia and nearby lymph nodes in chronic periaortitis [144].

Abdominal aortic aneurysms differ from aortic atherosclerosis by extensive degeneration of the elastic media with loss of elastin and smooth muscle cells, and adventitial inflammation. Recently, insight has been gained in the role of potential mediators of these degenerative and inflammatory processes. The inflammatory process appears to begin at the *vasa vasorum* in the adventitia, where numerous inflammatory cells are recognized around *vasa vasorum*. An accelerated reaction of inflammatory cytokines and chemokines, such as intercellular adhesion molecule-1 (ICAM-1), vascular cell adhesion molecule-1 (VCAM-1), monocyte chemoattractant protein-1 (MCP-1) and others were demonstrated in and around *vasa vasorum* [145]. In parallel with the appearance of these cytokines chemotactic activity of T-cells and macrophages appears to take place. Destruction of smooth muscle cells, elastophagia and collagenous fibrosis become more noticeable with cellular infiltration into the media and the intima.

Vasa vasorum capillaries may facilitate leukocyte entry into lesions, perfuse the vessel wall beyond diffusion limits from the artery lumen, or cause intraplaque hemorrhage [146]. *Vasa vasorum* are more prevalent as vessel wall layers increase, interruption of *vasa vasorum* results in medial necrosis, and diffusible tracers localize near these capillaries. This single function predicts that plaque neovascularization would correlate with lesion size and be distributed at the lesion base. Plaque neovascularization may also function as conduits for the entry of leukocytes and plasma components into the artery wall in addition to the endothelium on the artery surface. The endothelium of intimal capillaries shows increased E-selectin, ICAM-1, and VCAM-1 levels compared with the artery surface [146]. Recent work on adhesion molecules and human atherosclerosis showed that as aortic atherosclerosis develops, ICAM-1 expression is associated with intimal lymphocyte and macrophage populations, and that E-selectin and VCAM-1 expression in the aortic adventitia increases with the severity of the atheromatous plaque as well as the development of adventitial inflammatory cell infiltrates [147, 148]. Ramshaw *et al.* have shown that ICAM-1 and especially VCAM-1 correlated strongly with the adventitial mononuclear cell infiltrate suggesting its importance in the development of this B-cell dominant chronic inflammatory response [148]. The expression of these adhesion molecules are induced by pro-inflammatory cytokines such as IL-1α, IL-2, IL-4, IFNγ and IL-2 receptors [137].

In the media of abdominal aortic aneurysms, the density of smooth muscle cells is significantly decreased. Apoptosis with an increased expression of *p53*, which is itself a potential mediator of cell cycle arrest and programmed cell death, has been demonstrated in medial smooth muscle cells [149]. Another characteristic of abdominal aortic aneurysms is a change in the cellular composition of the outer aortic wall associated with infiltration of the media and adventitia by vascular dendritic cells that are similar to Langerhans cells and interdigitating cells [150]. They express both CD1a and S-100 protein, which are markers for their immunohistochemical identification, and like other dendritic cells, they also express HLA-DR, VCAM-1 and ICAM-1. This suggests that interactions between vascular dendritic cells and T cells might lead to the activation of T cells.

Structural alterations of the aortic wall seen in abdominal aortic aneurysms result in part from degradation of the macromolecules, collagen and elastin. These changes are associated with excessive production of matrix metalloproteinases (MMPs) [151-153], which are assumed to orchestrate the widespread matrix destruction. As with many chronic disease processes, descriptive human studies are enlightening but often fail to distinguish important causal factors from epiphenomena. Animal models are essential to precisely define to the mechanisms of aneurysm formation. Murine models are particularly useful because of the ability to produce and access a wide array of mice with targeted gene deletions. Recent work in transgenic mice has raised the possibility that MMPs may have proaneurysm activity [154]. The inflammatory infiltrate in human abdominal aortic aneurysm tissue is spatially related to destruction of extracellular matrix macromolecules. The inflammatory infiltrate is thought to play an etiologic role in aneurysm formation by direct local production of matrix-degrading enzymes and production of cytokines that induce resident mesenchymal cell production of MMPs [155]. Proinflammatory cytokines secreted from macrophages enhance MMP production by human vascular smooth muscle cells [155-157], and many of these cytokines are present within abdominal aortic aneurysm tissue [158]. Recent findings suggest that both the local mesenchymal cell expression and the macrophage expression of MMPs are required for aneurysm formation [159].

Both fibrillar collagen and elastin are highly organized in the lamellar structure of the aortic media. One potential mechanism for the complementary role of MMP-2 and MMP-9 is that MMP-2 is primarily acting as a collagenase initiating cleavage of the triple helix into one-quarter and three-quarter lengths [160]. The single α chains could then be degraded by MMP-9, releasing the coiled elastin and causing it to become fattened and attenuated. Rupture and expansion rates of abdominal aortic aneurysms have been linked to MMP-2 and MMP-9 levels in tissue [161] and plasma [162]. Such observations appear consistent with the increased medial atrophy observed within abdominal aortic aneurysms, because activated MMPs may weaken the media by causing destruction of elastic and collagen fibers and smooth muscle cells [163].

Cells of the immune system are known to be sources of mediators regulating fibroblast proliferation [61, 119]. As in other fibrotic disorders (e.g. sclerodermia, idiopathic pulmonary fibrosis, chronic graft-versus-host disease) [61, 164], the dramatic proliferative response of fibroblasts may be mediated by abnormal secretion or response to growth factors released at sites of chronic inflammation [61, 119]. Eosinophil-derived products, shown to be present in idiopathic RPF as well as in related disorders (sclerosing cholangitis, sclerosing mediastinitis and idiopathic pulmonary fibrosis), may also stimulate fibroblast proliferation [165].

Although these findings clearly demonstrate the inflammatory nature of RPF, several questions remain unanswered. Since only a small percentage of patients with atherosclerosis appear to develop clinical disease (only 5% of atherosclerotic aneurysms are inflammatory) [133, 166], there may be other factors such as intrinsic immune responsiveness, HLA genotype, antigen processing and localization of antigen, important in the expression of clinical disease. Although autoantibodies to ceroid have been demonstrated in patients with clinical and subclinical chronic periaortitis, they were also seen in a high percentage of elderly patients without demonstrable disease and in patients with atherosclerosis but without clinical disease, indicating that antigenic exposure is common whereas clinical disease is rare. This may reflect the heterogeneous response of a population to an antigenic challenge, or it may represent an epiphenomenon seen in advanced atherosclerosis with no pathophysiologic significance. On the other hand, the described association with systemic lupus erythematosus and other connective tissue disease supports the immunologic theories of RPF [16, 22, 167, 168]. These conditions have histopathologic similarities to chronic periaortitis, such as marked adventitial inflammation, typical atherosclerotic lesions, and the loss of smooth muscle fibers [14, 169]. Vasculitis of the aortic *vasa vasorum* and periaortic retroperitoneal vessels may lead to the development of chronic periaortitis, by promoting atherosclerosis and aneurysm formation, and its extension into the adjacent retroperitoneum could give rise to the fibroinflammatory reaction typical of chronic periaortitis. Moreover, the beneficial effect of corticosteroid treatment and sporadic reports of benefit from immunosuppressive agents such as mycophenolate also fit the hypothesis that chronic periaortitis represents an auto-allergic reaction to components of atheromatous plaques.

Management

To a clinician, the management of RPF remains a problem. Difficulties are encountered in securing the diagnosis, providing the most appropriate and effective treatment, assessing the prognosis, and devising methods to prevent the illness and its progression (Figure 4). It is important to know about a group of multisystem diseases of unknown cause that may involve the kidneys. Prompt diagnosis of RPF preserves renal function, prevent other organ involvement, and relieve symptoms. Treatment of RPF has traditionally been approached in a surgical manner. There are many reasons for this. First, the ureteral obstruction should be relieved mechanically as quickly as possible as there is a risk of severe renal impairment. Second, an open biopsy is useful to rule out malignant RPF. Nevertheless, surgical treatment should not be undertaken without an analysis of the RPF etiology and a careful evaluation of the opportunity to adjunct an immunosuppressive drug usually corticosteroids. Indeed, the therapeutic approach to RPF includes the removal of any identifiable inciting agents, preservation of renal function and suppression of inflammatory process. However, no controlled therapeutic trials have been performed and, although rare, spontaneous regression may occur.

Surgical Management

In cases of severe renal failure, the first approach consists of retrograde ureteral catheterization or percutaneous nephrostomy [170-172]. Although retrograde insertion of catheters is usually easy to achieve, great care should be taken to prevent retrograde infection in such cases. Percutaneous nephrostomy may be the preferred method as this technique is associated with less risk of infection and because evaluation of response to treatment is easily achieved by descending ureterography through the nephrostomy tube or subsequent clamping of the tube, which can be removed as soon as the ureter is found to be patent. The second approach consists of relieving the obstruction by placing an ureteral stent. The advantages of stenting and corticosteroids include avoiding surgery with its attendant risks and scar, and reducing or eliminating the need for inpatient care. A major disadvantage of the stent/corticosteroid approach is that corticosteroid therapy does not always sufficiently reduce the fibrotic mass to relieve the obstruction. Under these circumstances, repeated stent changes will be required and the likelihood is that the patient will receive prolonged, relatively high-dose corticosteroid therapy in vain. Beside the emergency cases, the standard approach for RPF conventionally consists of open biopsy and surgical relief of obstruction by ureterolysis, with or without omental wrapping of the displaced ureter or ureters followed or not by corticosteroid therapy aimed at shrinking the fibrotic mass [173-177]. More recently, several authors report successful laparoscopic ureterolysis and intraperitonealisation of the ureter [178, 179]. In a review analyzing 430 patients with RPF, Wagenknecht *et al.* showed that 70% of the cases were treated surgically by ureterolysis alone or associated with laterocolic transposition of the ureter (Table 6) [175]. When ureterolysis was performed, atonia was usually temporary, and the risk of partial necrosis varied around 5%. After three years follow-up 40% of the cases showed bilateral normalization of the ureteral stenosis, and renal function remained normal in 82% of the cases after 1-25 year's follow-up.

Table 6. Management of 430 patients with RPF [1]

Treatment	Primary cases	RPF %	Secondary cases	RPF %	Malignant cases	RPF %	**Total cases**	**%**
No treatment	3	1	52	26	0	0	**55**	**13**
Exploratory laparotomy	5	3	5	3	14	29	**24**	**6**
Corticosteroids therapy alone	21	11	28	14	0	0	**49**	**11**
Surgery and corticosteroids therapy	77	42	82	42	4	8	**163**	**38**
Surgery alone	79	43	30	15	30	63	**139**	**32**
Total	**185**	**100**	**197**	**100**	**48**	**100**	**430**	**100**

[1]According to Wagenknecht *et al.* [88].

However, the postoperative mortality was 4.6%, and the ureterolysis alone was of little effect, since 68% of the cases presented restenosis in the follow-up. Peritoneal flap plasty or peritoneal reduplication showed as good results as did laterocolic intraperitoneal transposition of the ureter. Overall, surgery alone was followed by recurrence in about 50% of the cases whereas the combination with long-term corticosteroids permitted a recurrence of 10% [175]. As proposed by Baker, high-risk patients should benefit from stenting with corticosteroid therapy rather than ureterolysis [179, 180]. If bilateral obstruction is present in a borderline patient, a reasonable option would be unilateral ureterolysis (preferably of the better functioning kidney) and corticosteroid treatment to relieve obstruction on the contralateral side. The patient's choice must naturally be considered once the pros and cons of each option have been fully explained. In cases of intrinsic involvement of a segment of the ureter surgical ureterolysis may not be enough to relieve the obstruction but more extensive procedures may be necessary, such as excision and anastomosis, replacement of the ureter or autotransplantation of the kidney [9]. The patient with symptomatic or asymptomatic periaortitis but no ureteric obstruction poses a particular problem. In all probability, corticosteroid or another immunosuppressive therapy and meticulous follow-up is probably the correct approach. However, surgical treatment is not without hazard. Ureteral devascularisation and ischemia, tears and strictures due to difficult surgical dissection of the ureter or urinary fistula are frequent complications [170, 176]. Other complications such as postoperative hypertension and thromboembolism have also been reported [181, 182]. Recurrence of ureteric obstruction after ureterolysis and development of contralateral obstruction after unilateral ureterolysis is relatively common if corticosteroid therapy is not used. Thus, since a few years, the use of corticosteroids to complete the surgical management of RPF has gained general acceptance [35, 57, 170, 173-177, 179, 180].

Medical Management

At present, treatment with corticosteroids remains the mainstay of medical therapy for RPF [14, 175, 183-188]. However, some authors are reluctant to use corticosteroids as the primary form of treatment, as they consider laparoscopic or open biopsies the only way to establish a definite diagnosis [40, 30, 177, 183]. Corticosteroids act through reduction of inflammation and edema, inhibition of fibroblastic proliferation, and immunosuppression. Although corticosteroids do not reverse established fibrosis, further fibroblastic proliferation may be slowed and symptomatology reversed. In a long-term follow-up study, Alexopoulos *et al.* showed that in 11 patients with idiopathic RPF, corticosteroids were of value in 100% of the cases [44]. All patients presented with moderate upper urinary dilation without significant uremic symptoms at the time of diagnosis. In the same study, six patients were treated by a combination of surgery and corticosteroid administration. They presented with severe hydronephrosis and had severely compromised renal function. Only one patient of this group developed end-stage renal failure. The value of corticosteroids in the postoperative periods is warranted. Concerning the duration of corticosteroid treatment, most authors suggest at least 6 months of therapy [44, 175, 184]. In recent study, Kardar *et al.* analyzed the dose and the duration of corticosteroid treatment in 12 patients with idiopathic RPF [184]. The authors used prednisolone at an initial dose of 60 mg on alternate days for 2 months. This dosage was then tapered during the following 2 months to a daily dose of 5 mg. The total duration of prednisolone use was 2 years. Eleven patients completed this treatment regimen and were followed for a duration of 26 to 132 months (median 63.1) after discontinuation of treatment. Good response in the form of relief of symptoms and regression of the mass occurred in 9 cases and there were 2 failures. The authors concluded that the regimen of corticosteroid proposed may be used as the primary mode of treatment for the majority of patients with idiopathic RPF with minimal complications. Furthermore, they added that each patient with idiopathic RPF should be followed periodically for the rest of their lives. As the etiology of this chronic inflammatory disease is unknown, the medical therapy may need to be continued for a period long enough to allow suppression of the inflammatory process and regression of the retroperitoneal mass. If the duration of treatment is short (3 to 6 months) idiopathic retroperitoneal fibrosis may recur and lead to renal damage. Despite the relief of symptoms and normalization of ESR, if the retroperitoneal mass does not regress, patients should be seriously considered for surgical treatment to prevent loss of renal function. Higgins *et al.* suggested that idiopathic RPF could be divided into 2 distinct groups [40]. A more seriously ill group of patients who responded poorly to surgery and corticosteroid therapy and a second group in which ureteral obstruction, often predominantly unilateral, develops earlier in the disease process should be more responsive to corticosteroid treatment. Other corticosteroid regimen may be used such as a pulse dose of méthylprednisolone (1gm/d intravenously for 3 days), which has been used along with azathioprine [189].

Once corticosteroids are initiated, pain and constitutional symptoms often disappear within a few days and a rapid fall of ESR is seen [131]. Recovery of the diuresis can be observed within ten days and frequently and frequently as early as 24 to 48 hours after starting treatment. Several authors have described CT scanner-documented regression of the retroperitoneal mass within weeks after starting treatment [187, 190].

In corticosteroid-resistant, or dependent cases, or contraindication of high-dose corticosteroid therapy, when there is no doubt as to the initial diagnosis, other forms of immunosuppression, either alone or in combination with low-dose corticosteroids, may be useful (Table 7) [175, 189, 191-195]. Some authors have suggested the use of immunosuppressive agents such as azathioprine [191], while others have reported good results using a combination of cyclophosphamide and corticosteroids [196]. Methotrexate, an immunosuppressive agent, is employed for its remarkable anti-inflammatory effects by inhibiting adenosine kinase and interfering the production of several inflammatory mediators and lymphocyte functions [193, 197, 198]. As idiopathic RPF may be the result of an auto-allergic reaction to atherosclerotic lipids, and on the basis of data indicating a T cell pathogenesis, cyclosporin and mycophenolate mofetil have been used with success in cases with idiopathic RPF [194, 195]. Treatment with tamoxifen has also been reported to have been of benefit in many isolated cases [199-202]. Tamoxifen is a non-steroidal anti-estrogen drug utilized for the treatment of breast cancer, desmoid tumors, and fibrotic disorders such as fibromatosis. The first successful treatment of RPF with tamoxifen was described by Clark *et al.* in 1991 [201]. Many authors suggest that it is not its anti-estrogenic property, but the induction of an increasing synthesis of tissue growth factor-beta (TGF-β) from the fibroblasts that is important for RPF treatment [202, 203]. Normally TGF-β is a trophic factor for mesenchymal tissue and is responsible for the fixing processes within the tissues. In fact, TGF-β induces angiogenesis and production of tissue extracellular matrix by collagen, fibronectin and proteoglycan synthesis. Tissue growth factor-beta is a chemotactic factor for monocytes and therefore has an important role in activating inflammation. It also blocks the IL-1 capacity to stimulate T cell proliferation with consequent depression of the immune system. Some authors suggest that fibroblasts in RPF may be of the fetal phenotype and therefore tamoxifen may induce the synthesis of an abnormal TGF-β that blocks the inflammatory and fibrogenetic process through a negative feedback mechanism within the macrophagic cells [204]. According to other authors, tamoxifen could also inhibit adenosine kinase or protein kinase C by blocking the calmodulin or the epidermal growth factor synthesis [201-203]. Tamoxifen has mild side effects that include hot flushes, vulval itching, vaginal leakage and bleeding. In addition, some serious side effects such as an increased risk of thromboembolism and ovarian cancer, have to be considered carefully for each patient. Due to the effectiveness, simplicity and safety of tamoxifen therapy, it must be considered as an alternative and attractive new choice of drug treatment for RPF.

Recently, Marcolongo *et al.* evaluated the efficacy of immunosuppressive therapy in a retrospective series of 26 patients with idiopathic RPF [205]. Fifteen patients (58%) were treated with azathioprine and prednisone, and the remaining patients were treated with cyclophosphamide and prednisone. Compared to other studies, the treatment failure rate was similar to other studies [30, 174, 206]. It was approximately 1 per 100 patient-years (95% confidence interval [CI]: 0.02 to 5 per 100 patient-years). This study suggests that immunosuppressive therapy of idiopathic RPF in combination with ureteral stenting in case of ureteral obstruction can permit remission of the clinical, biological and radiological signs of the disease. The results of this study support the immune origin for the disease and suggest that inflammation is relevant in its pathogenesis. The hypothesis of Th2-mediated immune reaction at the origin of the idiopathic RPF is supported by the diffuse eosinophilic infiltrate encountered in histological analyses. Indeed, Th2 cytokines such as IL-4 could activate fibroblast chemotaxis, increase matrix production, and reduce antigen clearance in fibrotic tissue [207]. As a consequence, immunosuppressive therapy might act by reducing the number and activity of Th2 cells and, indirectly, by downregulating release of IL-1 and IL-6. For these reasons, immunosuppressive therapy is likely to be more successful in early stage of the disease, when fibrotic tissue is rich in inflammatory cells. In later stages, the mass becomes mostly fibrous and is less likely to shrink with medical therapy [73].

Table 7. Medical Treatment of Non-Malignant Retroperitoneal Fibrosis

Immunosuppressive regimen
Corticosteroids
Azathioprine ± corticosteroids
Cyclophosphamide + corticosteroids
Mycophenolate mofetil ± corticosteroids
Cyclosporin ± corticosteroids
Mezhotrexate ± corticosteroids

Hormonal
Tamoxifen ± corticosteroids
Progesterone
Medroxyprogesterone acetate

Novel therapeutic combinations (e.g. tamoxifen with corticosteroids or immunosuppressive drugs) and drugs, which inhibit fibroblast proliferation or induce fibroblast apoptosis (e.g. interferon gamma) may also be attempted. If the mass does not decrease significantly or recurs, a repeat biopsy is required to rule out malignancy or infection. Recurrence may be controlled with the same drug alone or with additional drugs often required.

Prognosis and Follow-Up

Although natural history of RPF is not well studied, its prognosis depends upon several factors such as its etiology, renal damage at time of diagnosis, extension of the lesion, progressive or stable stage of RPF, and additional urinary infection. Indeed, different rates of progression have been reported. Spontaneous complete resolution is extremely rare. Renal impairment resolves or improves significantly in a majority of treated patients, regardless of whether treatment is surgical or medical. Some authors favoring medical treatment suggest that surgery may still be indicated in cases of radiographic ureteral obstruction, non-functioning kidneys or in the presence of severe renal failure [44]. Fearing adverse effects or a hidden underlying retroperitoneal malignancy, physicians are often reluctant to treat idiopathic RPF with immunosuppressive therapy or corticosteroids. However, CT scanner or MRI can be helpful to distinguish malignant from idiopathic fibrosis.

As mentioned, recurrences are not rare and occur within some years (usually less than five years) after diagnosis. However, in more extensive cases, recurrences are more unpredictable and may occur at any time. Therefore, long-term follow-up (years) is mandatory. The patients are monitored by clinical evaluation of symptoms, particularly pain, measurement of ESR and assessment of renal function. A CT scanner should be performed at 3 and 6 months and then yearly to assess the response to medical treatment. In only a small number (6% to 10%) of the patients the retroperitoneal mass did not regress and surgical ureterolysis should be required. However, for routine follow-up, abdominal and renal ultrasound are sufficient.

Excluding cases of malignant RPF, the prognosis is good [9, 35, 122]. In a large retrospective study, cumulative mortality was 9% [208]. A diagnosis of RPF, in itself, does not reduce life expectancy. In case of chronic periaortitis, the prognosis is guarded and depends on the severity of atherosclerosis. Despite many patients being elderly, cumulative actuarial survival in well-managed patients in the 1960s to the 1980s was reasonably satisfactory, being 86% at 1 year and 78% at 2 years after surgical treatment. Older patients and those more uremic at the time of presentation were more likely to die. Whether current results are equivalent, better or worse is not clear. The future lies with the prevention and treatment of atherosclerosis

Conclusion

Retroperitoneal fibrosis is an uncommon inflammatory disease, which leads to extensive fibrosis throughout the retroperitoneum. Since the signs and symptoms of the disease are nonspecific, the diagnosis should be suspected in presence of mild normochromic normocytic anemia and significantly elevated ESR or CRP. CT scanner and MRI represent the modalities of choice for imaging diagnosis and follow-up of patients with RPF. Once the diagnosis is suggested, the distinction between malignant and non-malignant RPF must be made. The majority of cases remain classified as idiopathic. The patients who are presumed to present idiopathic RPF are probably suffering from chronic periaortitis with severe aortic atherosclerosis. Evidence to date suggests that the pathogenesis of inflammatory component in RPF may be multifactorial in nature with some mechanism acting upon the resultant inflammatory tissue to produce striking fibrosis. Surgical biopsy remains the only way to definitively establish the diagnosis, because the prognosis is dismal for malignant RPF, but very good for other forms of the disease. Prompt recognition and treatment are of importance, as the therapy is effective and prevents further renal damage. Despite the preferred treatment of idiopathic RPF is uncertain, corticosteroids remain the first-line drug for RPF with mild ureteral obstructive signs. A combination of corticosteroids with surgery or ureteral stenting should be retained for patients with advanced renal failure, severe upper urinary dilatation or urinary tract sepsis. Immunosuppressive therapy or tamoxifen may be a treatment in some patients who are corticosteroid-resistant, or dependent, or in patients who are not suitable for surgery or when ureteral stenting can no longer be performed. Patients with RPF should be followed periodically for life.

References

[1] Albarran J. Retention rénale par périurétérite: Libération externe de l'uretère. *Assoc Fr Urol.* 1905.9:511-5

[2] Ormond JK. Bilateral ureteral obstruction due to envelopment and compression by inflammatory retroperitoneal process. *J Urol.* 1948,59:1072-79.

[3] Utz DC, Henry JD. Retroperitoneal fibrosis. *Med Clin North Am.* 1966 Jul;50(4):1091-9.

[4] Demko TM, Diamond JR, Groff J. Obstructive nephropathy as a result of retroperitoneal fibrosis: a review of its pathogenesis and associations. *J Am Soc Nephrol.* 1997 Apr;8(4):684-8.

[5] Davison A, Cameron J, Grünfeld J, Kerr D, Ritz E, Winearls C 1998 Oxford Textbook of Clinical Nephrology (2nd ed). *Oxford University Press,* Oxford

[6] Fletcher CD, Jarrett PE. Variable symptomatology in idiopathic retroperitoneal fibrosis. *J R Soc Med.* 1983 Dec;76(12):1023-5.

[7] Srinivas V, Dow D. Retroperitoneal fibrosis. Can J Surg. 1984 Mar;27(2):111-3.

[8] Jones JH, Ross EJ, Matz LR, Edwards D, Davies DR. Retroperitoneal fibrosis. *Am J Med.* 1970 Feb;48(2):203-8.

[9] Lepor H, Walsh PC. Idiopathic retroperitoneal fibrosis. *J Urol.* 1979 Jul;122(1):1-6.

[10] Gilkeson GS, Allen NB. Retroperitoneal fibrosis. A true connective tissue disease. *Rheum Dis Clin North Am.* 1996 Feb;22(1):23-38.

[11] Kottra JJ, Dunnick NR. Retroperitoneal fibrosis. *Radiol Clin North Am.* 1996 Nov;34(6):1259-75.

[12] Koep L, Zuidema GD. The clinical significance of retroperitoneal fibrosis. *Surgery.* 1977 Mar;81(3):250-7.

[13] Meier P, Gilabert C, Burnier M, Blanc E. Retroperitoneal fibrosis, an unrecognized inflammatory disease. Clinical observations and review of the literature. *Néphrologie.* 2003;24(4):173-80.

[14] Mitchinson MJ. The pathology of idiopathic retroperitoneal fibrosis. *J Clin Pathol* 1970; 23: 681-9.

[15] Mitchinson MJ. Retroperitoneal fibrosis revisited. *Arch Pathol Lab Med* 1986; 110: 784-6.

[16] Littlejohn GO, Keystone EC. The association of retroperitoneal fibrosis with systemic vasculitis and HLA-B27: a case report and review of the literature. *J Rheumatol.* 1981 Jul-Aug;8(4):665-9.

[17] Witten DM. Retroperitoneal fibrosis. In Pollack HM eds. *Clinical Urography.* Philadelphia: W.B. Saunders Co.,1990; 2469-83.

[18] Saxton HM, Kilpatrick FR, Kinder CH, Lessof MH, McHardy-Young S, Wardle DF. Retroperitoneal fibrosis. A radiological and follow-up study of fourteen cases. *Q J Med.* 1969 Apr;38(150):159-81.

[19] Larrieu AJ, Weiner I, Abston S, Warren MM. Retroperitoneal fibrosis. *Surg Gynecol Obstet.* 1980 May;150(5):699-702.

[20] Keith DS, Larson TS. Idiopathic retroperitoneal fibrosis. *J Am Soc Nephrol* 1993; 3: 1748-52.

[21] Leseche G, Schaetz A, Arrive L, Nussaume O, Andreassian B. Diagnosis and management of 17 consecutive patients with inflammatory abdominal aortic aneurysm. *Am J Surg* 1992; 164: 39-44.

[22] Lindell OI, Sariola HV, Lehtonen TA. The occurrence of vasculitis in perianeurysmal fibrosis. *J Urol.* 1987 Oct;138(4):727-9.

[23] Baker LRI, Croxson R, Khader N, Rezneck RH, Rukhaimi MA, Wickkam JEA. Rate of development of ureteric obstruction in idiopathic retroperitoneal fibrosis (peri-aortitis). *Br J Urol* 1992; 69: 102-5.

[24] Chan SL, Johnson HW, McLoughlin MG. Idiopathic retroperitoneal fibrosis in children. *J Urol.* 1979 Jul;122(1):103-4.

[25] Webb AJ, Dawson-Edwards P. Non-malignant retroperitoneal fibrosis. *Br J Surg.* 1967 Jun;54(6):508-18.

[26] Webb AJ, Dawson-Edwards P. Malignant retroperitoneal fibrosis. *Br J Surg.* 1967 Jun;54(6):505-8.

[27] Wicks IP, Robertson MR, Murnaghan GF, Bertouch JV. Idiopathic retroperitoneal fibrosis presenting with back pain. *J Rheumatol.* 1988 Oct;15(10):1572-4.

[28] Serra RM, Engle JE, Jones RE, Schoolwerth AC. Perianeurysmal retroperitoneal fibrosis. An unusual cause of renal failure. *Am J Med.* 1980 Jan;68(1):149-53.

[29] Byrd WE, Hunt RE, Burgess R. Retroperitoneal fibrosis as a cause of fever of undetermined origin. *West J Med.* 1981 Apr;134(4):357-61.

[30] Baker LR, Mallinson WJ, Gregory MC, Menzies EA, Cattell WR, Whitfield HN, Hendry WF, Wickham JE, Joekes AM. Idiopathic retroperitoneal fibrosis. A retrospective analysis of 60 cases. *Br J Urol.* 1987 Dec;60(6):497-503.

[31] Anwar N, Taylor PM, Carrol RN, Ramsden RT, Merchant M, Gokal R. An unusual case of retroperitoneal fibrosis. *Am J Kidney Dis.* 1993 Jul;22(1):57-9.

[32] de Sa J, Pimentel J, Carvalho M, Evangelista P, Martins P. Spinal cord compression secondary to idiopathic retroperitoneal fibrosis. Neurosurgery. 1990 Apr;26(4):678-81.

[33] Doi M, Uji Y. A case of uveitis associated with idiopathic retroperitoneal fibrosis. *Am J Ophthalmol.* 1994 Mar 15;117(3):358-62.

[34] Ewald EA, Gikas PW, Castor CW. Periarticular fibrosis associated with idiopathic retroperitoneal fibrosis. *J Rheumatol.* 1988 Sep;15(9):1443-6.

[35] Buff DD, Bogin MB, Faltz LL. Retroperitoneal fibrosis. A report of selected cases and a review of the literature. *N Y State J Med.* 1989 Sep;89(9):511-6.

[36] Arger PH, Stolz JL, Miller WT. Retroperitoneal fibrosis: an analysis of the clinical spectrum and roentgenographic signs. *Am J Roentgenol Radium Ther Nucl Med.* 1973 Dec;119(4):812-21.

[37] Cotsamire D, Ibrahim G, Robertson C. Clinical parameters and therapeutic outcome in patients with idiopathic retroperitoneal fibrosis. *Arthritis Rheum* 1991; 34: R34-R38.

[38] Gans RO, Hoorntje SJ, Rauwerda JA, Luth WJ, van Hattum LA, Donker AJ. The inflammatory abdominal aortic aneurysm. Prevalence, clinical features and diagnostic evaluation. *Neth J Med.* 1993 Oct;43(3-4):105-15.

[39] Todd GJ, DeRose JJ Jr. Retroperitoneal approach for repair of inflammatory aortic aneurysms. *Ann Vasc Surg.* 1995 Nov;9(6):525-34.

[40] Higgins PM, Bennett-Jones DN, Naish PF, Aber GM. Non-operative management of retroperitoneal fibrosis. *Br J Surg.* 1988 Jun;75(6):573-7.

[41] Klisnick A, Fourcade J, Ruivard M, Baud O, Souweine B, Boyer L, Deteix P. Combined idiopathic retroperitoneal and mediastinal fibrosis with pericardial involvement. *Clin Nephrol* 1999; 52: 51-5.

[42] Morad N, Strongwater SL, Eypper S, Woda BA. Idiopathic retroperitoneal and mediastinal fibrosis mimicking connective tissue disease. *Am J Med* 1987; 82: 363-6.

[43] Rault R, Kapoor W, Kam W. Perianeurysmal fibrosis and ureteric obstruction: case report and review of literature. *Clin Nephrol.* 1982 Sep;18(3):159-62.

[44] Alexopoulos E, Memmos D, Bakatselos S, Rombis V, Sakellariou G, Gaganakis J, Hadjidimitriou C, Papadimitriou M. Idiopathic retroperitoneal fibrosis : a long-term follow-up study. *Eur Urol* 1987; 13: 313-17.

[45] Faubert PF, Porush JG, Chou SY, Shapiro WB. Retroperitoneal fibrosis presenting as spontaneously reversible renal failure. *Am J Kidney Dis.* 1982 Sep;2(2):264-7.

[46] Wallach PM, Flannery MT, Adelman HM, PowSang J, Saba H, Altus P, Espinoza LR. Retroperitoneal fibrosis accompanying immune thrombocytopenia. *Am J Hematol.* 1991 Jul;37(3):204-5.

[47] Kurzel RB, Yoonesi M, Munabi A. Retroperitoneal fibrosis: a two decade experience and gynecologic manifestations. *Int J Gynaecol Obstet.* 1981 Aug;19(4):271-80.

[48] Bucci JA, Manoharan A. Methysergide-induced retroperitoneal fibrosis: successful outcome and two new laboratory features. *Mayo Clin Proc.* 1997 Dec;72(12):1148-50.

[49] Kaipiainen-Seppanen O, Jantunen E, Kuusisto J, Marin S. Retroperitoneal fibrosis with antineutrophil cytoplasmic antibodies. *J Rheumatol.* 1996 Apr;23(4):779-81.

[50] Sakemi T, Tomiyoshi Y, Yano H, Ikeda Y, Matsuo Y, Kudo S. Retroperitoneal fibrosis with perinuclear antineutrophil cytoplasmic antibodies and a longitudinally extended periaortic soft-tissue structure on CT. *Nephron.* 1998;78(2):218-20.

[51] Mitchinson MJ. Aortic disease in idiopathic retroperitoneal and mediastinal fibrosis. *J Clin Pathol.* 1972 Apr;25(4):287-93.

[52] Mulligan SA, Holley HC, Koehler RE, Koslin DB, Rubin E, Berland LL, Kenney PJ. CT and MR imaging in the evaluation of retroperitoneal fibrosis. *J Comput Assist Tomogr.* 1989 Mar-Apr;13(2):277-81.

[53] Wagenknecht LV, Auvert J. Symptoms and diagnosis of retroperitoneal fibrosis. Analysis of 31 cases. *Urol Int.* 1971;26(3):185-95.

[54] Lalli AF. Retroperitoneal fibrosis and inapparent obstructive uropathy. *Radiology.* 1977 Feb;122(2):339-42.

[55] Minford JE, Davies P. The urographic appearances in acute and chronic retroperitoneal fibrosis. *Clin Radiol* 1984; 35: 51-7.

[56] Triantopoulou C, Rizos S, Bourli A, Koulentianos E, Dervenis C. Localized unilateral perirenal fibrosis: CT and MRI appearances. *Eur Radiol* 2002 ; 12: 2743-6.

[57] Miles RM, Brock J, Martin C. Idiopathic retroperitoneal fibrosis. A sometime surgical problem. *Am Surg.* 1984 Feb;50(2):76-84.

[58] Persky L, Kursh ED, Feldman S, Resnick MI: Diseases of the retroperitoneum; Retroperitoneal fibrosis. In Campbell's Urology. Philadelphia, *WB Saunders,* 1986, pp 595-601.

[59] Halverstadt DB. Problems in the use of urography and lymphangiography in the diagnosis of idiopathic retroperitoneal fibrosis. *J Urol.* 1968 Apr;99(4):423-6.

[60] Clouse ME, Fraley EE, Litwin SB. Lymphangiographic criteria for diagnosis of retroperitoneal fibrosis. *Radiology.* 1964;83:1-5.

[61] Rubenstein WA, Gray G, Auh YH, Honig CL, Thorbjarnarson B, Williams JJ, Haimes AB, Zirinsky K, Kazam E. CT of fibrous tissues and tumors with sonographic correlation. *AJR Am J Roentgenol.* 1986 Nov;147(5):1067-74.

[62] Fagan CJ, Larrieu AJ, Amparo EG. Retroperitoneal fibrosis: ultrasound and CT features. *AJR* 1979; 133: 239-43.

[63] Erden A, Aytac S, Cumhur T, Yurdakul M, Calikoglu U. Retroperitoneal fibrosis: evaluation by ultrasonography and color Doppler imaging. *Urol Int.* 1995;55(2):111-4.

[64] Kikumori T, Imai T, Kaneko T, Sugimoto H, Shibata A, Hibi Y, Nakao A. Intracaval endovascular ultrasonography for large adrenal and retroperitoneal tumors. *Surgery.* 2003 Dec;134(6):989-93; discussion 993-4.

[65] Degesys GE, Dunnick NR, Silverman PM, Cohan RH, Illescas FF, Castagno A. Retroperitoneal fibrosis: use of CT in distinguishing among possible causes. *AJR Am J Roentgenol.* 1986 Jan;146(1):57-60.

[66] Sterzer SK, Herr HW, Mintz I. Idiopathic retroperitonial fibrosis misinterpreted as lymphoma by computed tomography. *J Urol.* 1979 Sep;122(3):405-6.

[67] Glynn TP Jr, Kreipke DL, Irons JM. Amyloidosis: diffuse involvement of the retroperitoneum. *Radiology.* 1989 Mar;170(3 Pt 1):726.

[68] Brooks AP, Reznek RH, Webb JA. Aortic displacement on computed tomography of idiopathic retroperitoneal fibrosis. *Clin Radiol.* 1989 Jan;40(1):51-2.

[69] Brun B, Laursen K, Sorensen IN, Lorentzen JE, Kristensen JK. CT in retroperitoneal fibrosis. *AJR Am J Roentgenol.* 1981 Sep;137(3):535-8.

[70] Pistolese GR, Ippoliti A, Mauriello A, Pistolese C, Pocek M, Simonetti G. Postoperative regression of retroperitoneal fibrosis in patients with inflammatory abdominal aortic aneurysms: evaluation with spiral computed tomography. *Ann Vasc Surg.* 2002 Mar;16(2):201-9. Epub 2002 Mar 15.

[71] Hricak H, Higgins CB, Williams RD. Nuclear magnetic resonance imaging in retroperitoneal fibrosis. *AJR Am J Roentgenol.* 1983 Jul;141(1):35-8.

[72] Arrivc L, Hricak H, Tavares NJ, Miller TR. Malignant versus nonmalignant retroperitoneal fibrosis: differentiation with MR imaging. *Radiology.* 1989 Jul;172(1):139-43.

[73] Barker CD, Brown JJ. MR imaging of the retroperitoneum. Top Magn Reson Imaging. 1995 Spring;7(2):102-11.

[74] Rominger MB, Kenney PJ. Perirenal involvement by retroperitoneal fibrosis: the usefulness of MRI to establish diagnosis. *Urol Radiol.* 1992;13(3):173-6.

[75] Bechtold RE, Dyer RB, Zagoria RJ, Chen MY. The perirenal space: relationship of pathologic processes to normal retroperitoneal anatomy. *Radiographics.* 1996 Jul;16(4):841-54.

[76] Rapezzi D, Racchi O, Ferraris AM. Perirenal extramedullary hematopoiesis in agnogenic myeloid metaplasia: MR imaging findings. *AJR Am J Roentgenol.* 1997 May;168(5):1388-9.

[77] Leibowich S, Tumeh SS. Gallium-67 imaging and computed tomography in early retroperitoneal fibrosis. *Clin Nucl Med.* 1988 Nov;13(11):829-30.

[78] Liebman RM. Positive gallium scan in retroperitoneal fibrosis. *AJR Am J Roentgenol.* 1983 Nov;141(5):949-50.

[79] Fink AM, Miles KA, Wraight EP. Indium-111 labelled leucocyte uptake in aortitis. *Clin Radiol.* 1994 Dec;49(12):863-6.

[80] Bar-Shalom R, Valdivia AY, Blaufox MD. PET imaging in oncology. *Semin Nucl Med.* 2000 Jul;30(3):150-85.

[81] Blockmans D, Stroobants S, Maes A, Mortelmans L. Positron emission tomography in giant cell arteritis and polymyalgia rheumatica: evidence for inflammation of the aortic arch. *Am J Med.* 2000 Feb 15;108(3):246-9.

[82] Drieskens O, Blockmans D, Van den Bruel A, Mortelmans L. Riedel's thyroiditis and retroperitoneal fibrosis in multifocal fibrosclerosis: positron emission tomographic findings. *Clin Nucl Med.* 2002 Jun;27(6):413-5.

[83] Blockmans D, Van Moer E, Dehem J, Feys C, Mortelmans L. Positron emission tomography can reveal abdominal periaortitis. *Clin Nucl Med.* 2002 Mar;27(3):211-2.

[84] Kubota K, Yamada K, Yoshioka S, Yamada S, Ito M, Ido T. Differential diagnosis of idiopathic fibrosis from malignant lymphadenopathy with PET and F-18 fluorodeoxyglucose. *Clin Nucl Med.* 1992 May;17(5):361-3.

[85] Levine MR, Kaye L, Mair S, Bates J. Multifocal fibrosclerosis. Report of a case of bilateral idiopathic sclerosing pseudotumor and retroperitoneal fibrosis. *Arch Ophthalmol.* 1993 Jun;111(6):841-3.

[86] Richards AB, Shalka HW, Roberts FJ, Flint A. Pseudotumor of the orbit and retroperitoneal fibrosis. A form of multifocal fibrosclerosis. *Arch Ophthalmol.* 1980 Sep;98(9):1617-20.

[87] de Boer WA, van Coevorden F, Wiersinga WM. A rare case of Riedel's thyroiditis, 6 years after retroperitoneal fibrosis: two diseases with one pathogenesis? *Neth J Med.* 1992 Apr;40(3-4):190-6.

[88] Julie C, Vieillefond A, Desligneres S, Schaison G, Grunfeld JP. Franc B. Hashimoto's thyroiditis associated with Riedel's thyroiditis and retroperitoneal fibrosis. *Pathol Res Pract* 1997; 193: 573-7.

[89] Bartholomew LG, Cain JC, Woolner LB, Utz DC, Ferris DO. Sclerosing cholangitis: its possible association with Riedel's struma and fibrous retroperitonitis. Report of two cases. *N Engl J Med.* 1963 Jul 4;269:8-12.

[90] De Luca S, Terrone C, Manassero A, Rocca Rossetti S. Aetiopathogenesis and treatment of idiopathic retroperitoneal fibrosis. *Ann Urol* (Paris). 1998;32(3):153-9.

[91] Alberti C, Sacchini P, Cortellini P, Rossi A. Retroperitoneal fibrosis: some new acquisitions about pathogenesis and diagnostics. *Arch Ital Urol Nefrol Androl.* 1991 Mar;63(1):23-35.

[92] Gonzalez C, Penado S, Llata L, Valero C, Riancho JA. The clinical spectrum of retroperitoneal hematoma in anticoagulated patients. *Medicine* (Baltimore). 2003 Jul;82(4):257-62.

[93] Iwahashi C, Nakajima H, Handa Y, Owada F, Nagai Y, Kawamura S. Retroperitoneal fibrosis and immune-complex glomerulonephritis. *Clin Nephrol.* 2001 May;55(5):400-3.

[94] de RS, Serratrice J, Granel B, Disdier P, Bartoli JM, Pache X, Astoul P, Garbe L, Branchereau A, Weiller PJ. Periaortitis heralding Wegener's granulomatosis. *J Rheumatol.* 2002 Feb;29(2):392-4.

[95] Wendling D, Toussirot E, Michel F. Spondyloarthropathy and retroperitoneal fibrosis: a case report. *Joint Bone Spine.* 2002 May;69(3):334-7.

[96] LeBlanc CM, Inman RD, Dent P, Smith C, Babyn P, Laxer RM. Retroperitoneal fibrosis: an extraarticular manifestation of ankylosing spondylitis. *Arthritis Rheum.* 2002 Apr 15;47(2):210-4.

[97] Braun J, Schuldes H, Berkefeld J, Zanella F, Jonas D, Usadel KH, Badenhoop K. Panhypopituitarism associated with severe retroperitoneal fibrosis. *Clin Endocrinol* (Oxf). 2001 Feb;54(2):273-6.

[98] Tang KH, Schofield JB, Powell-Jackson PR. Primary biliary cirrhosis and idiopathic retroperitoneal fibrosis: a rare association. *Eur J Gastroenterol Hepatol.* 2002 Jul;14(7):783-6.

[99] van Bommel E, Brouwers A, Makkus A, van Vliet A. Retroperitoneal fibrosis and p-ANCA-associated polyarteritis nodosa: coincidental or common etiology? *Eur J Intern Med.* 2002 Sep;13(6):392.

[100] Hamano H, Kawa S, Ochi Y, Unno H, Shiba N, Wajiki M, Nakazawa K, Shimojo H, Kiyosawa K. Hydronephrosis associated with retroperitoneal fibrosis and sclerosing pancreatitis. *Lancet.* 2002 Apr 20;359(9315):1403-4.

[101] Hosaka N, Ito M, Taki Y, Iwai H, Toki J, Ikehara S. Amyloid A gastrointestinal amyloidosis associated with idiopathic retroperitoneal fibrosis. Report of a rare autopsy case and review of the literature. *Arch Pathol Lab Med.* 2003 Jun;127(6):735-8.

[102] Bleumink GS, van der Molen-Eijgenraam M, Strijbos JH, Sanwikarja S, van Puijenbroek EP, Stricker BH. Pergolide-induced pleuropulmonary fibrosis. *Clin Neuropharmacol.* 2002 Sep-Oct;25(5):290-3.

[103] Graham JR, Suby HI, LeCompte PR, Sadowsky NL. Fibrotic disorders associated with methysergide therapy for headache. *N Engl J Med* 1966; 274: 359-68.

[104] Lewis CT, Molland EA, Marshall VR, Tresidder GC, Blandy JP. Analgesic abuse, ureteric obstruction, and retroperitoneal fibrosis. *Br Med J.* 1975 Apr 12;2(5962):76-8.

[105] Graham JR. Drug-induced localized systemic scleroses. *Trans Am Clin Climatol Assoc.* 1980;92:122-32.

[106] Silberstein SD. Methysergide. *Cephalalgia.* 1998 Sep;18(7):421-35.

[107] Kains JP, Hardy JC, Chevalier C, Collier A. Retroperitoneal fibrosis in two patients with Parkinson's disease treated with bromocriptine. *Acta Clin Belg.* 1990;45(5):306-10.

[108] Mondal BK, Suri S. Pergolide-induced retroperitoneal fibrosis. *Int J Clin Pract.* 2000 Jul-Aug;54(6):403.

[109] Lewis RV, McDevitt DG. Adverse reactions and interactions with beta-adrenoceptor blocking drugs. *Med Toxicol.* 1986 Sep-Oct;1(5):343-61.

[110] Pryor JP, Castle WM, Dukes DC, Smith JC, Watson ME, Williams JL. Do beta adrenoreceptor blocking drugs cause retroperitoneal fibrosis ? *BMJ* 1983; 287: 639-41.

[111] Comings DE, Skubi KB, Van Eyes J, Motulsky AG. Familial multifocal fibrosclerosis. Findings suggesting that retroperitoneal fibrosis, mediastinal fibrosis, sclerosing cholangitis, Riedel's thyroiditis, and pseudotumor of the orbit may be different manifestations of a single disease. *Ann Intern Med.* 1967 May;66(5):884-92.

[112] Scott J, Foster R, Moore A. Retroperitoneal fibrosis and nonmalignant ileal carcinoid. *J Urol.* 1987 Dec;138(6):1435.

[113] Leu HJ. Inflammatory abdominal aortic aneurysms: a disease entity? Histological analysis of 60 cases of inflammatory aortic aneurysms of unknown aetiology. *Virchows Arch A Pathol Anat Histopathol.* 1990;417(5):427-33.

[114] Lance NJ, Levinson DJ. Aortitis and periaortic fibrosis. *J Rheumatol.* 1991 Jul;18(7):1095-9.

[115] Parums DV, Choudhury RP, Shield SA, Davies AH. Characterization of inflammatory cells associated with « idiopathic retroperitoneal fibrosis ». *Br J Urol* 1991; 67: 564-8.

[116] Zabetakis PM, Novich RK, Matarese RA, Michelis MF. Idiopathic retroperitoneal fibrosis: a systemic connective tissue disease? *J Urol.* 1979 Jul;122(1):100-2.

[117] Mansell MA, Watts RW. Retroperitoneal fibrosis and scleroderma. *Postgrad Med J.* 1980 Oct;56(660):730-3.

[118] Rivlin ME, McGehee RP, Bower JD. Retroperitoneal fibrosis associated with carcinoma of the cervix: review of the literature. *Gynecol Oncol.* 1991 Apr;41(1):95-7.

[119] Fromowitz FB, Miller F. Retroperitoneal fibrosis as host response to papillary renal cell carcinoma. *Urology.* 1991 Sep;38(3):259-63.

[120] Jimenez SA. Other fibrosing syndromes. *Curr Opin Rheumatol.* 1989 Dec;1(4):516-22.

[121] Chapelon-Abric C, Godeau P, Piette JC. Fibroses systémiques idiopathiques. In Kahn MF, Peltier AP, Meyer O, Piette JC eds. Maladies et syndromes systémiques. Paris: *Flammarion Médecine-Science,* 2000; 1169-88.

[122] van Bommel EF. Retroperitoneal fibrosis. *Neth J Med.* 2002 Jul;60(6):231-42.

[123] Parums DV. The spectrum of chronic periaortitis. *Histopathology* 1990; 16: 423-31.

[124] Parums DV, Dunn DC, Dixon AK, Mitchinson MJ. Characterization of inflammatory cells in a patient with chronic periaortitis. *Am J Cardiovasc Pathol* 1990; 3: 121-9.

[125] Vaglio A, Corradi D, Manenti L, Ferretti S, Garini G, Buzio C. Evidence of autoimmunity in chronic periaortitis: a prospective study. *Am J Med.* 2003 Apr 15;114(6):454-62.

[126] Amis ES Jr. Retroperitoneal fibrosis. *AJR Am J Roentgenol.* 1991 Aug;157(2):321-9.

[127] Warkentin JH. An unusual manifestation of idiopathic retroperitoneal fibrosis. *Radiology.* 1969 Dec;93(6):1313-4.

[128] Ahsan N, Choudry AA, Berger A. Retroperitoneal fibrosis. *AFP* 1990; 41: 1775-80.

[129] Wu J, Catalano E, Coppola D. Retroperitoneal fibrosis (Ormond's disease): clinical pathologic study of eight cases. *Cancer Control.* 2002 Sep-Oct;9(5):432-7.

[130] Chim CS, Liang R, Chan AC. Sclerosing malignant lymphoma mimicking idiopathic retroperitoneal fibrosis: importance of clonality study. *Am J Med.* 2001 Aug 15;111(3):240-1.

[131] Osborne BM, Butler JJ, Bloustein P, Sumner G. Idiopathic retroperitoneal fibrosis (sclerosing retroperitonitis). *Hum Pathol.* 1987 Jul;18(7):735-9.

[132] Mitchinson MJ. Chronic periaortitis and periarteritis. *Histopathology.* 1984 Jul;8(4):589-600.

[133] Pennell RC, Hollier LH, Lie JT, Bernatz PE, Joyce JW, Pairolero PC, Cherry KJ, Hallett JW. Inflammatory abdominal aortic aneurysms: a thirty-year review. *J Vasc Surg.* 1985 Nov;2(6):859-69.

[134] Doolin EJ, Goldstein H, Kessler B, Vinocur C, Marchildon MB. Familial retroperitoneal fibrosis. *J Pediatr Surg.* 1987 Dec;22(12):1092-4.

[135] Duffy PG, Johnston SR, Donaldson RA. Idiopathic retroperitoneal fibrosis in twins. *J Urol.* 1984 Apr;131(4):746.

[136] Willscher MK, Novicki DE, Cwazka WF. Association of HLA-B27 antigen with retroperitoneal fibrosis. *J Urol.* 1978 Nov;120(5):631-3.

[137] Ramshaw AL, Roskell DE, Parums DV. Cytokine gene expression in aortic adventitial inflammation associated with advanced atherosclerosis (chronic periaortitis). *J Clin Pathol.* 1994 Aug;47(8):721-7.

[138] Dixon AK, Mitchinson MJ, Sherwood T. Computed tomographic observations in periaortitis: a hypothesis. *Clin Radiol.* 1984 Jan;35(1):39-42.

[139] Parums DV, Brown DL, Mitchinson MJ. Serum antibodies to oxidized low-density lipoprotein and ceroid in chronic periaortitis. *Arch Pathol Lab Med* 1990; 114: 383-7.

[140] Parums DV, Chadwick DR, Mitchinson MJ. The localisation of immunoglobulin in chronic periaortitis. *Atherosclerosis* 1986; 61: 117-23.

[141] Mitchinson MJ, Hothersall DC, Brooks PN, De Burbure CY. The distribution of ceroid in human atherosclerosis. *J Pathol.* 1985 Feb;145(2):177-83.

[142] Hughes D, Buckley PJ. Idiopathic retroperitoneal fibrosis is a macrophage-rich process. Implications for its pathogenesis and treatment. *Am J Surg Pathol.* 1993 May;17(5):482-90.

[143] Pasquinelli G, Preda P, Gargiulo M, Vici M, Cenacchi G, Stella A, D'Addato M, Martinelli GN, Pileri S. An immunohistochemical study of inflammatory abdominal aortic aneurysms. *J Submicrosc Cytol Pathol.* 1993 Jan;25(1):103-12.

[144] Mitchinson MJ. Insoluble lipids in human atherosclerotic plaques. *Atherosclerosis.* 1982 Oct;45(1):11-5.

[145] Hannson GK. Immune and inflammatory mechanisms in the pathogenesis of atherosclerosis. *J. Atheroscl et Thromb.* 1 suppl 1 (1993), pp. 6–9.

[146] O'Brien KD, McDonald TO, Chait A, Allen MD, Alpers CE. Neovascular expression of E-selectin, intercellular adhesion molecule-1, and vascular cell adhesion molecule-1 in human atherosclerosis and their relation to intimal leukocyte content. *Circulation.* 1996 Feb 15;93(4):672-82.

[147] Lopez-Candales A, Holmes DR, Liao S, Scott MJ, Wickline SA, Thompson RW. Decreased vascular smooth muscle cell density in medial degeneration of human abdominal aortic aneurysms. *Am J Pathol.* 1997 Mar;150(3):993-1007.

[148] Wood KM, Cadogan MD, Ramshaw AL, Parums DV. The distribution of adhesion molecules in human atherosclerosis. *Histopathology.* 1993 May;22(5):437-44.

[149] Ramshaw AL, Parums DV. The distribution of adhesion molecules in chronic periaortitis. *Histopathology.* 1994 Jan;24(1):23-32.

[150] Bobryshev YV, Lord RS, Parsson H. Immunophenotypic analysis of the aortic aneurysm wall suggests that vascular dendritic cells are involved in immune responses. *Cardiovasc Surg.* 1998 Jun;6(3):240-9.

[151] Freestone T, Turner RJ, Coady A, Higman DJ, Greenhalgh RM, Powell JT. Inflammation and matrix metalloproteinases in the enlarging abdominal aortic aneurysm. *Arterioscler Thromb Vasc Biol.* 1995 Aug;15(8):1145-51.

[152] Curci JA, Liao S, Huffman MD, Shapiro SD, Thompson RW. Expression and localization of macrophage elastase (matrix metalloproteinase-12) in abdominal aortic aneurysms. *J Clin Invest.* 1998 Dec 1;102(11):1900-10.

[153] Davis V, Persidskaia R, Baca-Regen L, Itoh Y, Nagase H, Persidsky Y, Ghorpade A, Baxter BT. Matrix metalloproteinase-2 production and its binding to the matrix are increased in abdominal aortic aneurysms. *Arterioscler Thromb Vasc Biol.* 1998 Oct;18(10):1625-33.

[154] Silence J, Collen D, Lijnen HR. Reduced atherosclerotic plaque but enhanced aneurysm formation in mice with inactivation of the tissue inhibitor of metalloproteinase-1 (TIMP-1) gene. *Circ Res.* 2002 May 3;90(8):897-903.

[155] Lee E, Grodzinsky AJ, Libby P, Clinton SK, Lark MW, Lee RT. Human vascular smooth muscle cell-monocyte interactions and metalloproteinase secretion in culture. *Arterioscler Thromb Vasc Biol.* 1995 Dec;15(12):2284-9.

[156] Keen RR, Nolan KD, Cipollone M, Scott E, Shively VP, Yao JS, Pearce WH. Interleukin-1 beta induces differential gene expression in aortic smooth muscle cells. *J Vasc Surg.* 1994 Nov;20(5):774-84.

[157] Galis ZS, Muszynski M, Sukhova GK, Simon-Morrissey E, Unemori EN, Lark MW, Amento E, Libby P. Cytokine-stimulated human vascular smooth muscle cells synthesize a complement of enzymes required for extracellular matrix digestion. *Circ Res.* 1994 Jul;75(1):181-9.

[158] Newman KM, Jean-Claude J, Li H, Ramey WG, Tilson MD. Cytokines that activate proteolysis are increased in abdominal aortic aneurysms. *Circulation.* 1994 Nov;90(5 Pt 2):II224-7.

[159] Longo GM, Xiong W, Greiner TC, Zhao Y, Fiotti N, Baxter BT. Matrix metalloproteinases 2 and 9 work in concert to produce aortic aneurysms. *J Clin Invest.* 2002 Sep;110(5):625-32.

[160] Aimes RT, Quigley JP. Matrix metalloproteinase-2 is an interstitial collagenase. Inhibitor-free enzyme catalyzes the cleavage of collagen fibrils and soluble native type I collagen generating the specific 3/4- and 1/4-length fragments. *J Biol Chem.* 1995 Mar 17;270(11):5872-6.

[161] Petersen E, Gineitis A, Wagberg F, Angquist KA. Activity of matrix metalloproteinase-2 and -9 in abdominal aortic aneurysms. Relation to size and rupture. *Eur J Vasc Endovasc Surg.* 2000 Nov;20(5):457-61.

[162] McMillan WD, Pearce WH. Increased plasma levels of metalloproteinase-9 are associated with abdominal aortic aneurysms. *J Vasc Surg.* 1999 Jan;29(1):122-7.

[163] Vine N, Powell JT. Metalloproteinases in degenerative aortic disease. *Clin Sci* (Lond). 1991 Aug;81(2):233-9.

[164] Wahl SM, Gately CL. Modulation of fibroblast growth by a lymphokine of human T cell continuous T cell line origin. *J Immunol.* 1983 Mar;130(3):1226-30.

[165] Noguchi H, Kephart GM, Colby TV, Gleich GJ. Tissue eosinophilia and eosinophil degranulation in syndromes associated with fibrosis. *Am J Pathol.* 1992 Feb;140(2):521-8.

[166] Moosa HH, Peitzman AB, Steed DL, Julian TB, Jarrett F, Webster MW. Inflammatory aneurysms of the abdominal aorta. *Arch Surg.* 1989 Jun;124(6):673-5.

[167] Lichon FS, Sequeira W, Pilloff A, Skosey JL. Retroperitoneal fibrosis associated with systemic lupus erythematosus: a case report and brief review. *J Rheumatol.* 1984 Jun;11(3):373-4.

[168] Hollingworth P, Denman AM, Gumpel JM. Retroperitoneal fibrosis and polyarteritis nodosa successfully treated by intensive immunosuppression. *J R Soc Med.* 1980 Jan;73(1):61-4.

[169] Numano F. Vasa vasoritis, vasculitis and atherosclerosis. *Int J Cardiol.* 2000 Aug 31;75 Suppl 1:S1-8.

[170] Hem E, Mathisen W. Retroperitoneal fibrosis. A follow-up study. Eur Urol. 1984;10(1):43-7.

[171] Denes FT, Arap S. Retroperitoneal fibrosis: an alternative therapy. *Eur Urol.* 1986;12(4):283-4.

[172] Slavis SA, Wilson RW, Jones RJ, Swift C. Long-term results of permanent indwelling wallstents for benign mid-ureteral strictures. *J Endourol.* 2000 Sep;14(7):577-81.

[173] Cooksey G, Powell PH, Singh M, Yeates WK. Idiopathic retroperitoneal fibrosis: A long-term review after surgical treatment. *Br J Urol* 1982; 54: 628-31.

[174] Tiptaft RC, Costello AJ, Paris AM, Blandy JP. The long-term follow-up of idiopathic retroperitoneal fibrosis. *Br J Urol* 1982; 54: 620-3.

[175] Wagenknecht LV, Hardy JC. Value of various treatments of retroperitoneal fibrosis. *Eur Urol* 1981; 7: 193-200.

[176] Osborn DE, Rao PN, Barnard RJ, Ackrill P, Ralston AJ, Best JJ. Surgical management of idiopathic retroperitoneal fibrosis. *Br J Urol.* 1981 Aug;53(4):292-6.

[177] Lindell OI, Lehtonen TA. Surgical treatment of ureteric obstruction in idiopathic retroperitoneal fibrosis. *Scand J Urol Nephrol Suppl.* 1988;110:299-302.

[178] Kavoussi LR, Clayman RV, Brunt LM, Soper NJ. Laparoscopic ureterolysis. *J Urol.* 1992 Feb;147(2):426-9.

[179] Demirci D, Gulmez I, Ekmekcioglu O, Sozuer EM, Keklik E. Intraperitonealization of the ureter during laparoscopic ureterolysis: a modification of the technique. *J Urol.* 2001 Jan;165(1):180-1.

[180] Baker LR. Auto-allergic periaortitis (idiopathic retroperitoneal fibrosis). *BJU Int.* 2003 Nov;92(7):663-5.

[181] Kinder CH. Retroperitoneal fibrosis. *J R Soc Med.* 1979 Jul;72(7):485-7.

[182] Mundy AR, Kinder CH, Flannery JF, Joyce MR. Hypertension and thromboembolism in idiopathic retroperitoneal fibrosis. *Br J Urol.* 1982 Dec;54(6):625-7.

[183] Cerfolio RJ, Morgan AS, Hirvela ER, Vaughan ED Jr. Idiopathic retroperitoneal fibrosis: is there a role for postoperative steroids? *Curr Surg.* 1990 Nov-Dec;47(6):423-7.

[184] Kardar AH, Kattan S, Lindstedt E, Hanash K. Steroid therapy for idiopathic retroperitoneal fibrosis: dose and duration. *J Urol.* 2002 Aug;168(2):550-5.

[185] Feild C, Arnold W, Gloster ES, Sharp G, Redman J. Steroid therapy as treatment for idiopathic fibrosis of the retroperitoneum and mediastinum. *Pediatrics.* 1986 Nov;78(5):936-8.

[186] Moody TE, Vaughan ED Jr. Steroids in the treatment of retroperitoneal fibrosis. *J Urol.* 1979 Jan;121(1):109-11.

[187] Ochsner MG, Brannan W, Pond HS, Goodlet JS Jr. Medical therapy in idiopathic retroperitoneal fibrosis. *J Urol.* 1975 Nov;114(5):700-4.

[188] Ross JC, Goldsmith HJ. The combined surgical and medical treatment of retroperitoneal fibrosis. *Br J Surg.* 1971 Jun;58(6):422-7.

[189] Harreby M, Bilde T, Helin P, Meyhoff HH, Vinterberg H, Nielsen VA. Retroperitoneal fibrosis treated with methylprednisolon pulse and disease-modifying antirheumatic drugs. *Scand J Urol Nephrol.* 1994 Sep;28(3):237-42.

[190] Smith SJ, Bosniak MA, Megibow AJ, Hulnick DH, Smiles S. CT demonstration of rapid improvement of retroperitoneal fibrosis in response to steroid therapy. *Urol Radiol.* 1986;8(2):104-7.

[191] McDougal WS, MacDonell RC Jr. Treatment of idiopathic retroperitoneal fibrosis by immunosuppression. *J Urol.* 1991 Jan;145(1):112-4.

[192] Cogan E, Fastrez R. Azathioprine. An alternative treatment for recurrent idiopathic retroperitoneal fibrosis. *Arch Intern Med* 1985; 145: 753-55

[193] Scavalli AS, Spadaro A, Riccieri V, Ricciuti GP, Taccari E, Marini M, Zoppini A. Long term follow-up of low-dose methotrexate therapy in one case of idiopathic retroperitoneal fibrosis. *Clin Rheumatol* 1995; 14: 481-4.

[194] Grotz W, von Zedtwitz I, Andre M, Schollmeyer P. Treatment of retroperitoneal fibrosis by mycophénolate mofétil and corticoids. *Lancet* 1998; 352: 1195.

[195] Marzano A, Trapani A, Leone N, Actis GC, Rizzetto M. Treatment of idiopathic retroperitoneal fibrosis using cyclosporin. *Ann Rheum Dis.* 2001 Apr;60(4):427-8.

[196] Kohler HP, Laeng RH, Egger C, Streuli R. Systemic fibrosis (generalized form of Ormond's disease). Report of a case which achieved complete remission with cyclophosphamide and corticosteroids. *Schweiz Med Wochenschr.* 1995 Nov 4;125(44):2131-6.

[197] Cronstein BN, Naime D, Ostad E. The antiinflammatory mechanism of methotrexate. Increased adenosine release at inflamed sites diminishes leukocyte accumulation in an in vivo model of inflammation. *J Clin Invest.* 1993 Dec;92(6):2675-82.

[198] Cronstein BN, Naime D, Firestein G. The antiinflammatory effects of an adenosine kinase inhibitor are mediated by adenosine. *Arthritis Rheum.* 1995 Aug;38(8):1040-5.

[199] Bourouma R, Chevet D, Michel F, Cercueil JP, Arnould L, Rifle G. Treatment of idiopathic retroperitoneal fibrosis with tamoxifen. *Nephrol Dial Transplant.* 1997 Nov;12(11):2407-10.

[200] Puce R, Porcaro AB, Curti P, Girelli D, Pantalena M, Malossini G, Tallarigo C. Treatment of retroperitoneal fibrosis with tamoxifen: case report and review of literature. *Arch Esp Urol.* 2000 Mar;53(2):184-90.

[201] Clark CP, Vanderpool D, Preskitt JT. The response of retroperitoneal fibrosis to tamoxifen. *Surgery.* 1991 Apr;109(4):502-6.

[202] Spillane RM, Whitman GJ. Treatment of retroperitoneal fibrosis with tamoxifen. *AJR Am J Roentgenol.* 1995 Feb;164(2):515-6.

[203] Colletta AA, Wakefield LM, Howell FV, van Roozendaal KE, Danielpour D, Ebbs SR, Sporn MB, Baum M. Anti-oestrogens induce the secretion of active transforming growth factor beta from human fetal fibroblasts. *Br J Cancer.* 1990 Sep;62(3):405-9.

[204] Benson JR, Baum M. Tamoxifen for retroperitoneal fibrosis. *Lancet* 1993 ; 341: 836.

[205] Marcolongo R, Tavolini IM, Laveder F, Busa M, Noventa F, Bassi P, Semenzato G. Immunosuppressive therapy for idiopathic retroperitoneal fibrosis: a retrospective analysis of 26 cases. *Am J Med.* 2004 Feb 1;116(3):194-7.

[206] Carini M, Selli C, Rizzo M, Durval A, Costantini A. Surgical treatment of retroperitoneal fibrosis with omentoplasty. *Surgery.* 1982 Feb;91(2):137-41.

[207] Selman M, King TE, Pardo A. Idiopathic pulmonary fibrosis: prevailing and evolving hypotheses about its pathogenesis and implications for therapy. *Ann Intern Med.* 2001 Jan 16;134(2):136-51.

[208] Dedeoglu F, Rose CD, Athreya BH, Conard K, Grissom L, Magnusson M. Successful treatment of retroperitoneal fibrosis with tamoxifen in a child. *J Rheumatol.* 2001 Jul;28(7):1693-5.

In: Progress in Inflammation Research
Editor: James A. Pitzer, pp. 39-93

ISBN 1-59454-277-5

Chapter II

Involvement of Invading Macrophage Derived Prostaglandins in the Pathogenesis of Neuropathic Pain Caused by Nerve Injury

Weiya Ma[*]
Douglas Hospital Research Center, McGill University, 6875 LaSalle Boulevard, Verdun, Montreal, Quebec, Canada H4H 1R3

Abstract

Neuropathic pain is a serious clinical concern, arising from various diseases as well as physical damage of the central and peripheral nervous systems. Neuropathic pain is usually manifested as spontaneous pain, hyperalgesia and allodynia. Due to unclear mechanisms, the treatment is largely unsatisfactory. Therefore, it adversely affects the life quality of the patients. Damage of a nerve is inevitably followed by infiltration of blood-borne inflammatory cells into degenerating axons, of which macrophages are the principal effecter cells. Macrophages not only clean myelin debris, but also produce pro-inflammatory cytokines, growth factors and pain inducing mediators including prostaglandins (PGs). The role of this inflammatory event in the pathogenesis of neuropathic pain is yet to be determined. The purpose of the book chapter is to address morphological and pharmacological evidence that invading macrophage derived PGs are involved in the pathogenesis of neuropathic pain following nerve injury.

In this chapter, we demonstrate that PG synthesizing enzyme cyclooxygenase 2 (COX2) is dramatically up-regulated in invading macrophages in injured nerve of rats following partial sciatic nerve ligation (PSNL), chronic constriction injury of sciatic nerve (CCI) and spinal nerve ligation (SNL). COX2-IR cells appear as early as 3 days postlesion,

[*] Correspondent address: Douglas Hospital Research Center, McGill University, 6875 LaSalle Boulevard, Verdun, Montreal, Quebec, Canada H4H 1R3; Tel.: (514) 761-6131, ext 2935; Fax: (514) 762-3034; e-mail: weiya.ma@douglas.mcgill.ca

reach a peak by 2 to 4 weeks, then gradually decrease and completely disappear by 7 month postlesion. PGE2 released from injured nerve explants is significantly increased compared to that from intact nerve explants. Both non-selective and selective COX inhibitors suppress the release of PGE2 from injured nerve explants. Perineural and intraplantar injection of a non-selective COX inhibitor ketorolac effectively relieves mechanical allodynia in rats treated with PSNL, CCI and SNL. Local ketorolac achieved maximum anti-allodynia during 2-4 weeks postlesion. Seven months after lesion, the anti-allodynia induced by local ketorolac completely disappears. Two and 4 weeks following PSNL, cell profiles expressing EP1, EP2, EP3, and EP4 receptors are dramatically increased in injured nerve. EP4 up-regulation in these cells is the most prominent and widespread among other EP receptors. About half of macrophages express EP1 and EP4, only small fraction of macrophages express EP2 and EP3. Local ketorolac significantly suppress the phosphorylation of cAMP responsive element binding protein and the expression of pain-related neuropeptide substance P, calcitonin gene-related peptide and dynorphin in the dorsal horn. The hypothesis that macrophage derived PGE2 is involved in the up-regulation of pro-inflammatory cytokine interleukin-6 (IL-6) in injured nerve was tested. PSNL increased IL-6 IR cell profiles in injured nerves and most of them were identified as invading macrophages. PGE2 and IL-6 releases from cultured cells derived from injured nerves are significantly increased and suppressed by both non-selective and selective COX2 inhibitors. Treatment with PGE2 further enhanced IL-6 release in a concentration- and time-dependent manner. A selective EP4 receptor antagonist and a protein kinase C inhibitor suppressed IL-6 release, suggesting that IL-6 induction by PGE2 is mediated through EP4 receptor and PKC signaling pathway.

All above data suggest that PG over-production in invading macrophages in injured nerve is a common event following peripheral nerve injury, which contributes to the plasticity in signal transduction events and neuropeptide expression in primary sensory neurons and dorsal horn neurons and to the development of neuropathic pain during initial several months. Up-regulation of EP receptors in invading macrophages suggests that, through autocrine or paracrine pathways, over-produced PGE2 may influence macrophage functions, including pro-inflammatory cytokine production, which indirectly contributes to the development of neuropathic pain.

Abbreviations

CCI	chronic constriction injury;
CGRP	calcitonin gene-related peptide;
COX	cyclooxygenase 2;
CREB	cAMP responsive element binding protein;
CSNT	complet sciatic nerve transaction;
DAB	diaminobenzidine;
IR	immunoreactive or immunoreactivity;
IL	interleukin;
iNOS	inducible nitric oxide synthase;
i.p.	intraperitoneal injection;
i.pl.	intraplantar injection;
NGF	nerve growth factor;

NGS	normal goat serum;
NO	nitric oxida;
LPS	lipopolysaccharide;
PB	phosphate buffer;
PBS	phosphate buffered saline;
PBS+T	phosphate buffered saline containing 0.3% Triton X-100;
PG	prostaglandin;
PSNL	partial sciatic nerve ligation;
SNL	spinal nerve ligation;
SP	substance P;
TBS	Tris buffered saline;
TBS+T	Tris buffered saline containing 0.05% Tween 20;
TNF	tumor necrosis factor.

I. Introduction

1.1. Overview

Neuropathic pain refers to the pain caused by disease or physical damage to both central and peripheral nerve tissues. However, the pain elicited by peripheral nerve injury is often used synonymously with "neuropathic pain". The spectrum of partial damage to total destruction of peripheral nerves is associated with a variety of syndromes including spontaneous pain (burning pain), an increase in the sensitivity to noxious stimuli (hyperalgesia) and a painful response to normally innocuous mechanical and cold stimuli (allodynia). Neuropathic pain is usually chronic (lasts for many years) and refractory to treatment with opiates and other conventional analgesics. Hence, it severely deteriorates quality life of the patients.

In the past decade, our understanding of neuropathic pain caused by peripheral nerve injury has been advanced by the characterization of three animal models: chronic constriction injury of the sciatic nerve (CCI) (Bennett and Xie, 1988), partial sciatic nerve ligation (PSNL) (Seltzer et al., 1990) and spinal nerve ligation (SNL) (Kim and Chung, 1992). All three models involve partial damage of peripheral nerves, which evokes more severe neuropathic pain symptoms than complete transection of the nerves. Although the mechanisms underlying the generation and maintenance of neuropathic pain are complicated and unclear, peripheral as well as central mechanisms are generally thought to be involved (Millan, 1999). Most of the current research has focused on the role of the plastic changes in dorsal root ganglion (DRG) neurons and spinal dorsal horn neurons. In contrast, the role of peripheral inflammatory reactions in the injured nerve in the pathogenesis of neuropathic pain has been relatively ignored (Tracey and Walker, 1995).

1.2 The Role of Inflammatory Reaction in the Development of Neuropathic Pain Caused by Nerve Injury

Increasing evidence suggests inflammatory reaction in the injured nerve following initial damage as an important contributing factor in the development of neuropathic pain (Levine et al., 1990; Frisen et al., 1993; Clatworthy et al., 1995; Tracey and Walker, 1995). When a nerve is damaged, distal axons undergo Wallerian degeneration, which recruits inflammatory cells from the circulation into the degenerating axons (Brown et al., 1991; Frisen et al., 1993; Cui et al., 2000). Inflammatory cells (macrophages, lymphocytes, and neutrophils) not only clear up nerve debris but also facilitate axon regeneration by producing and releasing growth factors, pro- or anti-inflammatory cytokines and mediators. In addition to promoting regeneration, most of these Wallerian degeneration products are pro-nociceptive and sensitize both injured and intact axons to innocuous and noxious mechanical stimuli (Michaelis et al., 1998).

Wallerian degeneration can be regarded as an injury-induced inflammatory response initiated by cytokines. During the early stage, Schwann cells release pro-inflammatory cytokines including tumor necrosis factor (TNFα), interleukin-1β (IL-1β) and interleukin 6 (IL-6), which chemoattract blood-borne macrophages to migrate into injury sites. Macrophages not only ingest degrading myelin debris but also release cytokines, growth factors and algesic agents such as prostaglandins (PGs). Macrophage released products are usually pro-nociceptive, sensitizing peripheral nociceptors. Greater research attention has been drawn to the role of pro-inflammatory cytokines in the pathogenesis of neuropathic pain. Levels of TNFα (Wagner and Myers, 1996b; Wagner et al., 1998; Cui et al., 2000), IL-6 (Bourde et al., 1996) and IL-1β (Lindholm et al., 1987) are increased in injured sciatic nerve following injuries. Local injection of TNFα (Wagner and Myers, 1996a) and IL-1β (Fukuoka et al., 1994) produces hyperalgesia and mechanical allodynia. Macrophages are the major producer of IL-6 (Reichert et al., 1996; Cui et al., 2000). In IL-6 knockout mice, hyperalgesia and allodynia are attenuated following SNL (Ramer et al., 1998). Thus, depletion of cytokine producers, macrophages (Liu et al., 2000) and neutrophils (Perkins and Tracey, 2000), attenuates hyperalgesia following PSNL. As inflammation advances, macrophages begin to switch from producing pro- to producing anti-inflammatory cytokines or agents such as transforming growth factor β1, platelet activating factor and interleukin 10 (Kiefer et al., 2001). The mechanism underlying this switch is that macrophages ingesting necrotic cells produce pro-inflammatory cytokines, and when ingesting apoptotic cells, they produce anti-inflammatory cytokines (Fadok et al., 1998).

1.3. The Role of Peripheral Prostaglandin in the Development of Neuropathic Pain Caused by Nerve Injury

In addition to cytokines, recruited inflammatory cells also produce pro-nociceptive mediators including serotonin, bradykinin, and prostaglandins in the injured nerve. Although the role of these inflammatory mediators has been well characterized during acute inflammatory pain (Davies and MacIntyre, 1992; Dray and Perkins, 1993; Levine and

Reichling, 1999), their role in the underlying peripheral mechanisms of chronic neuropathic pain is poorly understood (Tracey and Walker, 1995).

PGs belong to a large family of arachidonic acid oxygenation products existing in practically every mammalian tissue and mediating a wide array of physiologic and pathological events. PGs, especially the major product, PGE2, are well known algesic agents and abundantly produced during inflammation. Cyclooxygenase 1 (COX1) and cyclooxygenase 2 (COX2), two isoenzymes in the pathway of PG synthesis, convert arachidonic acid into PGH2 (Davies and MacIntyre, 1992). COX1 and COX2 exist in both the central and peripheral nervous systems. COX2 is usually regarded as inducible while COX1 is considered as a 'housekeeping' isoenzyme. Macrophages are known to synthesize PGE2 in response to pro-inflammatory stimuli such as IL-1, TNF and bacterial lipopolysaccharide (LPS) (Reddy and Herschman, 1994; Levi et al., 1998). COX2 enzyme, which drives PGE2 production, is also synthesized *de novo* upon pro-inflammatory stimulation (Lee et al., 1992). PGE2 is well known to mediate a wide range of biological effects and plays an important role in multiple pathological processes, such as inflammation, angiogenesis and tumor growth. All PGE2 effects are mediated through specific receptors present in the target cells. Four subtypes of PGE2 receptor, EP1, EP2, EP3, and EP4, have been identified and differ in their signal transduction pathways (Coleman et al., 1994; Ichikawa et al., 1996). All these receptors belong to the G protein-coupled receptor superfamily. EP1 receptor mediates an increase in intracellular calcium, thus facilitating neurotransmitter release. EP2 and EP4 receptors stimulate adenylyl cyclase and increase cAMP concentrations. EP3 receptor has been traditionally thought to inhibit adenylyl cyclase (Vanegas and Schaible, 2001). mRNA of four EP receptors was found in DRG neurons (Oida et al., 1995). More than one EP receptor is involved in mediating PGE2 induced hyperalgesia, predominantly via the cAMP second messenger system, in the rat hindpaw (Khasar et al., 1995). Nuclear EP receptors are also characterized as functional (Bhattacharya et al., 1998).

Similar to macrophages, PGE2 acts in a Janus fashion, with both pro- and anti-inflammatory effects, partly dependent on the array of EP receptor subtypes with opposing signal transduction pathways. PGE2 contributes to immune suppression and inflammation termination by inhibiting B and T lymphocyte proliferation, as well as various macrophage functions (Taffet and Russell, 1981; Chouaib et al., 1985; Simkin et al., 1987). Released PGE2 acts on macrophages, thus forming a negative feedback loop in macrophage activation. PGE2 inhibits the production of various cytokines such as TNFα, IL-1β and IL-12 by macrophages (Zhong et al., 1995; Yamane et al., 2000; Shinomiya et al., 2001), but increases the production of IL-6 (Yamane et al., 2000; Repovic and Benveniste, 2002) and IL-10 (Shinomiya et al., 2001). These effects on cytokines are mediated through EP4 and EP2 receptors (Katsuyama et al., 1998; Yamane et al., 2000) which are also increased in macrophages stimulated by inflammatory agents (Katsuyama et al., 1998; Kurihara et al., 2001). Overall, these lines of evidence suggest that PGE2 plays both pro- and anti-inflammatory roles during inflammation. However, all these studies were done *in vitro* and in an arthritis model, conditions that are considerably different from Wallerian degeneration after partial nerve injury, where injured and spared axons are exposed to PGE2 released from invading macrophages.

In contrast to these *in vitro* studies, we and others have suggested that, in vivo peripherally produced PGE2 by macrophages is a pro-inflammatory or pro-nociceptive player following nerve injury. Intraplantar injection of non-selective and selective COX inhibitors and a EP1 antagonist alleviates hypersensitivity caused by PSNL (Syriatowicz et al., 1999). The selective EP1 receptor antagonist (ONO-8711) reduces allodynia and c-fos expression in the dorsal horn of CCI rats (Kawahara et al., 2001). PGI2 enhances ectopic activity in rat sensory neurons following neuropathic injury (Omana-Zapata and Bley, 2001).

Recently, we have demonstrated that up-regulation of COX2 in infiltrating macrophages is a common event following various types of nerve injury (Ma and Eisenach, 2002; Ma and Eisenach, 2003a). PGE2 (Schafers et al., 2004) and 4 PGE2 EP receptors (Ma and Eisenach, 2003b) are increased in injured nerve. We also showed that both local and systemic injection of a non-selective COX inhibitor ketorolac significantly relieves neuropathic pain caused by various types of partial nerve injury and the anti-allodynia induced by COX inhibitors is closely associated with the abundance of COX2 expressing macrophages in injured nerve (Ma and Eisenach, 2002; Ma and Eisenach, 2003a). We further demonstrated that peripherally over-produced PGs are involved in nerve injury induced plasticity in signaling molecules (Ma and Eisenach, 2002) and in neuropeptide expression in DRG neurons and in the dorsal horn neurons (Ma and Eisenach, 2003c). Finally, we further explored the underlying mechanisms how macrophage derived PGE2 affects macrophage functions, such as production of pro-inflammatory cytokine IL-6, via an autocrine or paracrine mechanism (Ma and Quirion, 2005).

All obtained data indicate that infiltrating macrophage over-produced PGs contribute to the pathogenesis of neuropathic pain. In this chapter, the major data were reviewed and perspective future research directions were proposed regarding PGE2 in macrophage functions and neuropeptide expression and axonal regeneration and sprouting of injured DRG neurons.

II. Materials and Methods

2.1. Nerve Injury Elicited Neuropathic Pain Models

Sprague-Dawley rats (male, 200-250g, Harlan Industries, Indianapolis, IN) were used in this study. All surgery and animal care procedures were in accordance with the protocol approved by the Animal Care and Use Committee of Wake Forest University School of Medicine. In all types of surgery, rats were under inhalation anesthesia of 4% halothane in oxygen and air. *Partial sciatic nerve ligation (PSNL):* The left sciatic nerve was exposed at the upper thigh level. One-third to one-half of the nerve was tightly ligated with silicon-treated silk suture (size 6-0) as previously described (Seltzer et al., 1990). Then muscle and skin layers were closed. *Spinal nerve ligation (SNL):* SNL was performed as described previously (Kim and Chung, 1992). The left L5 and L6 spinal nerves were isolated adjacent to the vertebral column and tightly ligated with 6-0 silk sutures distal to the dorsal root ganglion. *Chronic constriction injury (CCI):* CCI was performed as described previously (Bennett and Xie, 1988). At the middle thigh level of the sciatic nerve, four chromic gut sutures (size 4-0) were loosely tied around the sciatic nerve. The distance between each ligation was approximately 1mm. *Complete sciatic nerve transection (CSNT):* A 5mm-long nerve segment was removed from the left sciatic nerve at the middle thigh level. All rats had free access to food and water and were allowed to survive for different periods of time (3 days, 1, 2, 4 weeks, 3 and 7 months).

2.2. Behavioral Testing and Drug Treatment

The paw withdrawal threshold in response to mechanical stimulation was measured at different time points before and after surgery or drug treatment. The pre-lesion baseline value for each rat was obtained one day before nerve injury. Thirty minutes before testing, rats were placed in individual plastic enclosures with a mesh floor and allowed to explore and groom until they settled. After accommodation to the environment, a series of von Frey filaments with bending forces ranging from 1-30g were applied perpendicularly to the plantar surface of the hind paw and pressed to the point of bending 5 times over approximately 5 seconds. Withdrawal threshold was determined using an up-down method previously described (Chaplan et al., 1994). Three measurements of the withdrawal threshold were determined for each paw, with testing separated by 5-10 min, and the mean withdrawal threshold from each group was analyzed using one-way repeated measures ANOVA with *post hoc* Dunnett's multiple comparison method. The significance level was set at $p<0.05$.

At different time points, under a brief anesthesia with 4% halothane in oxygen and air, ketorolac (0.5%, 0.2ml, Syntex Inc., Palo Alto, CA, USA) was injected subcutaneously into the ipsilateral plantar surface of the hindpaw of rats using a 30-gauge needle. For intraperitoneal administration, 0.2ml ketorolac (5%) was injected in the abdominal cavity of rats under brief halothane anesthesia. Perineural injection was done as previously described (Thalhammer et al., 1995). Briefly, the rat was held in lateral recumbency with the limb to be injected forming a right angle with the longitudinal axis of the trunk. The greater trochanter and ischial tuberosity were localized by palpation. On an imaginary line from the greater trochanter to the ischial tuberosity, about one third of the distance caudal to the greater trochanter, a 25 gauge injection needle was advanced from dorsolateral direction at a 45^0 angle until the tip encountered the ischium. A total volume of 0.2ml was injected in a fanning motion along the path of the sciatic nerve.

2.3. COX2, EP Receptor, IL-6 Immunostaining and Quantification of COX2 Expressing Cells in Injured Nerve

After various survival periods, under deep anesthesia with sodium pentobarbital (100 mg/kg), all rats were perfused intracardially with cold phosphate buffered saline (PBS) containing 1% sodium nitrite and subsequently with 4% paraformaldehyde in 0.1M phosphate buffer (PB, pH 7.4). Nerve segments containing the lesion site were removed from the ipsilateral and contralateral sciatic nerve (PSNL, CCI and CSNT rats) or spinal nerve

(SNL rats) and postfixed in the same fixative for 3 to 6 hours. Then all tissues were transferred to 30% sucrose in 0.1M PB at 4°C for cryoprotection.

Both ipsilateral and contralateral nerve segments were mounted in the same block using O.C.T. mounting media. Ten-µm-thick sections were cut on a cryostat and thaw-mounted on precleaned Superfrost/plus slides (Fisher Scientific, Pittsburgh, PA, USA), and kept at –80°C until used. After pretreatment in 0.3 % H_2O_2 and 10% normal goat serum (NGS) in 0.1M Tris buffered saline (TBS), sections were incubated in polyclonal rabbit antibodies raised against COX2 (1:1000), EP1 (1:1000), EP2 (1:20,000), EP3 (1:20,000), EP4 (1:20,000) and goat anti-IL-6 antibody (Santa Cruz Biotechnology, Inc., Santa Cruz, CA, USA) diluted in TBS containing 10% NGS. Except IL-6 antibody, all other antisera were purchased from Cayman Chemical Inc., Ann Arbor, MI, USA. Subsequently, the sections were incubated in biotinylated goat anti-rabbit IgG (Vector Laboratories, Inc.) and further processed using Elite Vectastain ABC kit (Vector) according to the instructions of the manufacturer. Finally, the immunoprecipitates were developed by 3, -3' diaminobenzedine (DAB) and the chromogen was enhanced by the glucose oxidase-nickel-DAB method (Shu et al., 1988). Sections were washed in TBS containing 0.05% Tween-20 (5 min twice) between incubations.

Omission of all primary antibodies resulted in negative staining in all tested sections. For EP4 and IL-6, commercially available blocking peptides at concentration of 10 folds higher than antibodies were used to pre-absorb the antibodies. Incubation of sections with pre-absorbed antibodies produced negative staining.

For the quantification of COX2-IR cells, 5 sections of injured nerve (PSNL, CCI and CSNT: sciatic nerve; SNL: L5 or L6 spinal nerve) that were processed with COX2 immunostaining were selected randomly from each rat. In each section, one image (435µm x 445µm) was captured in an area immediately adjacent to the lesion site, while another image (435µm x 445µm) was taken in an area that was approximately 5mm distal from the lesion site. All COX2-IR cells with clear cell profiles were counted per area (435µm x 445µm). The cell number from the five sections was averaged for each rat. Eventually, the mean number ±SEM of COX2-IR cells was obtained for each group. The mean number of COX2-IR cells per area at the two locations was compared among SNL, CCI and CSNT rats, using one-way ANOVA with post hoc Student-Newman-Keuls multiple comparison method. Significance level was set at $P < 0.05$.

2.4. Immunostaining and Quantification of Pcreb, SP, CGRP, and Dynorphin in the Dorsal Horn of PSNL Rats

Tissue was obtained from rats with PSNL 5 days after saline or ketorolac injection (n=4 in each group at each time point). Under deep anesthesia with sodium pentobarbital (100 mg/kg), rats were perfused intracardially with cold PBS containing 1% sodium nitrite and subsequently with 4% paraformaldehyde in 0.1 M PB (pH 7.4). L4 to L6 spinal cord segments were removed and postfixed in the same fixative for 3 to 6 hours. Then all tissues were transferred to 30% sucrose in 0.1 M PB at 4°C for cryoprotection.

The spinal cord segments were cut on a cryostat at the thickness of 40 µm. The free-floating sections were collected in PBS. After being pretreated with 0.3% H_20_2 and 10%

NGS, spinal cord sections were incubated for 36 hours at 4°C in rabbit polyclonal antibodies raised against phospho-(p)CREB (1:1,000, New England Biolabs, Beverly, MA, USA), SP (1:4,000), CGRP (1:4,000) or dynorphin (1:12,000) diluted in PBS containing 0.3% Triton-X 100 (PBS+T) and 10% NGS. Anti-SP, CGRP and dynorphin antiserum were purchased from Peninsula Laboratories, Inc., Belmont, CA, USA. Subsequently, the sections were incubated in biotinylated goat anti-rabbit IgG (Vector Laboratories, Inc.) and further processed using Elite Vectastain ABC kit (Vector) according to the instructions of the manufacturer. Sections were washed in PBS+T (15 min twice) between incubations. Finally, the immunoprecipitates were developed by DAB, and the chromogen was enhanced by the glucose oxidase-nickel-DAB method. Omission of primary antibodies (SP, CGRP and dynorphin) resulted in negative staining in all tested sections.

Five L4-6 spinal cord sections were randomly selected from each rat. Images of both ipsilateral and contralateral dorsal horns were captured at X250 magnification using a digital CCD camera (SPOT, Diagnostic Instruments, Inc., Sterling Heights, Michigan, USA). The number of digitized pixels overlying IR axons or cells in the fixed area on each side of the dorsal horn was measured automatically using an image analysis software (SigmaScan, Jandel Scientific Inc., San Rafael, CA, USA). In a fixed area (235µm x 235µm) that covered the entire LI to LIII region in depth and was located in the middle one-third of the mediolateral extent of the dorsal horn, a threshold at which all IR axons or cells were overlaid by digitized pixels was applied to all sections measured. The more intense and abundant IR axons or cells were, the greater the number of digitized pixels which would cover the cell profile images. Values are expressed as mean ± SEM. The mean values from all groups were compared statistically using one-way ANOVA with *post hoc* Student-Newman-Keuls multiple comparison method. Significance level was set at $P < 0.05$.

2.5. Double Immunostaining

2.5.1 Double Immunostaining of COX2 and EP Receptors with ED1

Since most COX2-IR cells in injured nerve of rats exhibited macrophage-like morphology, we examined whether COX2 expressing cells also co-express macrophage marker ED1 in injured nerve of SNL and CCI rats at 2 weeks postlesion. Sections were incubated in 10% NGS in 0.1M TBS for 2 hours and then polyclonal rabbit antibodies raised against COX2 (1:500), EP1 (1:100), EP2 (1:2000), EP3 (1:2000) and EP4 (1:2000) diluted in TBS containing 10% NGS. All antibodies were purchased from Cayman Chemical Inc. The incubation lasted for 18 hours at 4°C. After thorough rinsing with TBS+T, sections were then incubated in a goat anti-rabbit IgG conjugated with Alexa Fluor 488 (1:400, Molecular Probes, Eugene, OR, USA) diluted in TBS containing 10% NGS for 1 hour. After rinsing with TBS+T, sections were further incubated in a mouse monoclonal antibody raised against ED1 (1:500, Serotec, Raleigh, NC, USA) for 18 hours at 4°C and then in biotinylated goat anti-mouse IgG (Vector) for 1 hour. Finally, sections were incubated in StreptAvidin conjugated with Alexa Fluor 568 (1:400, Molecular Probes).

2.5.2. Double Immunostaining of IL6 with COX2 and ED1

Sciatic nerve sections were incubated in 10% normal donkey serum (NDS) in 0.1M TBS for 2 hours and then in goat polyclonal antibody raised against IL-6 (1:200, source as mentioned above) diluted in TBS containing 10% NDS. The incubation lasted for 18 hours at 4°C. After thorough rinsing with TBS+T, sections were then incubated in a donkey anti-goat IgG conjugated with fluorescein (FITC, 1:50, Jackson ImmunoResearch Inc., Toronto, Ontario, Canada), diluted in TBS containing 10% NDS for 1 hour. After rinsing with TBS+T, sections were further incubated in a rabbit polyclonal antibody raised against COX2 (1:500, Cayman Chemical, Inc.) or in a mouse monoclonal antibody raised against ED1 (1:500, DAKO Corp., Carpinteria, CA, USA) for 18 hours at 4°C and then incubated in a donkey anti-rabbit or a donkey anti-mouse IgG conjugated with Texas Red (TR, 1:50, Jackson InnunoResearch Inc.) diluted in TBS containing 10% NDS.

Between incubations, sections were rinsed thoroughly with TBS+T. Finally, sections were cover-slipped with anti-fading mounting material (Vector) and examined under a laser confocal microscope (LSM 510, Carl Zeiss Microscopy, Jena, Germany).

2.6. Primary Cell Culture Derived from Intact and Injured Nerve Segments

Sprague Dawley rats (male, 150-200g) were used. All surgery and animal care procedures were in accordance with the protocol approved by Institutional Animal Care and Use Committee. Under the anesthesia with 2% halothane in oxygen, partial ligation of the left sciatic nerve at the high thigh level was made as mentioned above. Rats were allowed to survive for another one or two weeks. Under deep anesthesia with halothane inhalation, rats were decapitated. The injured sciatic nerve segment (approximately 1cm proximal and distal to the ligation site, total length = 2cm) was removed and immersed in Hank's balanced buffered saline (HBSS). The equivalent segment of intact sciatic nerve was also removed and immersed in HBSS in another well. Three to 6 rats are needed for each session.

Nerve segments were cut into 1mm long pieces in HBSS and incubate in 0.25% collagenase type II in Ham's F12 medium at 37^0C for 30min. After rinsing in HBSS, nerve segments were incubated in 0.25% trypsin at 37^0C for 10 min. Tissue was trituated with flame-polished glass pipette in Dulbecco Modified Eagle Medium (DMEM) containing 1% HEPES buffer solution, penicillin/streptomycin (1:200) and 10% heat inactivated fetal bovine serum (FBS). Cells were next subjected to density gradient centrifugation at 2000rpm, 4^0C for 10 min. The resulting pellet was resuspended with freshly prepared DMEM. The cell suspension was filtered through a cell strainer (70μm nylon, Becton Dickinson Labware, Franklin Lakes, NJ USA). Cells were seeded in 24-well culture plate, yielding a cell density of 5×10^5 cells per well, and cultured in a humid incubator at 37^0C with 5% CO2 and 95% air. All solutions and reagents were purchased from Invitrogen Life Technologies, Carlsbad, CA, USA.

2.7. Drug Treatments of Nerve Derived Cell Culture and Nerve Explants

Three days after seeding, cultured cells derived from intact or injured sciatic nerve segments were treated with PGE2 (PGE2, 1-30μM, Sigma, Oakville, Ontario, Canada) for 3, 6 12, 24 and 48 hours. The cultured cells were also treated with the following chemicals for 24 hours: non-selective COX inhibitor ketorolac (50μM, Syntex Inc., Palo Alto, CA, USA), selective COX2 inhibitor NS-398 (20μM, Cayman Chemical, Ann Arbor, MI, USA), DuP-697 (20μM, Cayman), Nimesulide (30μM, Cayman), EP1 receptor antagonist SC19220 (100μM, Cayman). A selective EP4 receptor antagonist L-161,982 ([4'- [3-butyl-5-oxo-1-(2-trifluoromethyl-phenyl)-1,5-dihydro- [1,2,4] triazol-4-ylmethyl]-biphenyl-2-sulphonic acid (3-methyl-thiophene-2-carbonyl)-amide]) (1μM) was generously provided by Dr. Robert Young (Merck Frosst Canada & Co., Kirkland, Montreal, Canada). A potent inhibitor of protein kinase A H-89 (50μM, Biomol Research Laboratory Inc., Plymouth Meeting, PA, USA), potent inhibitor of protein kinase C calphostin C (10μM, Biomol) and calcium chelator EGTA (3mM, Sigma) were also used. All chemicals were dissolved in ethanol. The final concentration of ethanol was less than 0.001%, which did not produce any change on the cultured cells. Each treatment was performed in triplicate and each experiment was repeated at least 3 times.

One to 2 weeks following PSNL, injured sciatic nerve segments (1cm proximal and distal to the ligation site) and uninjured nerve segments (at the same level) were dissected. Nerve segments were minced into 1mm-long pieces in Dulbecco Modified Eagle Medium (DMEM) containing 1% HEPES buffer solution, penicillin/streptomycin (1:200) and 10% heat inactivated fetal bovine serum (FBS). Small nerve segments were exposed to each of the following treatments for 24 hours: vehicle, non-selective COX inhibitor ketorolac (50μM, Allergan), selective COX2 inhibitor NS-398 (20μM), DuP-697 (20μM), Nimesulide (30μM). Following treatment, culture medium was collected in pyrogen-free eppendorf tubes and was frozen at -80^{0}C or underwent ELISA immediately.

2.8. Immunocytochemistry for Cultured Cells Derived from Intact and Injured Sciatic Nerve

Three days after seeding, cultured cells were fixed in 4% paraformaldehyde in 0.1MPB for 30min and then pretreated with 0.3%H_2O_2 and 10% NGS in 0.01M phosphate buffered saline containing 0.3% Triton-X 100 (PBS+T). Cultured cells were subsequently incubated in rabbit anti-COX2 (1:2000, source as above), goat anti-IL-6 (1:1000, source as above) and mouse anti-ED1 (1:1000, source as above) antisera for 18 hours at 4°C. Next, the sections were incubated with biotinylated linking IgG (Vector) and further processed using Elite Vectastain ABC kit (Vector) according to the instructions of the manufacturer. Between incubations, sections were rinsed in PBS+T. Finally, the immunoprecipitates were developed using DAB and the chromogen was enhanced by the glucose oxidase-nickel-DAB method.

2.9. Enzyme Linked Immunoassay (ELISA) for PGE2 and IL-6

Following treatment, culture medium, in which injured nerve derived cells and intact nerve derived cells were cultured, was collected in pyrogen-free eppendorf tubes and was frozen at -80^{0}C or underwent ELISA immediately. An IL-6 Immunoassay Kit (Biosource International, Inc. Camarillo, CA, USA) and a PGE2 High Sensitivity ELISA Kit (R&D Systems Inc., Minneapolis, MN, USA) were used. For measurement of PGE2 released from both injured and intact nerve explants, the culture medium, in which nerve explants were incubatedwas, was collected and used for PGE2 ELISA. All procedures were done following the manufacturer's instructions. Finally, the microplate was read on a microplate reader (BioTek FL600, Bio-Tek Instruments, Inc, Winooski, VT, USA). The mean value of PGE2 or IL-6 (pg/ml) released in culture medium was compared using one-way ANOVA with Student-Newman-Keuls multiple comparison methods, injured nerve vs. intact nerve, or vehicle vs. treatments. The significance level was set at $p<0.05$.

III. Results

3.1. COX2 is Up-Regulated in Invading Macrophages in Injured Nerve Following Never Injury

In the sciatic nerve of normal rats (not shown) and in the contralateral sciatic nerve of rats 2 and 4 weeks after PSNL, CCI, SNL and CSNT, there were no visible COX2-IR cell profiles. Only some axons were COX2-IR (Fig. 1A, arrows, Fig. 2A, 2C and 2E), likely reflecting the observations that some DRG neurons are COX2 containing (Ma, unpublished data). In striking contrast to the contralateral sciatic nerve, numerous intense COX2-IR cell profiles were observed in the ipsilateral sciatic nerve within a range approximately 1 cm proximal and distal to the ligation site (Fig. 1B, Fig. 2B, 2D and 2F, arrows). These COX2-IR cells exhibited characteristics of macrophages, e.g., foamy fatty vacuoles in the cytoplasm. At the ligation site of PSNL rats (Fig. 1C), more abundant and very intensely stained COX2-IR cells (arrows) were seen around the sutures. In the epineural connective tissues (Fig. 1D), some small size intense COX2-IR cells (arrows) were also observed. Some of them were adjacent to the small blood vessels.

Although numerous COX2-IR cells were localized in both the proximal and distal stumps of transected sciatic nerve of CSNT rats (Fig. 2F, arrows), COX2-IR cells were less abundant and the distribution range was much narrower than seen in SNL and CCI rats.

Table 1 illustrates the quantification of COX2-IR cell profiles in injured nerve of SNL, CCI and CSNT rats. The mean number of COX2-IR cells per area at the lesion site and in the stump 5 mm distal to the lesion site from both SNL rats and CCI rats was not significantly different (Table 1). However, the mean number of COX2-IR cells per area in the two locations was significantly lower in injured nerve of CSNT rats than in SNL and CCI rats (Table 1, $p<0.01$).

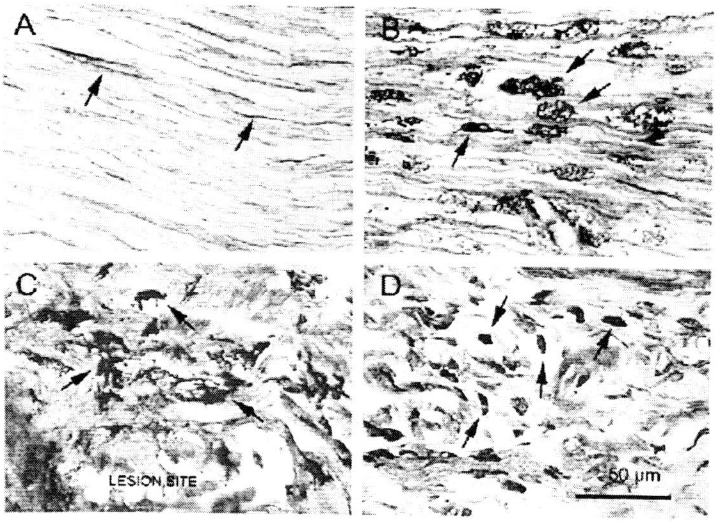

Figure 1. Photomicrographs of COX2 immunoreactivity in the sciatic nerve of a rat 4 weeks after PSNL. A shows the contralateral sciatic nerve at the high thigh level. COX2 immunoreactivity was localized in some axons (arrows), since COX2 was expressed in most of the DRG neurons (data not shown). B shows the ipsilateral sciatic nerve adjacent to the ligation site. Note that numerous COX2-IR cell profiles (arrows) were distributed among axons. The morphology of these labeled cells appears like macrophages due to foamy structures in the cytoplasm. C shows the ligation site. Intensely stained COX2-IR cells were observed at the lesion site (arrows). D. Numerous small size intensely stained COX2-IR cells were also visible in the epineural tissue in the ipsilateral sciatic nerve at high thigh level. Scale bar = 50μm.

3.2. The Time Course of COX2 Up-Regulation in Injured Nerve

Three days after PSNL, COX2-IR cells were observed in the injured sciatic nerve (Fig. 3A, arrows). By then, COX2-IR cells were mainly localized around the ligation site. One to 4 weeks after PSNL, COX2-IR cells had rapidly increased in abundance (Fig. 3B, 3C and 3D, arrows, area close to the lesion site) and expanded their distribution in both proximal and distal directions. However, 3 months after PSNL the abundance of COX2-IR cells had considerably declined in injured nerve (Fig. 4A, arrows). At the same time, the ligation site was surrounded by macrophages as well as connective tissue that formed a sheath (Fig. 4B, arrowheads). Similarly, 3 months after SNL (Fig. 4C) and CCI (Fig. 4D), COX2-IR cells were also evidently reduced in injured L5 and L6 spinal nerves and sciatic nerve, respectively. In the intact contralateral sciatic nerve, no COX2-IR cells were observed (not shown). Seven months after PSNL, no macrophage-like COX2-IR cells could be seen in the contralateral nerve (Fig. 5A) or in the injured nerve (Fig. 5B). The background staining in the ipsilateral nerve was also higher than in the contralateral side. However, in the ligation site ensheathed by connective tissue, some small size cells were COX2-IR (Fig. 5C and 5D).

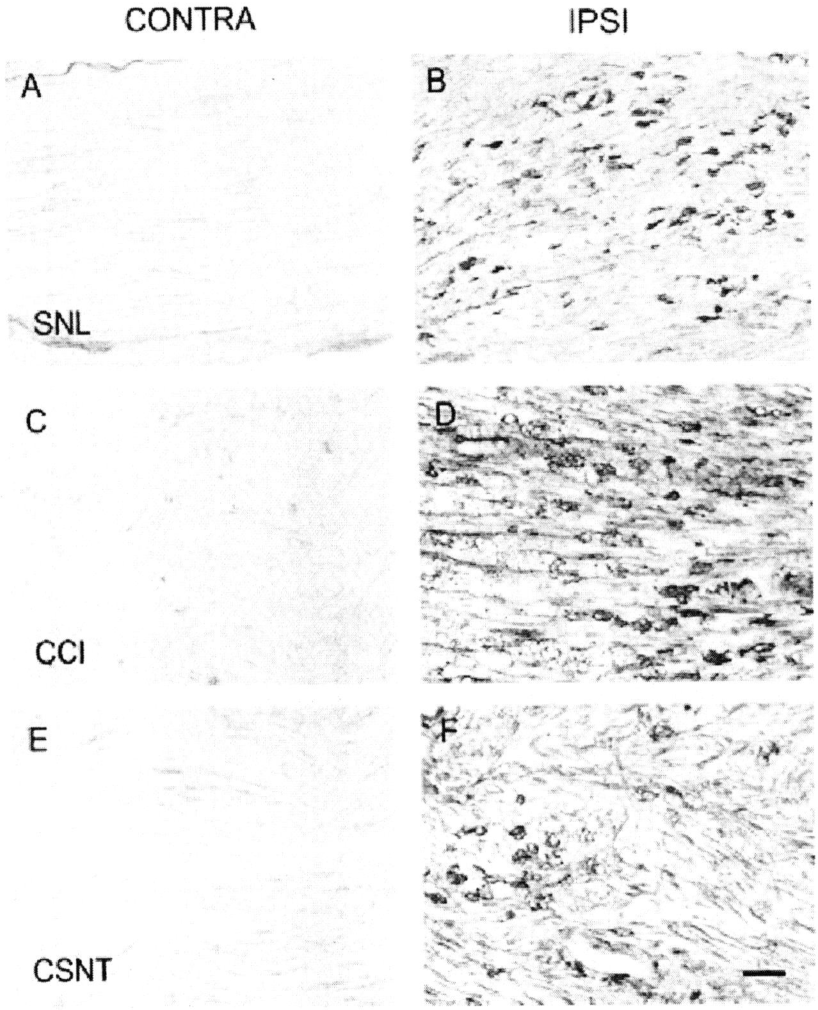

Figure 2. Photomicrographs of COX2 immunostaining in the contralateral and ipsilateral sciatic nerves 2 weeks following SNL (**A** and **B**), CCI (**C** and **D**) and CSNT (**E** and **F**). In the contralateral sciatic nerves of SNL (**A**), CCI (**B**) and CSNT (**C**) rats, no COX2-IR cell profiles were observed. In remarkable contrast, abundant COX2-IR cell profiles were observed in the ipsilateral sciatic nerves of SNL (**B**, arrows), CCI (**D**, arrows) and CSNT (**F**, arrows) rats. Morphologically, COX2-IR cell profiles were macrophage-like, with multiple foamy fatty vacuole-like structures existing in the cytoplasm. Much more abundant COPX2-IR cell profiles were seen in injured nerve of SNL and CCI rats than in CSNT rats. Scale bar = 50μm.

Table 1. The Mean Number±SEM of COX2-IR Cells at the Lesion Site and in the Distal Stump 5 mm from the Lesion Site in SNL Rats, CCI Rats and CSNT Rats

	SNL	CCI	CSNT
Lesion site	120±17	135±20	72±15*
Distal stump	122±18	130±29	52±11*

*, p<0.01.

One-way ANOVA with *post hoc* Student-Newman-Keuls multiple comparison method, n=4 in each group.

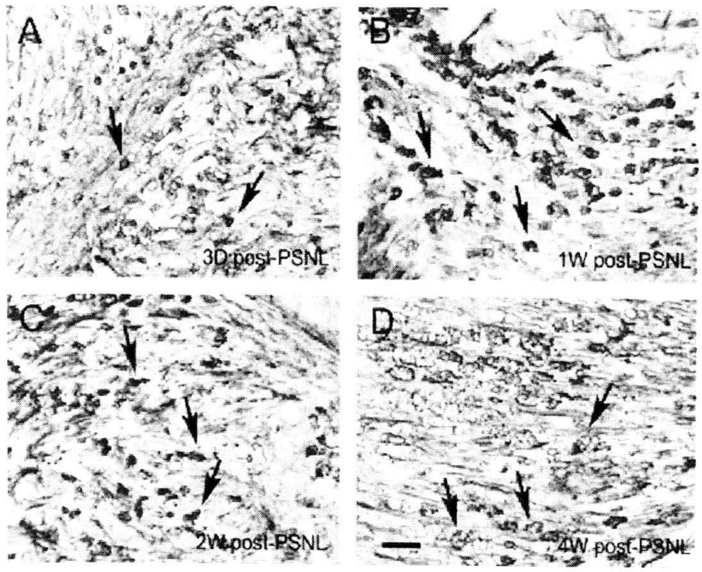

Figure 3. COX2 immunostaining in the area immediately adjacent to the injury site of PSNL rats at 3 days (**A**), 1 week (**B**), 2 weeks (**C**) and 4 weeks (**D**) post-lesion. In **A**, 3 days after PSNL numerous COX2-IR cell profiles were only seen in immediate regions adjacent to ligation site. One, 2 and 3 weeks after PSNL, COX2-IR cell profiles were increased in abundance and expanded to more proximal and distal regions from regions adjacent to the lesion site (**B**, **C** and **D**, arrows). Most COX2-IR cell profiles exhibited typical macrophage-like morphology, with numerous vacuoles in the cytoplasm. No COX2-IR cell profiles were observed in the contralateral sciatic nerve at any time points examined (not shown). Scale bar = 50μm.

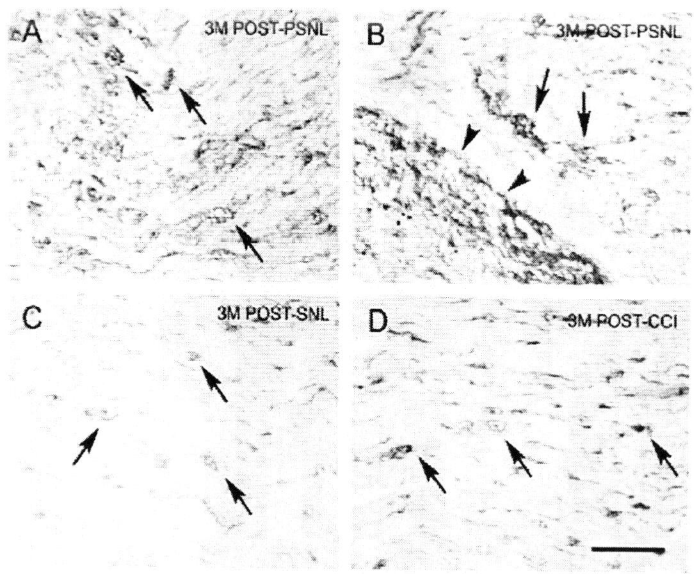

Figure 4. COX2 immunostaining in the ipsilateral sciatic nerve 3 months after PSNL (A and **B**), SNL (**C**) and CCI (**D**). Three months after PSNL, SNL and CCI, COX2-IR cells (**A-D**, arrows) in the ipsilateral sciatic nerve were evidently decreased compared with those 2 and 4 weeks after nerve injury. In the ligation site of PSNL rats (**B**), a sheath (arrowheads) was formed to surround the area immediately adjacent to the ligation suture in which some COX2-IR cells were visible. Scale bar = 50μm.

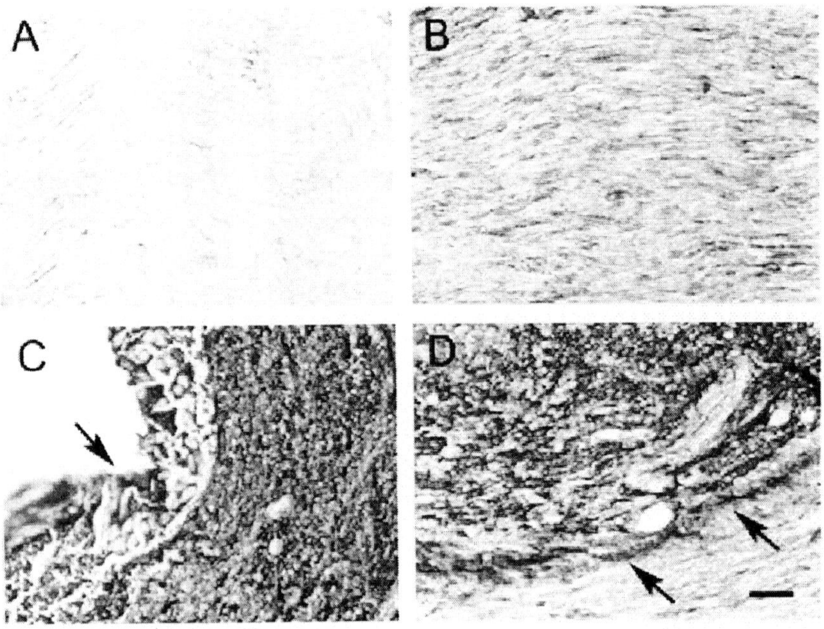

Figure 5. COX2 immunostaining in the contralateral (A) and ipsilateral (B, C and D) sciatic nerve 7 months after PSNL. No COX2-IR cell profiles were seen in the contralateral sciatic nerve (A). In the ipsilateral sciatic nerve outside the ensheathed area surrounding the ligation site, COX2-IR cell profiles completely disappeared (B). However, inside the ensheathed area close to the ligation site (C), some COX2-IR cell profiles were still seen around the ligation suture (large arrow). In D, arrows indicate the boundary between the ensheathed area and the rest of the ipsilateral sciatic nerve. Scale bar = 50μm.

Table 2 shows the mean number±SEM of COX2-IR cell profiles at the lesion site as well as in the distal stump approximately 5 mm from the lesion site in PSNL rats at different time points after lesion. Two to 4 weeks after PSNL, the mean number of COX2-IR cell profiles per area at the two locations was at a maximum, while it was dramatically decreased 3 months after lesion (Table 2). Seven months after PSNL, the mean number of COX2-IR cells in injured nerve was negligible (Table 2).

Table 2. The Mean Number±SEM (n=4) of COX2-IR Cells at the Lesion Site and in the Distal Stump 5 mm from the Lesion Site in PSNL Rats at Different Time Points After Lesion

	3 days	1 week	2 weeks	4 weeks	3 months	7 months
Lesion site	127±50	139±35	167±45	158±35	57±18	4±2.5
Distal stump	36±16	120±29	145±37	132±25	32±12	2.5±1.2

3.3. Majority of COX2-IR Cells Co-Expressing Invading Macrophage Marker ED1

Since COX2-IR cells appear like foamy macrophages, we employed an antibody raised against invading macrophage marker ED1 to conduct double immunostaining of COX2 (Fig. 6A and 6D) and ED1 (Fig. 6B and 6E) in the ipsilateral sciatic nerve of CCI rats (Fig. 6A-C) and in the ipsilateral spinal nerve of SNL rats (Fig. 6D-F). A majority of COX2-IR cells co-expressed ED1 (Fig. 6C and 6F, yellow, arrows). Single COX2-IR (Fig. 6C and 6F, green, small arrows) and ED1-IR (Fig. 6C and 6F, red, arrowheads) cells were also observed.

3.4. PGE2 Released from Injured Sciatic Nerve Segments is Significantly Increased Compared with that from Intact Nerve Segments

Figure 7 illustrates the content of PGE2 released from both intact and injured sciatic nerve segments following PGE2 ELISA assay. PGE2 release from the injured nerve segment was significantly increased compared with that from intact nerve segments (Fig. 7, $p<0.001$). The increased release of PGE2 from injured nerve segments was significantly attenuated following the treatment of non-selective COX inhibitor ketorolac as well as COX2 inhibitors NS398, DuP697 and Nimesulide for 24 hours compared with vehicle treatment (Fig. 7, $p<0.01$).

3.5. Peripheral Nerve Injury Induces the Up-Regulation of PGE2 EP Receptors in Inflammatory Cells in Injured Nerve

Two and 4 weeks following PSNL, no EP1-, EP2-, EP3-, and EP4- (Fig. 8A) IR cell profiles could be detected in the contralateral sciatic nerve. Only some EP4-IR axons were observed (Fig. 8A, arrows). In contrast, dramatically increased EP4-IR cells were observed in the ipsilateral sciatic nerve (Fig. 8B and 8C). EP4 immunoreactivity was localized in the nuclei of IR cell profiles; no explicit staining was seen in the cytoplasm. The distribution of EP4-IR cells ranged approximately 1cm proximal and distal to ligation site. Some large EP4-IR cell profiles appeared in the region immediately adjacent to the ligation site (Fig. 8B and 8C, arrows). EP4-IR cells were found in both the epineural and endoneural regions. In addition, numerous EP1- (Fig. 8D, arrow), EP2- (Fig. 8E, arrow) and EP3- (Fig. 8F, arrow) IR cell profiles were observed in the ipsilateral sciatic nerve 2 and 4 weeks following PSNL. However, these EP1-, EP2- and EP3-IR cell profiles only appeared in regions immediately close to ligation site. In other regions of the ipsilateral as well as in the contralateral sciatic nerve, we failed to observe these EP-IR cells. Similar to EP4, all EP1-, EP2- and EP3-IR were also localized in the nuclei of these positive cells.

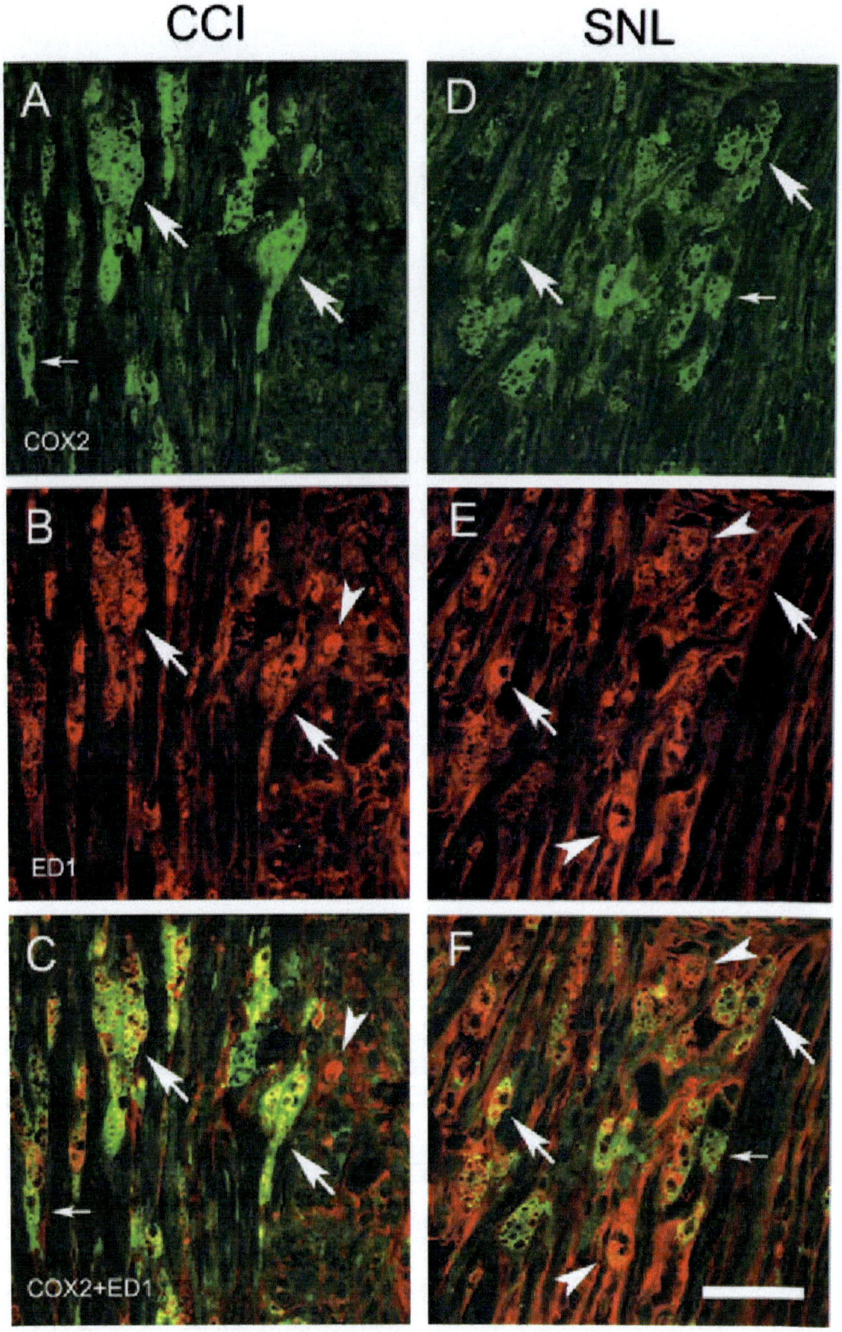

Figure 6. Color confocal photomicrographs of double immunofluorescent staining of COX2 with macrophage marker ED1 in the ipsilateral sciatic nerve 2 weeks after CCI (A, B and C) and in the ipsilateral L5 spinal nerve sciatic nerve 2 weeks after SNL (B, E and F). A and D show COX2-IR cells (green) while B and E show ED1-IR cells (red). C and F show the combined images of A and B, D and E. Note that most COX2-IR cells co-expressed ED1(C and F, yellow, arrows). However, some cells were either COX2-IR only (A, C, D, F, small arrows) or ED1-IR only (B, C, E, F, arrowheads). Note that foamy fatty structures, characteristic of macrophages, appeared in these cells co-expressing both COX2 and ED1 or ED1 alone. Scale bar = 50μm.

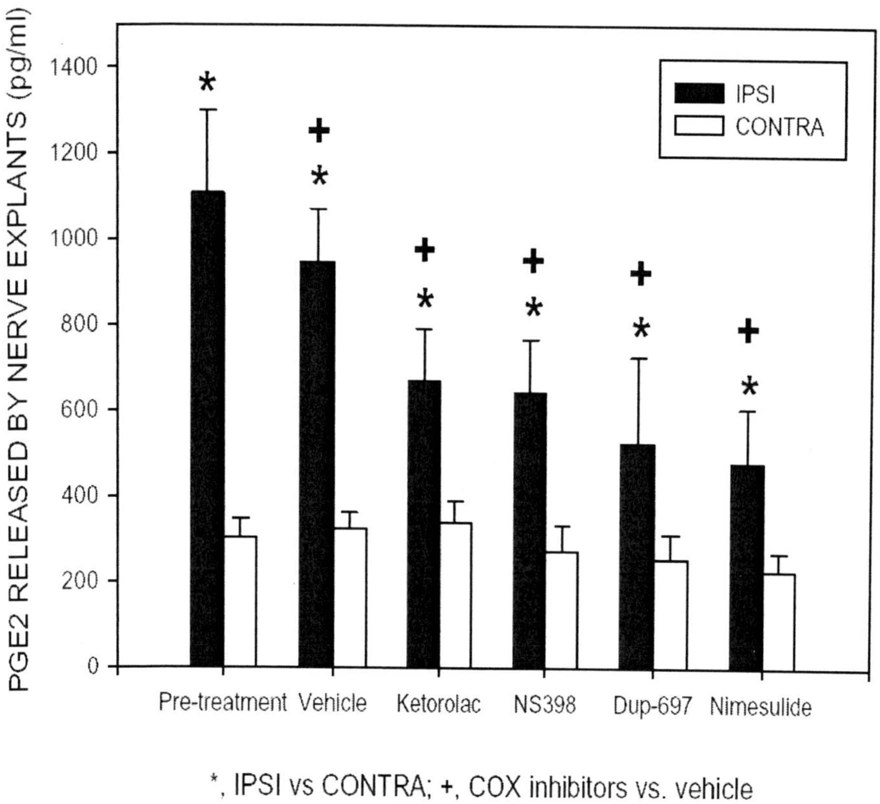

Figure 7. The content of PGE2 released from both intact and injured sciatic nerve segments following PGE2 ELISA assay. PGE2 released from the injured nerve segment was significantly increased compared with that released from intact nerve segments (***, $p<0.001$). The increased release of PGE2 from injured nerve segments was significantly attenuated following the treatment of ketorolac, NS-398, DuP-697 and Nimesulide for 24 hours compared with vehicle treatment (**,$p<0.01$). Mean±SEM, one-way ANOVA with *post hoc* Student-Newman-Keuls multiple comparison method, n=3.

In order to determine the identity of these EP-IR cell profiles, double immunostaining of EP receptor and macrophage marker ED1 was performed. Both EP2- (Fig. 9A, green, arrows) and EP3- (Fig. 9B, green, arrows) IR cells were found rarely to co-express ED1 (Fig. 9A and 9B, red). By contrast, most EP1-IR cells (Fig. 9C, green, arrows) also co-express ED1 (Fig. 9C, red, arrows), 4 weeks following PSNL. Similar to EP1, numerous EP4-IR cells (Fig. 9D, green, arrows) co-expressed ED1. Some EP1- or EP4-IR and ED1-IR single labeled cells were also observed.

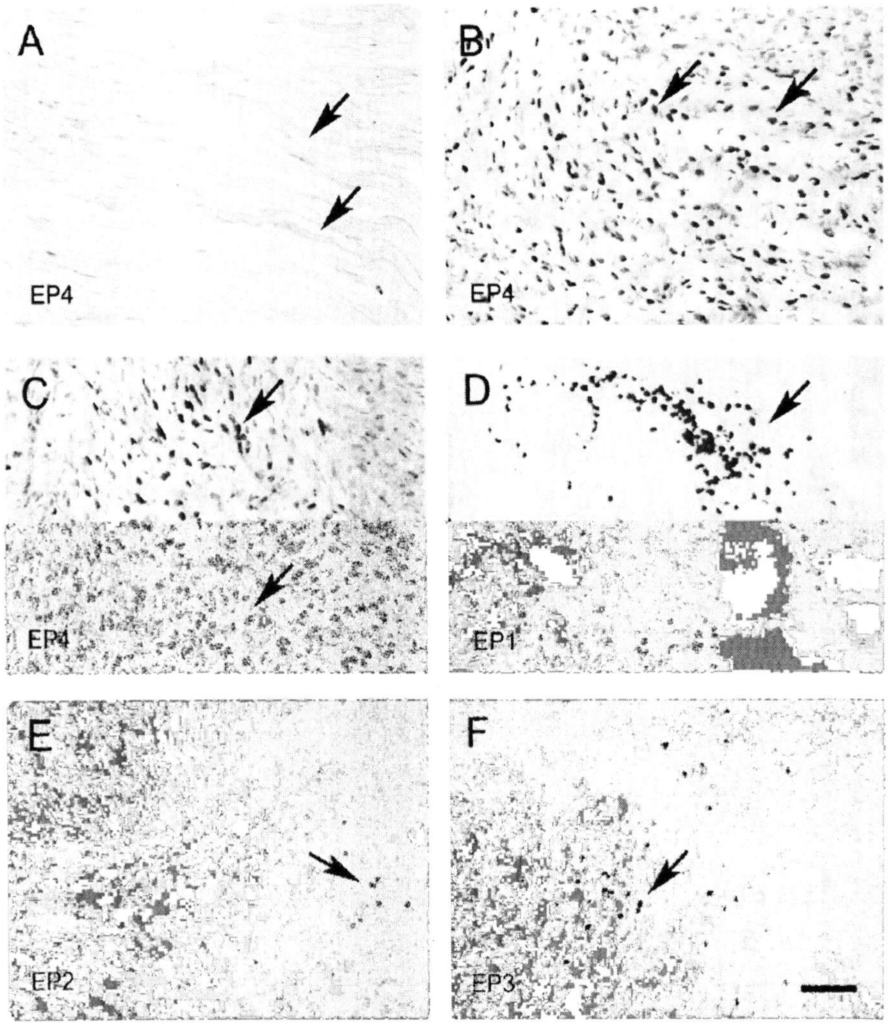

Figure 8. Photomicrographs of 4 EP receptor immunostaining in the contralateral and ipsilateral sciatic nerves 2 and 4 weeks following PSNL. EP1-, EP2-, EP3- (not shown) and EP4 (A) IR cell profiles were never observed in the contralateral sciatic nerve. Two (B) and 4 (C) weeks following PSNL, abundant EP4-IR cells (arrows) appeared in a region immediately adjacent to the ligation site in the ipsilateral sciatic nerve. EP4-IR was exclusively localized in the nuclei of these cells. Numerous EP1- (D, arrow), EP2- (E, arrow) and EP3- (F, arrow) IR cells were also observed in a region close to the ligation site. Similarly, all EP1-, EP2- and EP-3 IR were only localized in the nuclei of these cells. Scale bar = 50μm.

3.6. Relieve of Allodynia by Local Ketorolac is Closely Associated with the Abundance of COX2-IR Cell Profiles in Injured Nerve of SNL, CCI and PSNL Rats

Three weeks after PSNL, the mean withdrawal threshold in both ipsilateral and contralateral hindpaws was significantly lower than the pre-lesion baseline value (Fig. 10A and 10B, p<0.05-0.01). Two hours, 3 and 5 days after intraplantar injection of ketorolac, the mean withdrawal threshold in both hindpaws was reversed to the pre-lesion baseline value (Fig. 10A). Three and 5 days after perineural injection of ketorolac, the mean withdrawal threshold in both hindpaws returned to the pre-lesion baseline value (Fig. 10B). Two months after PSNL, the mean withdrawal threshold in both hindpaws was still significantly lower than pre-lesion baseline value (Fig. 10C, $p<0.01$). Two and 24 hours after injection, the mean withdrawal threshold in both ipsilateral and contralateral hindpaws was reversed to a level insignificantly different from the pre-lesion baseline value (Fig. 10C). However, the mean withdrawal threshold was significantly lower thereafter (Fig. 10C, $p<0.01$). Seven months after PSNL, the mean withdrawal threshold in both hindpaws remained significantly lower than baseline (Fig. 10D, $p<0.01$). Two and 24 hours after intraplantar injection, ketorolac failed to reverse the mean withdrawal threshold in both hindpaws, which was still significantly lower than pre-lesion baseline (Fig. 10D, $p<0.01$).

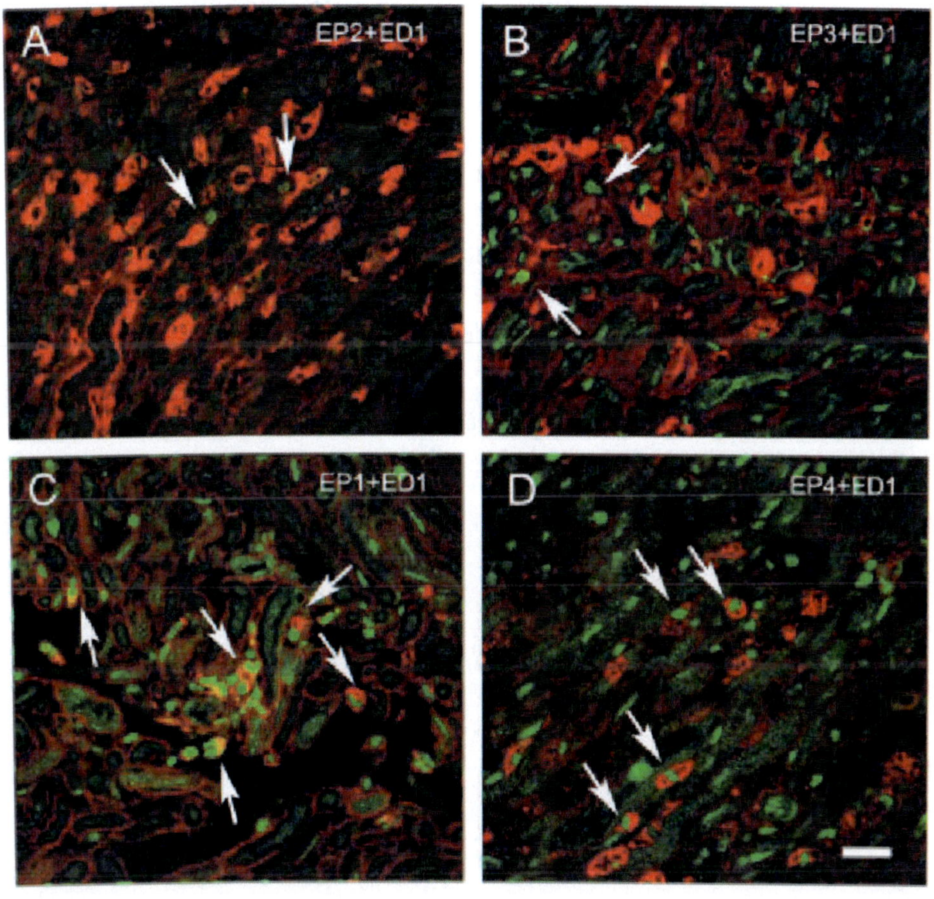

Figure 9. Color confocal photomicrographs of double immunofluorescent staining of EP1, EP2, EP3 and EP4 in the ipsilateral sciatic nerve 4 weeks following PSNL. Note that few EP2- (A, green, arrows) and EP3- (B, green, arrows) IR was co-localized in ED1-IR cells (A and B, red). However, majority of EP1-IR cells (C, green, arrows) and EP4-IR cells (D, green, arrows) also co-express ED1-IR (C and D, red, arrows). Scale bar = 50μm.

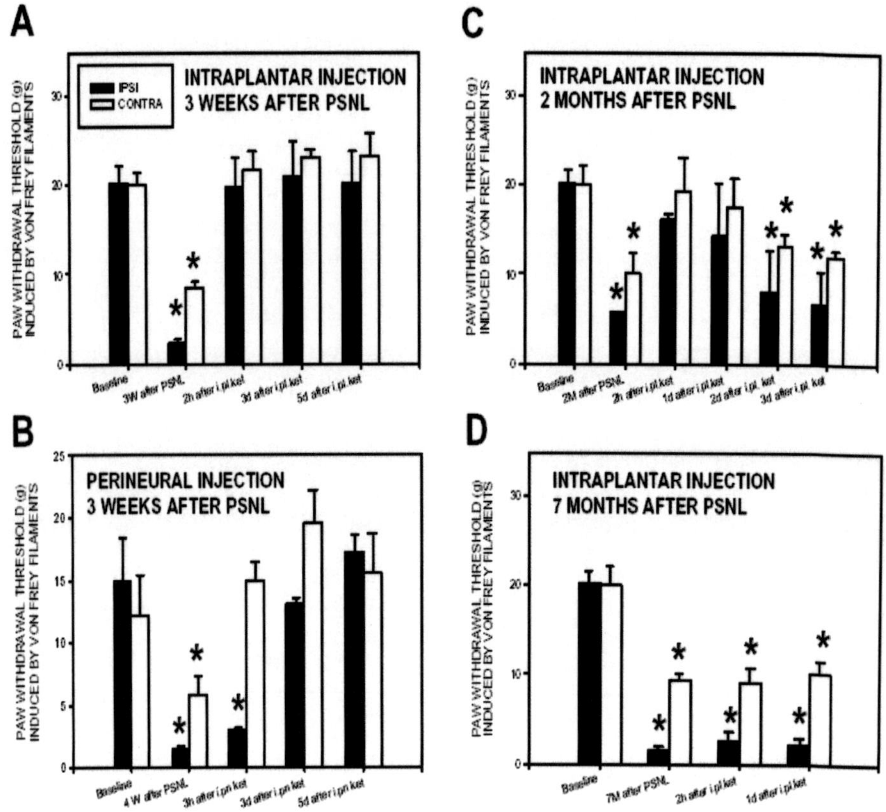

Figure 10. Mean paw withdrawal threshold (mean±SEM, n=4 in each group) in the ipsilateral and contralateral hindpaws 3 weeks (A and B), 2 (C) and 7 (D) months after PSNL. Two weeks, 2 and 7 months after PSNL, the mean withdrawal threshold in both hindpaws was significantly decreased compared with the pre-lesion baseline value (A-D, *, $p<0.05-0.01$). Two hours to 5 days after i.pl. ketorolac injection or 3 to 5 days after i.pn. ketorolac injection to PSNL rats at 3 weeks post-lesion, 2 to 24 hours after i.pl. ketorolac injection to PSNL rats at 2 months post-lesion, the mean withdrawal threshold in both hindpaws was reversed to the pre-lesion baseline level. Two and 3 days after i.pl. ketorolac injection to PSNL rats at 2 months post-lesion, the mean withdrawal threshold in both hindpaws was decreased again to a significantly lower level than pre-lesion baseline (C, *, $p<0.05$). Two hours and 1 day after i.pl. ketorolac injection to PSNL rats at 7 months post-lesion, the mean withdrawal threshold in both hindpaws remained significantly lower than pre-lesion baseline (D, *, $p<0.05$).

Two weeks after SNL, the mean withdrawal threshold in the ipsilateral hindpaw was significantly decreased compared to the pre-lesion baseline value (Fig. 11A and 11B, $p<0.01$). Two hours, 1, 2 and 3 days after intraplantar injection of ketorolac, the mean withdrawal threshold in the ipsilateral hindpaw was reversed to the pre-lesion level. However, the value was decreased significantly 5 days after injection (Fig. 11A, $p<0.01$), indicating the restoration of tactile allodynia. Two months after SNL, the mean withdrawal threshold in the ipsilateral hindpaw was still significantly lower than the pre-lesion value (Fig. 11 B, $p<0.01$). Two hours after intraplantar injection of ketorolac, the mean withdrawal threshold in the ipsilateral hindpaw was reversed to the pre-lesion baseline value. However, 1 to 3 days after injection the mean withdrawal threshold in the ipsilateral hindpaw was significantly lower than the pre-lesion baseline value (Fig. 11B, p<0.05-0.01). No significant difference in the mean withdrawal threshold in the contralateral hindpaw was detected after SNL and injection (Fig. 11A and 11B).

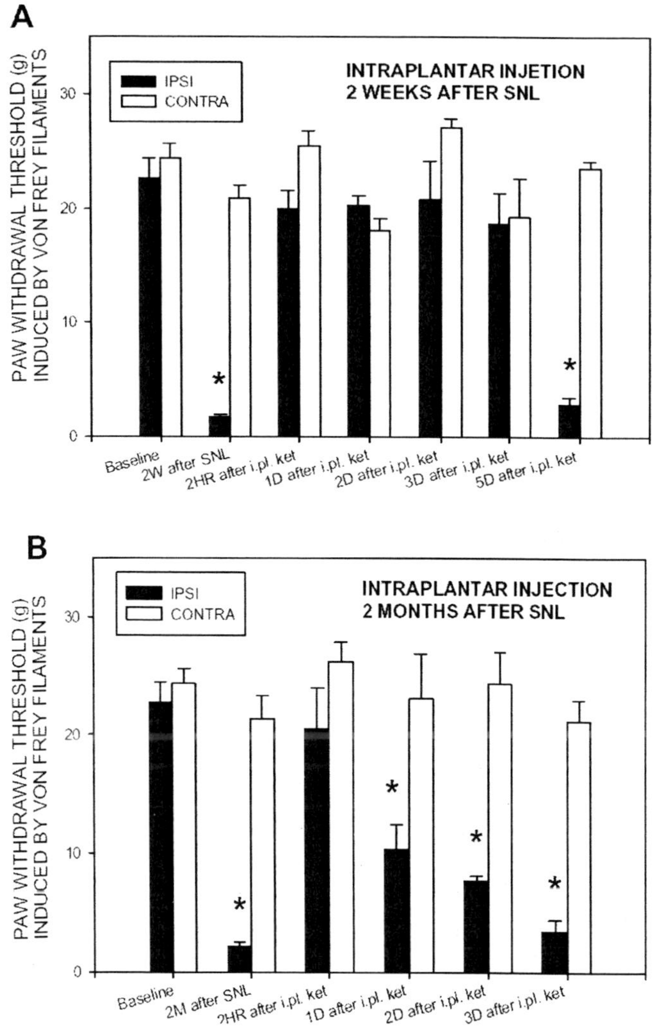

Figure 11. Mean paw withdrawal threshold (mean±SEM, n=4 in each group) in the ipsilateral and contralateral hindpaws 2 weeks and 2 months after SNL. Two weeks and 2 months after SNL, the mean withdrawal threshold in the ipsilateral hindpaw was significantly decreased compared with the pre-lesion baseline value (A and B, *, p<0.01). In A, 2 hours to 3 days after i.pl.injection of ketorolac, the mean withdrawal threshold in the ipsilateral hindpaw was reversed to the pre-lesion baseline level. Five days after i.pl. injection of ketorolac, the mean withdrawal threshold in the ipsilateral hindpaw returned to a significantly lower level than the pre-lesion baseline value (A, *, p<0.01). The mean withdrawal threshold in the contralateral hindpaw was not significantly different from the pre-lesion baseline value. In B, 2 hours after i.pl. injection of ketorolac, the mean withdrawal threshold in the ipsilateral hindpaw was reversed to the pre-lesion baseline level. One day after i.pl. injection, the mean withdrawal threshold in the ipsilateral hindpaw was decreased significantly compared to the pre-lesion baseline value (B, *, p<0.01). The mean withdrawal threshold in the contralateral hindpaw was not significantly different from the pre-lesion baseline value.

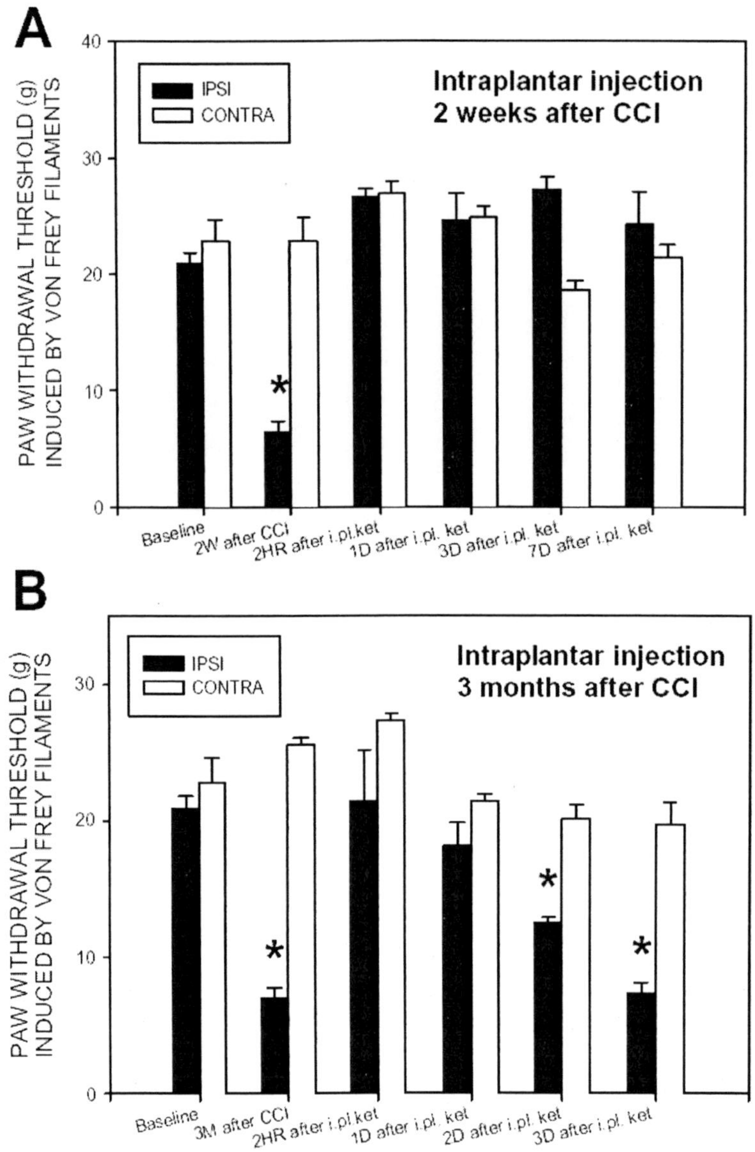

Figure 12. Mean paw withdrawal threshold (mean±SEM, n=4 in each group) in the ipsilateral and contralateral hindpaws of CCI rats. Two weeks (**A**) and 3 months (**B**) after CCI, the mean withdrawal threshold in the ipsilateral hindpaw was significantly decreased compared with the pre-lesion baseline value (**A** and **B**, *, $p<0.05$). Two hours to 1 week after i.pl. ketorolac injection in CCI rats at 2 weeks post-lesion (**A**), or 2 hours and 1 day after i.pl. ketorolac injection to CCI rats at 2 months post-lesion (**B**), the mean withdrawal threshold in the ipsilateral hindpaw was reversed to the pre-lesion baseline level. Two days after i.pl. ketorolac injection to CCI rats at 2 months post-lesion, the mean withdrawal threshold in the ipsilateral hindpaw was decreased significantly compared to the pre-lesion baseline value (**B**, *, $p<0.05$). The mean withdrawal threshold in the contralateral hindpaw was not significantly different from the pre-lesion baseline value.

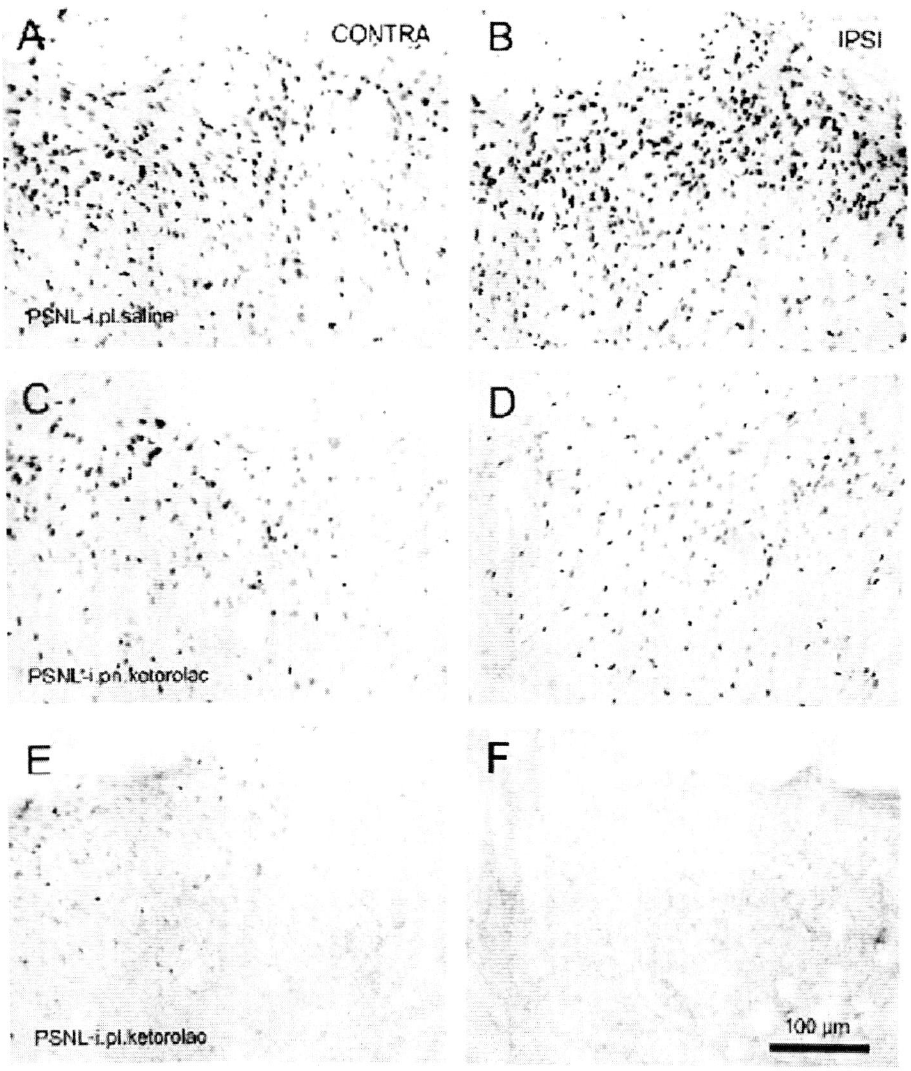

Figure 13. Photomicrographs of pCREB-IR cells in the superficial laminae of the dorsal horn of L4-5 spinal cord of PSNL rats receiving intraplantar saline injection (A and B), perineural ketorolac injection (C and D), and intraplantar ketorolac injection (E and F). Three weeks after PSNL and 5 days after intraplantar saline injection, the number of pCREB-IR cells in the ipsilateral dorsal horn (B) was obviously more abundant than the contralateral side (A). However, 3 weeks after PSNL and 5 days after perineural ketorolac injection (C and D) and after intraplantar ketorolac injection (E and F), the number of pCREB-IR cells in both ipsilateral (D and F) and contralateral (C and E) dorsal horn was dramatically decreased compared to the saline injected PSNL rats (A and B). The decrease in the number of pCREB-IR cells in the dorsal horn of PSNL rats receiving intraplantar ketorolac injection (E and F) was more evident than in PSNL rats receiving perineural ketorolac injection (C and D). Scale bar = 100 μm.

Two weeks after CCI, the mean withdrawal threshold in the ipsilateral hindpaw was significantly lower than pre-lesion baseline value (Fig. 12A, $p<0.05$). Two hours to 7 days after intraplantar injection of ketorolac, the mean withdrawal threshold in the ipsilateral hindpaw was reversed to pre-lesion baseline value. Three months after CCI, the mean withdrawal threshold in the ipsilateral hindpaw was still significantly lower than the pre-lesion baseline value (Fig. 12B, $p<0.05$). Two and 24 hours after intraplantar injection of ketorolac, the mean withdrawal threshold in the ipsilateral hindpaw was reversed to the pre-lesion level. However, 2 and 3 days after injection, the value was decreased to a significantly lower level than the pre-lesion baseline (Fig. 12B, $p<0.05$). No significant difference in the mean withdrawal threshold in the contralateral hindpaw was detected after CCI and injection (Fig. 12A and 12B).

3.7. Local Injection of Ketorolac Suppresses Phosphorylated CREB and Decreases SP, CGRP and Dynorphin Content in the Dorsal Horn of Neuropathic Rats

We previously showed that the phosphorylation of CREB was increased in the ipsilateral dorsal horn neurons 3 weeks after PSNL (Ma and Quirion, 2001) and phosphorylated CREB in the lumbar dorsal horn is involved in the development of neuropathic pain (Ma et al., 2003). In this study, we attempted to determine if local injection of ketorolac, which reversed tactile allodynia for more than 5 days, suppressed the increased number of pCREB in the dorsal horn of PSNL rats. The number of pCREB expressing cells in the ipsilateral dorsal horn of PSNL rats intraplantarly and perineurally injected saline (Fig. 13B) was significantly increased compared with the contralateral side (Fig. 13A). However, following intraplantar and perineural injection of ketorolac, the number of pCREB expressing cells in the ipsilateral dorsal horn was dramatically reduced (Fig. 13D and 13F). More interestingly, local injection of ketorolac also reduced the number of pCREB-IR cells in the contralateral dorsal horn (Fig. 13C and 13E) when compared with that observed in saline injected PSNL rats (Fig. 13A). It appeared that the increased phosphorylation of CREB in the dorsal horn of PSNL rats was more dramatically suppressed by intraplantar than by perineural injection of ketorolac.

Table 3 shows the quantification of pCREB expression in the dorsal horn of PSNL rats receiving either saline or ketorolac intraplantar injection. As we reported previously (Ma and Quirion, 2001), the mean number of pixels in a fixed area occupied by pCREB-IR cells in the ipsilateral superficial dorsal horn of PSNL rats with saline injection was significantly increased compared to the contralateral side (Table 3, $p<0.001$). However, no significant difference in the mean optical density in a fixed area occupied by pCREB-IR cells was detected between both sides of the dorsal horn. In PSNL rats with intraplantar ketorolac injection, the mean optical density in both the ipsilateral and contralateral dorsal horn was significantly decreased compared with that found in the respective counterparts obtained from saline injected rats (Table 3, $p<0.01$).

Furthermore, we examined whether local injection of ketorolac affects the expression of pain-related neuropeptide SP, CGRP and dynorphin in the dorsal horn. Four weeks after PSNL, SP- and CGRP-IR axons were not evidently altered between the contralateral and ipsilateral dorsal horn of saline injected rats (Fig. 14A and 14B, 15A and 15B). However, SP- and CGRP-IR axons in both contralateral and ipsilateral dorsal horns of ketorolac-injected rats (Fig. 14C and 14D, 15C and 15D) were dramatically decreased compared with saline injected rats. No obvious difference in SP- and CGRP-IR axons was observed between the contralateral and ipsilateral dorsal horn of ketorolac injected rats. Four weeks after PSNL, dynorphin-IR cells and axons in the ipsilateral dorsal horn (Fig. 16B) of saline injected rats were dramatically increased compared with the contralateral side (Fig. 16A). Dynorphin-IR axons were predominantly localized in laminae I and II while dynorphin-IR cells were distributed throughout all laminae of the dorsal horn. Five days after intraplantar ketorolac injection, dynorphin-IR cells and axons in both ipsilateral and contralateral dorsal horn were markedly decreased compared with saline injected rats (Fig. 16C and 16D).

Table 3. Quantitative Measurement of the Mean Area Occupied by pCREB-IR Cells and the Mean Optical Density of pCREB-IR Cells in the Dorsal Horn of PSNL Rats with Intraplantar Saline or Ketorolac Injection

	Area (Mean±SEM, n= 4)		Optical Density (Mean±SEM, n= 4)	
	Contra	Ipsi	Contra	Ipsi
Saline	53.46±2.95	73.32±3.16*	206.33±2.64	205.18±2.77
ketorolac	24.12±5.41++	25.89±8.75++	182.01±2.54+	184.25±5.40+

*, $p<0.001$, contralateral vs. ipsilateral;
+, $p<0.01$, ++, $p<0.001$, saline vs. Ketorolac.
One-way ANOVA with *post hoc* Student-Newman-Keuls multiple comparison method, n=4 in each group.

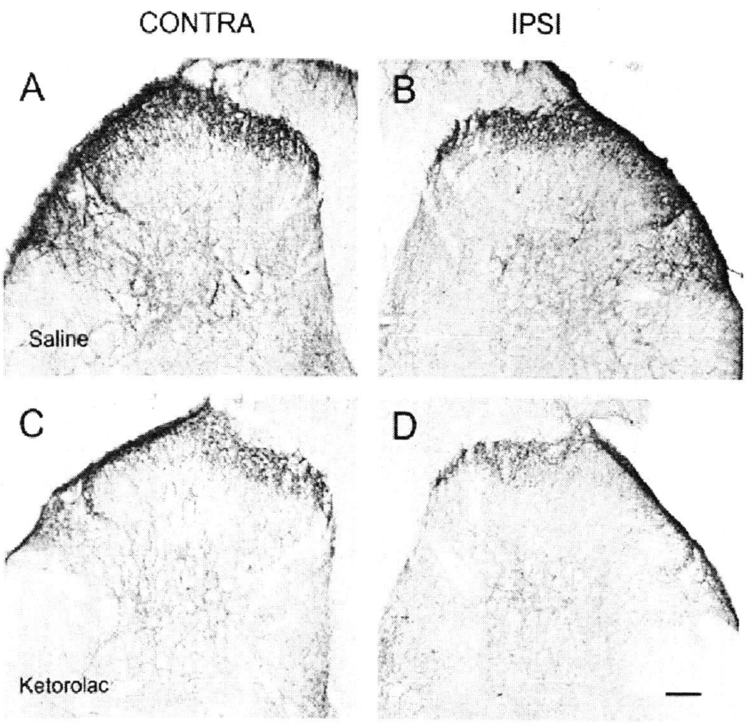

Figure 14. Photomicrographs of SP immunostaining in the dorsal horn of saline (A and B) and ketorolac (C and D) injected PSNL rats. In saline injected rats, SP-IR in the ipsilateral dorsal horn (B) was slightly decreased but not dramatically different from the contralateral side (A). In ketorolac injected rats, SP-IR in both contralateral and ipsilateral dorsal horn (C and D) was markedly reduced compared, respectively, with saline injected rats (A and B). Scale bar = 100μm.

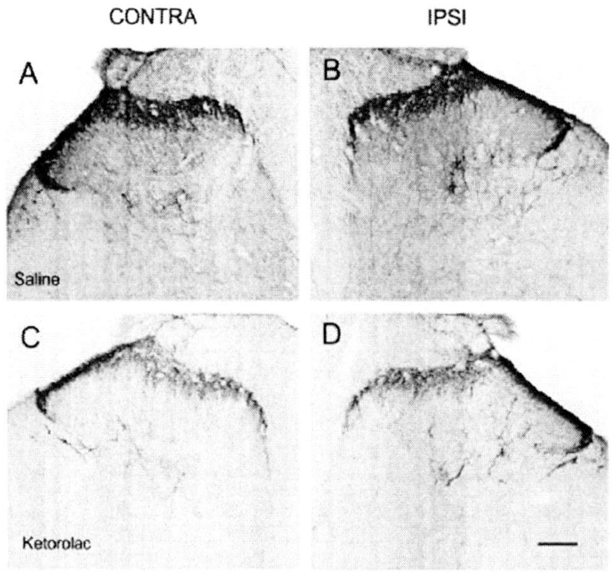

Figure 15. Photomicrographs of CGRP immunostaining in the dorsal horn of saline (A and B) and ketorolac (C and D) injected PSNL rats. In saline injected rats, CGRP-IR was not evidently different between the contralateral and ipsilateral dorsal horn (A and B). In ketorolac injected rats, CGRP-IR in contralateral and ipsilateral dorsal horn (C and D) was markedly reduced compared, respectively, with saline injected rats (A and B). Scale bar = 100μm.

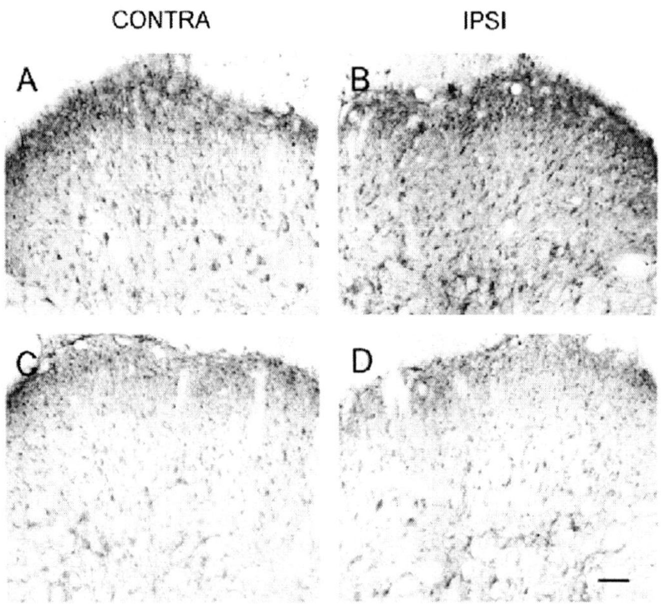

Figure 16. Photomicrographs of dynorphin immunostaining in the dorsal horn of saline (A and B) and ketorolac (C and D) injected PSNL rats. In saline injected rats, dynorphin-IR in the ipsilateral dorsal horn (B) was markedly increased compared with the contralateral side (A). In ketorolac injected rats, dynorphin-IR in both contralateral and ipsilateral dorsal horn (C and D) was evidently reduced compared, respectively, with saline injected rats (A and B). Scale bar = 100μm.

Quantitatively, no significant difference in the mean number of pixels per area occupied by SP- and CGRP-IR axons was detected between the ipsilateral and contralateral dorsal horn of naïve, saline and ketorolac injected rats (Table 4). However, the mean number of pixels per area occupied by SP- and CGRP-IR axons in both contralateral and ipsilateral dorsal horn of ketorolac injected rats was significantly decreased compared with saline injected rats (Table 4, $p<0.01$). The mean number of pixels per area occupied by dynorphin-IR axons and cells in the ipsilateral dorsal horn of naïve and saline-injected rats was significantly greater than the contralateral side (Table 4, $p<0.05$). Five days after ketorolac injection, the mean number of pixels per area occupied by dynorphin-IR axons and cells in both contralateral and ipsilateral dorsal horn was significantly lower than that for their counterparts in saline injected rats (Table 4, $p<0.05$-0.01). No significant difference was seen between the contralateral and ipsilateral dorsal horn in ketorolac injected rats.

Table 4. Pixel Number (Mean±SEM) of the Area Occupied by Substance P, CGRP and Dynorphin IR in the Dorsal Horn of Rats 4 Weeks After PSNL

	Substance P		CGRP		Dynorphin	
	Contra	Ipsi	Contra	Ipsi	Contra	Ipsi
Naive	33725±786	36245±359	35912±678	36727±591	8128±520	19236±870*
Saline	31887±636	35757±1070	37922±281	33059±225	7918±708	17071±637*
Ketorolac	17435±2103⁺	17381±1694⁺	5829±509⁺	8151±634⁺	5247±233⁺	7139±413⁺⁺

*, $p<0.05$, comparison of the ipsilateral vs. the contralateral;
++, $p<0.01$, +, $p<0.05$, comparison of ketorolac vs. saline.
One-way ANOVA with *post hoc* Student-Newman-Keuls multiple comparison method, n=4 in each group.

3.8. Macrophage Derived PGE2 is Involved in the Up-Regulation of Pro-Inflammatory Cytokine IL-6

IL-6 expression was examined in both injured and uninjured sciatic nerves of neuropathic rats 2 weeks after PSNL. In the sciatic nerve of normal rats and in the contralateral uninjured sciatic nerve of PSNL rats, there were no cells or axonal profiles immunoreactive for IL-6 (Fig. 17A). In contrast, in the injured sciatic nerve (Fig. 17B-17F), a large number of IL-6-IR cells were observed about 1 cm proximal and 2 cm distal to the ligation site. These IL-6-IR cells were distributed along axons and exhibited the morphology of macrophages, namely, the presence of foamy fatty vacuoles in the cytoplasm (Fig. 17B-17E). Numerous IL-6-IR cells were adjacent to small blood vessels (Fig. 17C and 17E), suggestive of their hematogenous origin. Incubation of injured nerve sections with antigen pre-absorbed IL-6 antibody resulted in dramatic decrease in immunostained cells (Fig. 17F).

In order to identify these IL-6-IR cells, we conducted double immunostaining of IL-6 and invading macrophage marker ED1, as well as IL-6 and COX2 in the injured nerve. We found that most IL-6-IR cells co-expressed ED1 (Fig. 18A-18C) and COX2 (Fig. 18D-18F).

In order to investigate further the role of prostaglandins, particularly PGE2, in the up-regulation of IL-6 in invading macrophages, we developed an *in vitro* injured nerve derived macrophage culture model. ED1-, COX2- and IL-6-IR cells were exclusively observed in cultures derived from injured nerve segments (Fig. 19B, 19D and 19F). No positive immunoreactive cell profiles were found in cultures derived from contralateral uninjured nerve segments (Fig. 19A, 19C and 19E). We examined next PGE2 release from cultured cells derived from both injured and uninjured nerve segments. PGE2 release from injured

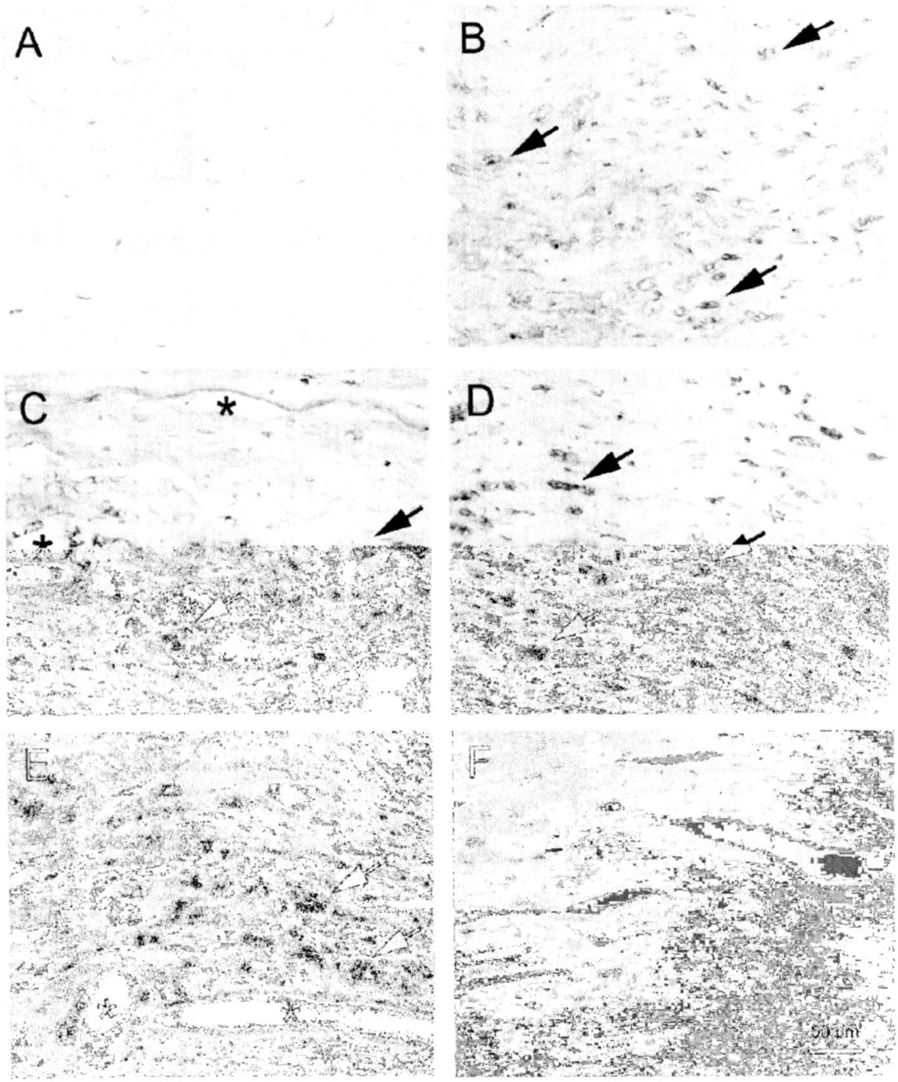

Figure 17. Photomicrographs of IL-6 immunostaining in both contralateral and ipsilateral sciatic nerve of a PSNL rat. In the sciatic nerve of normal rats (not shown) and in the contralateral sciatic nerve of PSNL rats (A), no convincing IL-6-IR cell profiles were observed. However, 2 (B and C) and 4 (D and E) weeks following PSNL, abundant IL-6-IR cells were observed in the injured nerve. B and D were from the proximal stump while C and E were from the distal stump of injured nerve. These IL-6-IR cells were distributed along axons and exhibited macrophages-like morphology (foamy fatty vacuoles in the cytoplasm). Numerous IL-6-IR cells were adjacent to small blood vessels (*, C and E) suggestive of their hematogenous origin. F shows the immunostaining with IL-6 antibody pre-absorbed with 10 folds higher concentration of the blocking peptide. IL-6 immunostained cells were very weak and decreased in number. Scale bar = 50µm.

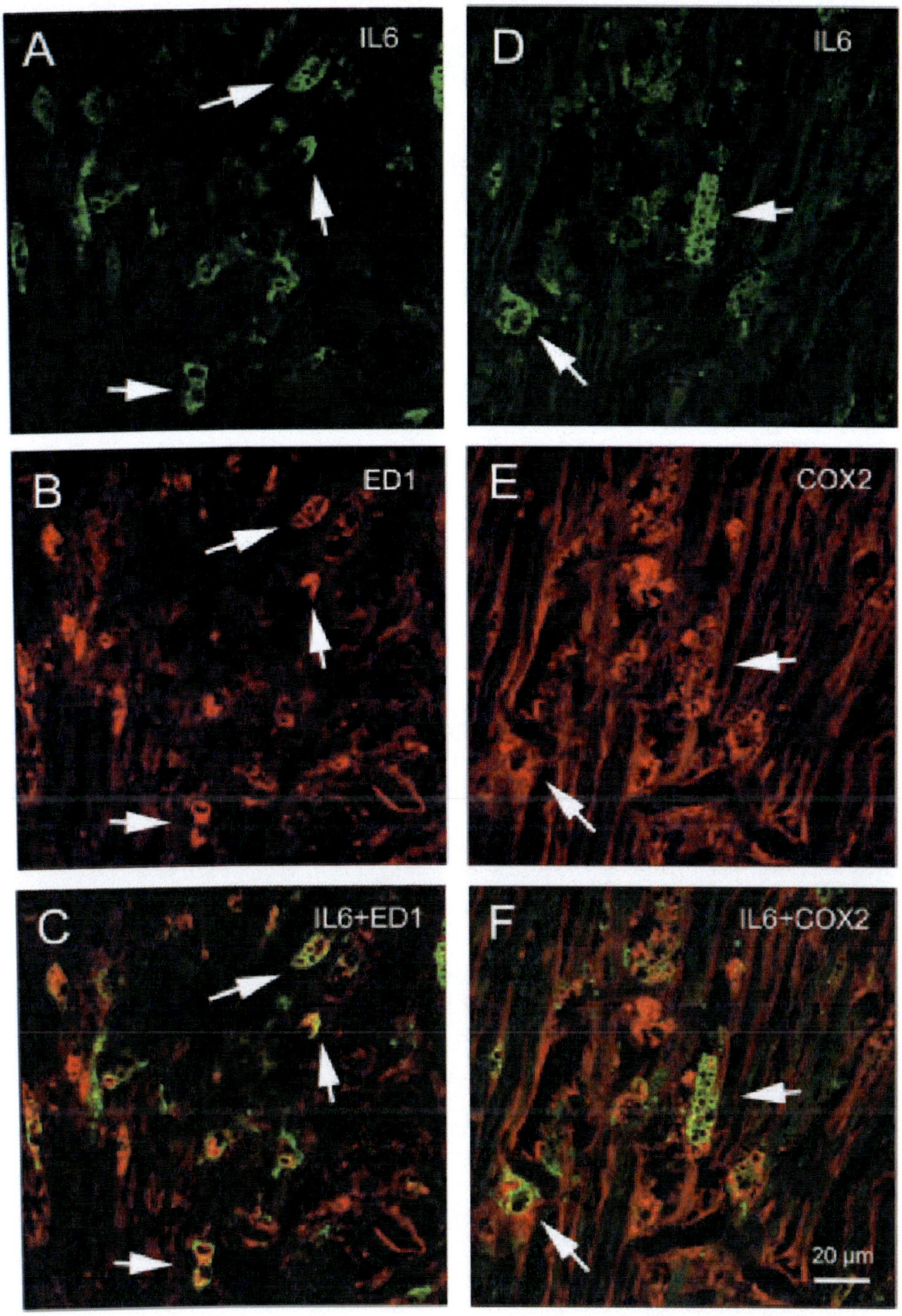

Figure 18. Color confocal photographs showing the co-localization of IL-6 with ED1 (A-C) and with COX2 (D-F) in infiltrating macrophages in injured nerve of PSNL rats. In injured nerve, IL-6 (A, arrow, green) and macrophage marker ED1 (B, arrow, red) were co-expressed in the same cells (C, arrows, yellow). Similarly, in injured nerve, IL-6 (D, arrows, green) and COX2 (E, arrows, red) were co-expressed in the same cells (F, arrows, yellow). Scale bar = 20 μm.

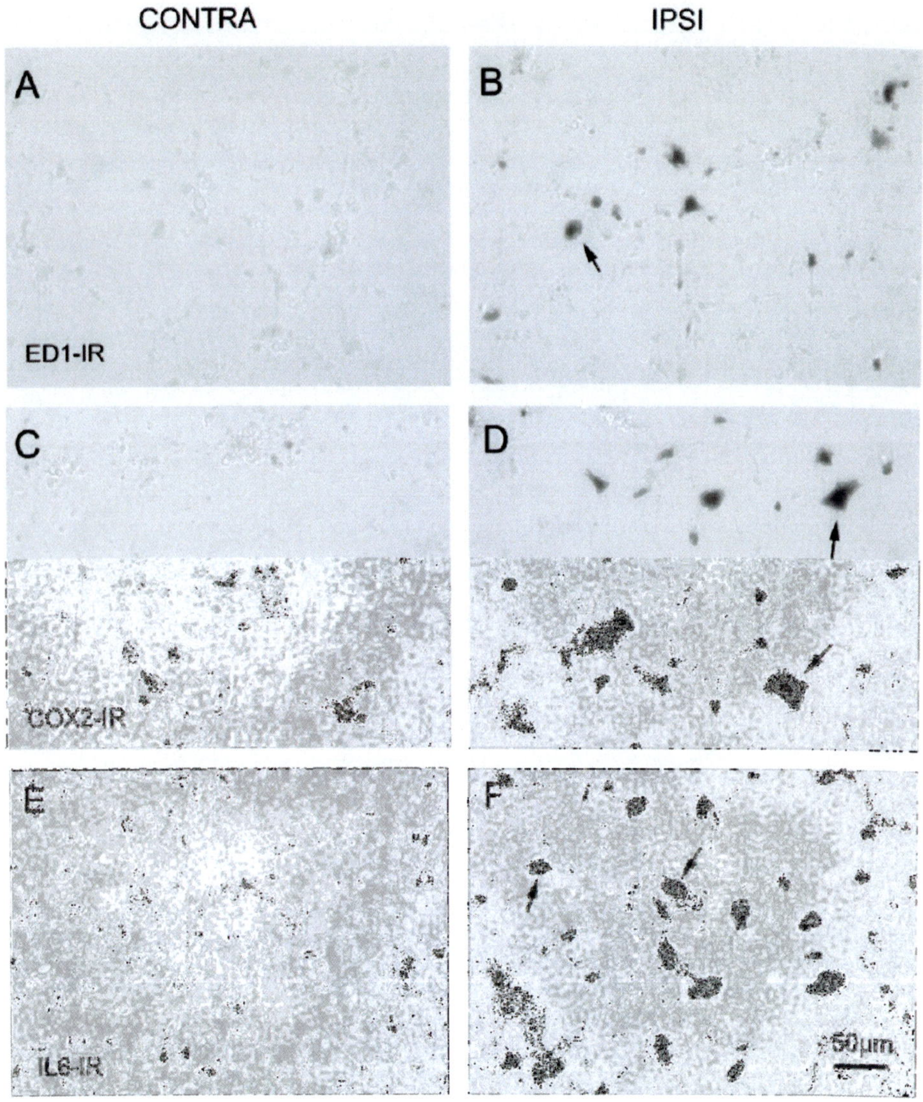

Figure 19. ED1, COX2 and IL-6 immunostaining of cultured cells derived from intact and injured sciatic nerve segments of rats one week after PSNL. Three days after seeding, no convincing ED1- (A), COX2- (C) and IL-6- (E) IR cells were observed in cultured cells obtained from the contralateral sciatic nerve segments. However, numerous cells in cultures derived from injured sciatic nerve segments were immunoreactive for ED1- (B), COX2- (D) and IL-6- (F). Foamy fatty vacuoles were clearly seen in some of these cells at higher magnification (B, D and F, arrows). Scale bar = 50 μm.

nerve cultures was highly significantly increased compared to intact nerve cultures (Fig. 20, $p<0.001$). Treatments of cultured cells with the non-selective COX inhibitor ketorolac or selective COX2 inhibitors such as NS398, DuP-697 and nimesulide dramatically suppressed PGE2 release (Fig. 20, $p<0.01$). IL-6 release from cultured cells of both injured and uninjured nerve segments was performed next. Prior to any treatment, the content of IL-6 released from injured nerve derived-cultures was significantly higher than from intact nerve-derived cultures (Fig. 21, $P<0.01$). Cultured cells derived from injured or intact nerve was further treated with vehicle, PGE2, ketorolac, NS-398, DuP-697 and nimesulide for 24 hours. Following vehicle treatments, IL-6 released by cultured cells derived from injured nerves was significantly increased compared to that release from cells derived from intact nerves (Fig. 21, $p<0.001$). Following PGE2 treatment, the level of IL-6 released by injured nerve derived cells was significantly higher than that released by intact nerve derived cells (Fig. 21, $p<0.001$) or injured nerve derived cells treated with vehicle (Fig.21, $p<0.01$). PGE2 treatment did not induce any significant increase in IL-6 release from cultured cells derived from uninjured nerve (Fig. 21). Following ketorolac and NS-398 treatments, IL-6 release from injured nerve-derived cells was still higher than that released by intact nerve derived cells (Fig.21, $p<0.05$). However, treatments with these two inhibitors significantly suppressed IL-6 release when compared with released from vehicle treated and injured nerve derived-cultured cells (Fig. 21, $p<0.001$). Following treatments with DuP-697 and nimesulide, IL-6 released by injured-nerve derived cells was significantly decreased compared to release from intact-nerve derived cells (Fig. 21, $p<0.05$) or vehicle treated, injured-nerve derived cells (Fig. 21, $p<0.001$).

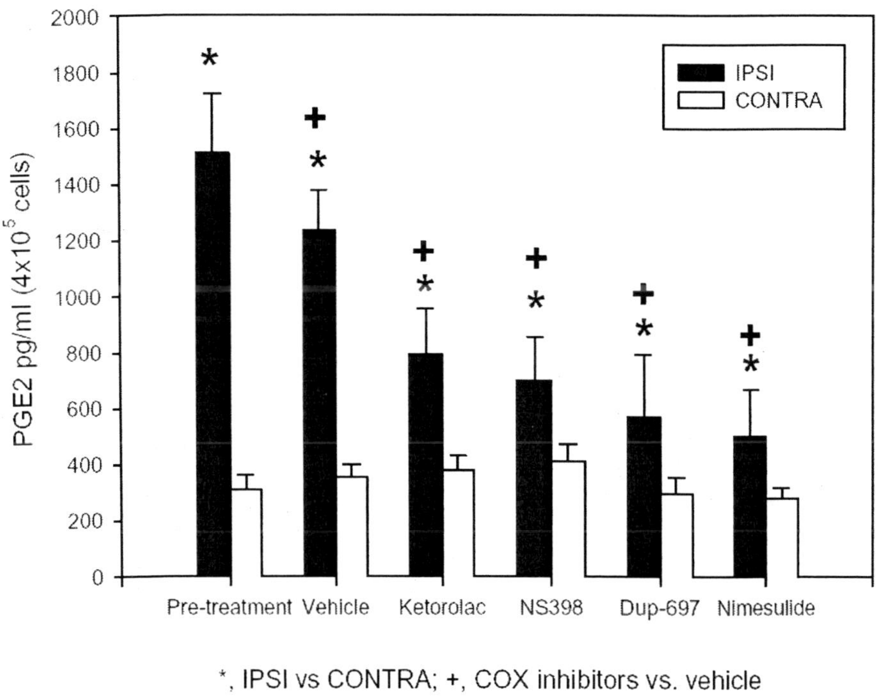

Figure 20. Levels of PGE2 in medium released by cultured cells derived from both intact and injured nerve segments. One week after PSNL and 3 days after seeding, the levels of PGE2 released from cultured cells derived from injured nerve was significantly increased compared with PGE2 released by cultured cells from intact nerve (*, $p<0.001$). Following treatments with ketorolac, NS398, DuP-697 and nimesulide for 24 hours, PGE2 release from injured nerve derived cultures was significantly suppressed compared with PGE2 release from vehicle treated and injured nerve derived cultures (+, $p<0.01$), but was significantly higher than PGE2 release from inhibitor treated intact nerve cultures (*, $p<0.01$). Mean±SEM, n=3.

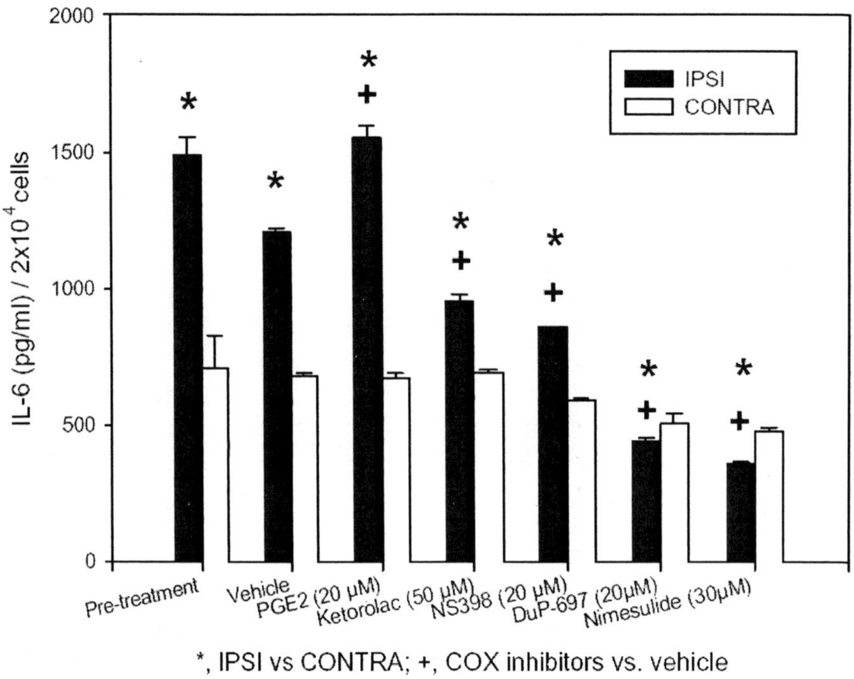

Figure 21. Levels of IL-6 in culture medium released by cultured cells derived from injured and intact sciatic nerve segments. One week following PSNL and 3 days after seeding, IL-6 release was dramatically increased from injured nerve derived cultures compared to release from intact nerve derived cultures (pre-treatment, *, $p<0.01$) . Cultured cells derived from injured nerve or intact nerve were further treated with vehicle, PGE2, ketorolac, NS-398, DuP-697 and nimesulide for 24 hours. Following vehicle treatments, IL-6 released by cultured cells derived from injured nerve was significantly increased compared to that released by cells derived from intact nerve (*, $p<0.001$). Following PGE2 treatment, IL-6 released by injured nerve derived cells was significantly higher than release by intact nerve derived cells (* $p<0.001$) and was also higher than release from injured nerve-derived cells treated by vehicle (+, $p<0.01$). Following ketorolac and NS-398 treatments, IL-6 content released by injured nerve derived cells was still higher than release from intact nerve derived cells (*, $p<0.05$). However, compared to vehicle treatment, IL-6 content was significantly decreased (+, $p<0.001$). Following the treatments with DuP-697 and nimesulide, IL-6 released by injured nerve derived cells was significantly decreased compared with release from intact nerve derived cells (*, $p<0.05$) and compared with vehicle treated injured-nerve derived cells (+, $p<0.001$). Mean±SEM, n=3.

We determined next the concentration-response relationship and time course of PGE2 treatment for 24 hours on the release of IL-6 from both injured and uninjured nerve segments. Compared with vehicle treatment, PGE2 concentration-dependently increased IL-6 release from injured nerve-derived cells (Fig. 22A, $p<0.001$). IL-6 release by cells treated with 20 and 30μM PGE2 was significantly higher than release induced by 10μM PGE2 (Fig. 22A, $p<0.05$) while 1μM PGE2 was ineffective. At the concentration of 20μM, PGE2 treatments for 3, 6, 12 and 24 hours significantly increased IL-6 release from injured nerve derived cells (Fig. 22B, $p<0.01$). However, a longer treatment (48 hours, 20μM) led to decrease in IL-6 release compared to vehicle treatment (Fig. 22B, $p<0.001$).

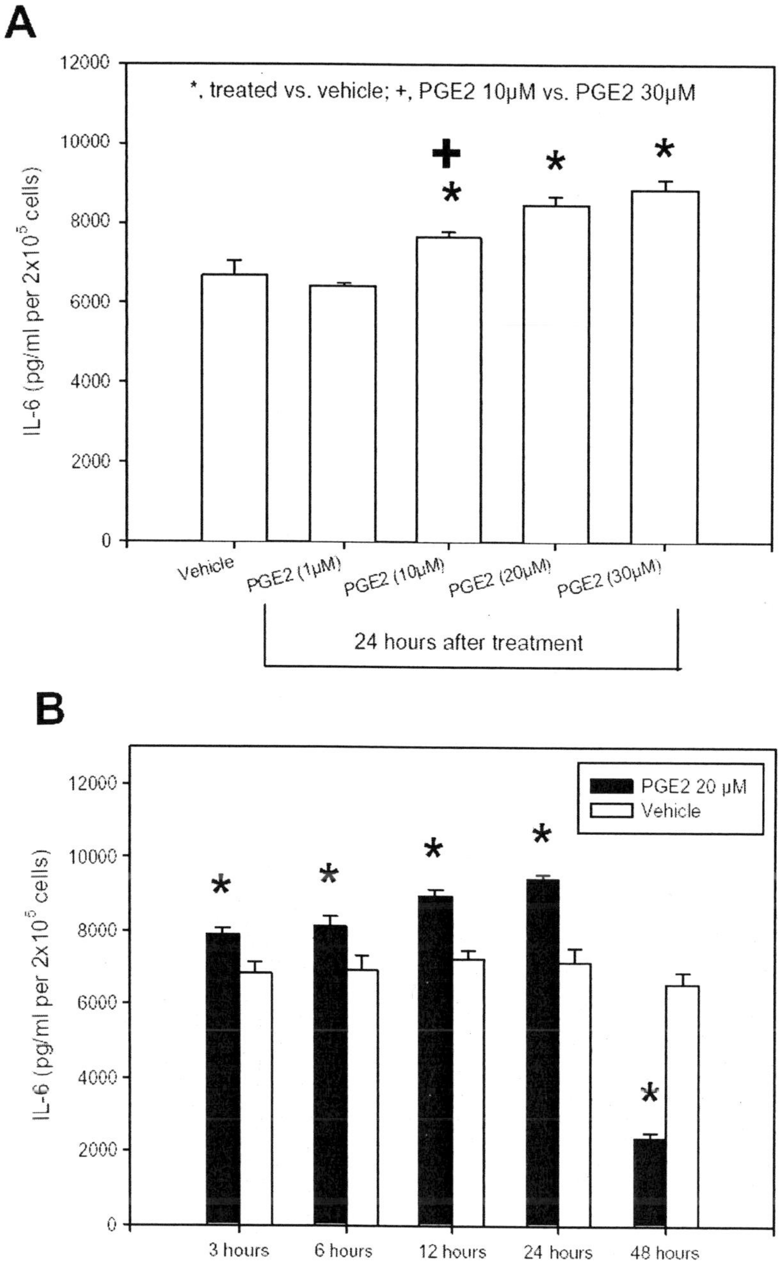

Figure 22. A. Concentration-response relationship between IL-6 content and PGE2 concentration. Following treatment with 10, 20 or 30μM PGE2 for 24 hours, IL-6 released by injured nerve derived cells was significantly increased compared with vehicle treatment (*, $p<0.001$). IL-6 released by cells treated with 20 and 30μM PGE2 was significantly higher than release from cells treated with 10μM PGE2 (+, $p<0.05$). IL-6 released by cells treated with 1μM PGE2 was not significantly different from release by cells treated with vehicle. B. Time course of IL-6 released by injured nerve derived cells treated with 20μM PGE2. Following 20μM PGE2 treatment for 3, 6, 12 and 24 hours, IL-6 was significantly increased compared to vehicle treatment (*, $p<0.01$). However, following 20μM PGE2 treatment for 48 hours, IL-6 released by injured nerve derived cells was highly, significantly decreased compared with vehicle treatment (*, $p<0.001$). Mean±SEM, n=3.

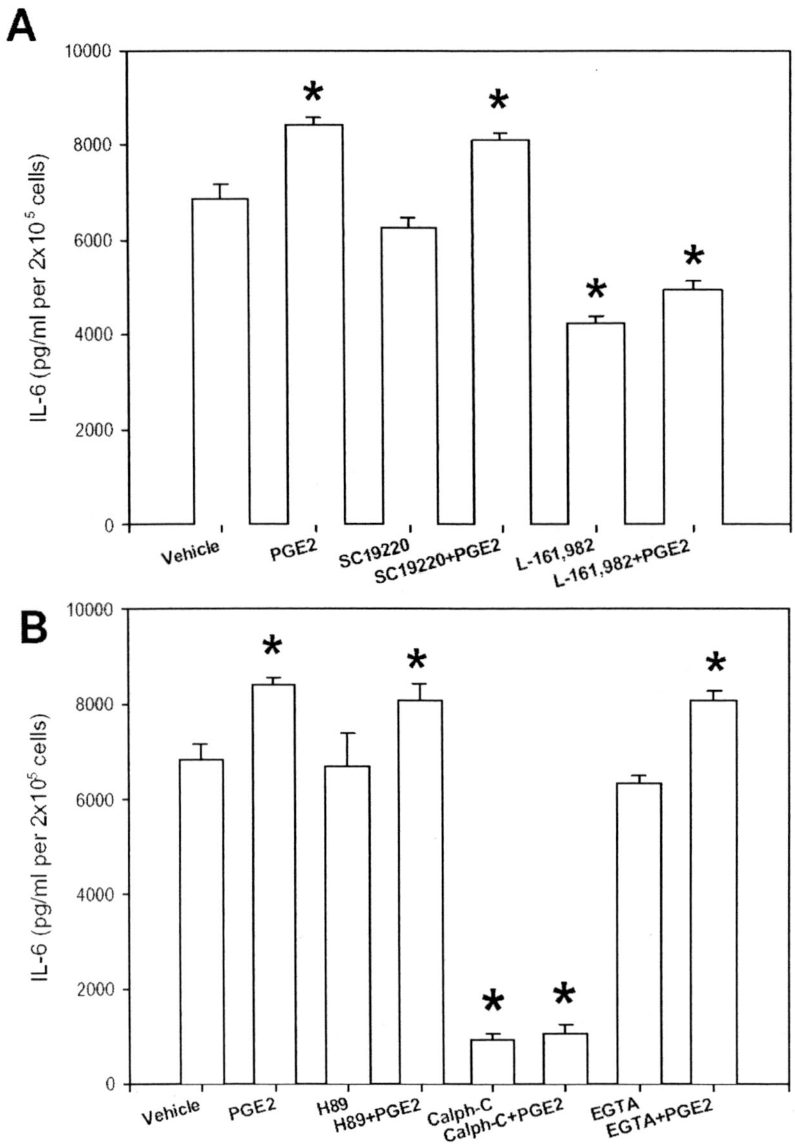

Figure 23. A. IL-6 release by injured nerve derived cells following treatment with vehicle, PGE2, selective EP1 receptor antagonist SC19220 and selective EP4 receptor antagonist L-161,982 for 24 hours. Following 20μM PGE2 treatment, IL-6 was significantly increased compared with vehicle treatment (*, $p<0.01$). Following treatments with SC19220, IL-6 release was not significantly different from vehicle treatments. SC19220, when co-treated with PGE2, did not suppress PGE2 induced significant increase in LI6 release (*, $p<0.05$). In contrast, compared with vehicle treatment, L-161,982 alone remarkably suppressed IL-6 release (*, $p<0.01$). When co-treated with PGE2, L-161,982 significantly inhibited PGE2 induced IL-6 release (*, $p<0.05$). B. IL-6 release by injured nerve derived cells following treatments with vehicle, PGE2, PKA inhibitor H-89, PGE2+H-89, PKC inhibitor calphostin C, PGE2+calphostin, Ca^{++} chelator EGTA and PGE2+EGTA. Following 24 hour treatment with 20μM PGE2, IL-6 content was significantly increased compared to vehicle treatment (*, $p<0.01$). Following treatments with calphostin C and PGE2+calphostin C, IL-6 release was significantly decreased compared with vehicle treatment (*, $p<0.001$). However, treatments with H-89, PGE2+H-89, EGTA and PGE2+EGTA failed to reduce IL-6 release or PGE2 enhanced IL-6 release compared with vehicle treatment (*, $p<0.01$). Mean±SEM, n=3.

The class of receptors involved in the PGE2 modulated IL-6 release was studied next. The EP4 receptor is the most likely candidate since it has been shown to be dramatically up-regulated in invading macrophages (Ma and Eisenach, 2003b). To test this hypothesis, we used a selective EP4 receptor antagonist L-161, 982, which has been shown to successfully block PGE2 induced effects (Takayama et al., 2002). Another candidate could be the EP1 receptor, since about 80% of EP1 expressing cell profiles in injured nerves are macrophages despite their restricted distribution in the vicinity of the injury site (Ma and Eisenach, 2003b). Following treatments with SC19220, a well established EP1 receptor antagonist (Rakovska and Milenov, 1984), IL-6 release was not significantly different from vehicle treatment (Fig. 23A). Moreover, when used in the presence of PGE2, SC19220 failed to suppress PGE2 induced up-regulation of IL-6 release, suggesting the lack of a role for the EP1 subtype. In contrast, compared with vehicle treatment, L-161,982 alone significantly attenuated IL-6 release (Fig. 23A). L-161,982 also significantly inhibited PGE2 induced IL-6 release when co-treated with PGE2 (Fig. 23A).

In order to dissect the intracellular signal transduction pathway(s) involved in PGE2 induced IL-6 release, various inhibitors were used. Treatments with H-89 (PKA inhibitor) or PGE2 and H-89 failed to suppress increased IL-6 release or PGE2 augmented IL-6 release in cultured cells derived from injured nerve segments (Fig. 23B). Similarly, treatment with EGTA failed to alter IL-6 release under these two conditions (Fig. 23B). In contrast, calphostin C (PKC inhibitor) treatment reduced IL-6 release from injured nerve cell cultures as well as significantly reduced PGE2 enhanced IL-6 release (Fig. 23B, $p<0.001$).

IV. Discussion

4.1. Major Findings

Following various types of peripheral nerve injury, COX2 expressing cells are dramatically increased in injured nerve. Majority of these cells are identified as invading macrophages. PGE2 released from injured nerve segments are significantly increased compared to that from uninjured nerve segments. COX2 expressing cells in injured nerve appear as early as 3 days after lesion, reach the maximum during 2 to 4 weeks, gradually decrease thereafter and completely disappear 7 months after lesion. Four PGE2 EP receptors are dramatically increased in inflammatory cells in injured nerve. Up-regulation of EP4 is the most abundant. Half of macrophages express EP4 receptors. Perineural and intraplantar injection of non-selective COX inhibitor ketorolac effectively relieves neuropathic pain. The anti-allodynia induced by local ketorolac is closely associated with the abundance of COX2 expressing cells in injured nerve. Local injection of ketorolac markedly suppresses increased phosphorylation of CREB and expression of SP, CGRP and dynorphin in the dorsal horn. Numerous IL-6 IR cells were found in the injured nerve of PSNL rat and most of them were invading macrophages. IL-6 release from cultured cells derived from injured nerve segments was significantly increased compared with release from intact nerve cultures. Moreover, exogenous PGE2 treatment, in concentration- and time-dependent manner, enhanced further IL-6 release but only from injured nerve cell cultures. Both non-selective and selective COX2 inhibitors significantly suppressed IL-6 release from injured nerve cell cultures. Finally, the PKC signaling pathway is likely involved as a key intracellular event in mediating the effects of PGE2 on IL-6 release from invading macrophages.

4.2. COX2 Up-Regulation and PGE2 Over-Production in Invading Macrophages in Injured Nerve are Universal Phenomena Following Peripheral Nerve Injury

When a peripheral nerve is damaged, the distal axons will undergo Wallerian degeneration, which is characterized by myelin breakdown and the recruitment of inflammatory cells such as macrophages, lymphocytes, mast cells and neutrophils to invade the degenerating regions (Brown et al., 1991; Frisen et al., 1993; Cui et al., 2000). Of these recruited inflammatory cells, macrophages are the principal effecter cells involved in the process. Macrophages not only clear up degraded nerve debris but also facilitate axonal regeneration by producing and releasing growth factors, cytokines and pro-inflammatory mediators. However, in addition to the beneficial effects in promoting axonal regeneration, most products of Wallerian degeneration are also pro-nociceptive. It has been shown that inflammatory mediators including PGE2, serotonin, bradykinin and histamine sensitize both injured and intact axons to mechanical innocuous and noxious stimuli following nerve injury (Michaelis et al., 1998). Thus, depletion of macrophages (Liu et al., 2000) and neutrophils (Perkins and Tracey, 2000) attenuate thermal hyperalgesia and tactile allodynia following partial sciatic nerve injury.

It has been shown in both *in vitro* and *in vivo* studies that macrophages up-regulate inducible COX2 expression when stimulated with inflammatory agents such as bacterial LPS, TNFα and IL-1β (Lee et al., 1992; Reddy and Herschman, 1994; Levi et al., 1998; Schiltz and Sawchenko, 2002) and thus over-produce PGE2. TNFα (Wagner and Myers, 1996b; Cui et al., 2000) and IL-1β (Lindholm et al., 1987) are increased in Schwann cells in injured nerve at an early stage during Wallerian degeneration. These two factors possibly not only chemoattract macrophages to migrate into the degenerating zone, but also stimulate macrophages to up-regulate COX2 expression. Since macrophage invasion of the degenerating nerve is a common event following peripheral nerve injury, we therefore hypothesized that up-regulation of COX2 or over-production of PGs occurs universally in injured nerve. In the current study, we tested this hypothesis in various nerve injury models and observed that 2 and 4 weeks following PSNL, SNL, CCI and CSNT, COX2 was markedly up-regulated in cell profiles in injured nerves and the majority of COX2-IR cell profiles were identified as macrophages. PGE2 released from injured nerve segment is increased significantly, suggesting that up-regulation of COX2 in invading macrophages leads to the over-production of PGE2 in injured nerve. We also noticed that some COX2 expressing cells did not co-express ED1, suggesting that other types of inflammatory cells may up-regulate COX2 expression as well. It has been shown in *in vitro* studies that mast cells produce PGs including PGD2 and PGE2 (Schmauder-Chock and Chock, 1989; Reddy et al., 1997). Mast cells are among the inflammatory cells that infiltrate the degenerating nerve following nerve injury. Further study is warranted to address whether mast cells are another source of PG over-production following nerve injury.

Our findings strongly indicate that peripheral nerve injury results in the up-regulation of COX2 or PG over-production in inflammatory cells in injured nerve and peripheral PG over-production is a universal phenomenon following various types of nerve injury.

4.3. The Anti-Allodynic Effect Induced by Local Injection of the COX Inhibitor Ketorolac Parallels the Abundance of COX2 Expressing Cells in the Injured Nerve Following Nerve Injury

Infiltrating blood-borne macrophages are present in injured nerve 3 days after lesion. Thereafter they increase in abundance to reach a maximum 2 to 4 weeks after lesion (Frisen et al., 1993). Macrophage infiltration lasts for several months (Deleo et al., 1996). PSNL induced neuropathic pain can be observed as early as 1 to 2 days post-lesion, reaches a peak at 2 to 4 weeks and lasts as long as 7 months post-lesion (Seltzer et al., 1990). Hence, the time course of PSNL elicited neuropathic pain parallels the initial time course of macrophage infiltration. We thus hypothesized that in parallel with macrophage recruitment, COX2 up-regulation or increased PG production by macrophages is closely associated with the time course of neuropathic pain elicited by PSNL.

We tested this hypothesis by examining the abundance of COX2 expression in injured nerve associated with various types of nerve injury and the abundance of COX2 expression in injured nerve at different time points following PSNL, SNL and CCI. The greatest COX2 expression, in terms of distribution region and the number of cells expressing COX2, was observed in injured sciatic nerve of CCI rats. CCI results in a much wider injury region due to 4 loose ligatures. Thus, injured nerve of CCI rats likely produces the greatest production of PGs and the anti-allodynic effect induced by local ketorolac lasts more than 1 week when given 2 weeks after lesion. In SNL and PSNL rats, with a relatively limited injury region where COX2 expressing macrophages infiltrate, the anti-allodynic effect induced by local ketorolac lasts shorter than in CCI rats when given 2 and 4 weeks after lesion. In contrast, far fewer COX2-IR cell profiles were observed in both proximal and distal stumps of injured sciatic nerve of CSNT rats, compared with those in SNL, CCI and PSNL rats. Behaviorally, we failed to observe any tactile allodynia occurring in these CSNT rats when the dermatome of L3-L5 spinal nerve in the hindpaw was stimulated with von Frey filaments (data not shown). The observation that there are fewer COX2 expressing cells in injured nerve of CSNT rats is consistent with a previous report that complete sciatic nerve axotomy results in far less macrophage infiltration in the degenerating nerve than partial nerve injuries (Cui et al., 2000). Our data suggest that the abundance of COX2 expression in injured nerve is closely associated with neuropathic pain behaviors and with the lasting duration of ketorolac elicited anti-allodynia. All these observations further support the hypothesis that COX2 up-regulation or PG over-production in injured nerve is involved in the maintenance of neuropathic pain and that local ketorolac likely exerts its anti-allodynic effect by suppressing peripheral PG over-production. The mechanism underlying the long-lasting effect of ketorolac is not clear. The anti-allodynic effect of ketorolac has outlasted its short half-life

(5.5 hours). We speculate that ketorolac may directly decrease PGs, particularly PGE2, in the hindpaw. The sensitizing effect of over-produced PGE2 on nociceptors may diminish immediately. PGE2 has an up-regulating effect on IL6 and other pain-inducing mediators, a process taking more time and lasting longer. Thus, decreasing PGE2 may indirectly inhibit the production of pain inducing substances, causing a prolonged anti-allodynia.

In the time course study of COX2 expression in injured nerve of PSNL rats, we observed that COX2-IR cells appeared in injured nerve as early as 3 days postlesion. However, they were only present in a region immediately adjacent to the ligation site. The abundance of COX2 expressing cells increased rapidly 1 week after PSNL and the most abundant COX2-IR cell profiles were detected by 2 to 4 weeks postlesion. However, 3 months after PSNL, the abundance of COX2 expressing cells was obviously decreased. By 7 months postlesion, COX2 expressing cells were only present in an ensheathed area surrounding the ligation site, but entirely disappeared from the other area of the injured nerve where COX2-IR cells existed during the initial 3 months after PSNL. Consistently, local ketorolac induced anti-allodynia lasted longest (>5 days) when given during a period of 2 to 4 weeks post-lesion, shorter than 2 days when given at 2 months postlesion and disappeared when given 3 and 7 months after PSNL. Similarly, the anti-allodynic effect of local ketorolac lasted longer in CCI and SNL rats when given 2 weeks than given 2 to 3 months after lesion. All these observations further suggest that the effectiveness of local ketorolac is closely associated with the abundance of COX2 expression or PG over-production in injured nerve at different time points.

It has been reported that the analgesic effect of ketorolac can be achieved through the central mechanism, i.e., by inhibiting the NMDA glutamate receptor in the wide dynamic range neurons in the dorsal horn (Sotgiu et al., 1998). Therefore, we must point out that the possibility cannot be excluded that local or systemic ketorolac may achieve its anti-allodynia through other mechanisms than inhibiting the synthesis of prostaglandins.

Our data also indicate that COX2 up-regulation in injured nerve is significant only during the initial several months after nerve injury. In other words, macrophage derived PGs, PGE2 in particular, are important in the maintenance of neuropathic pain only in the acute phase of Wallerian degeneration. By 7 months postlesion, we failed to observe convincing COX2-IR cell profiles in injured nerve except in the ensheathed area surrounding the ligation site. However, more than half of PSNL rats still exhibited explicit tactile allodynia. We hence postulate that, at a later stage of partial nerve injury, other mechanisms (central sensitization?) than peripherally over-produced PGs may underlie the maintenance of neuropathic pain.

4.4. Over-Produced PGE2 in Injured Nerve May Modulate the Functions of Infiltrating Macrophages Via Up-Regulation of EP Receptors

It has been well documented that PGE2 directly or indirectly sensitizes DRG neurons and facilitates the release of excitatory glutamate, substance P and CGRP from primary sensory neurons (Vanegas and Schaible, 2001). The sensitivity of both injured and uninjured axons and DRG neurons to innocuous and noxious mechanical stimuli is enhanced when exposed to

PGE2 (Michaelis et al., 1998). Thus, it is highly possible that over-produced PGE2 in injured nerve following PSNL acts directly on sensitized injured and uninjured primary afferents and contributes to the maintenance of tactile allodynia. Both *in vivo* and *in vitro* studies showed that more than one EP receptor is involved in mediating the behavioral hyperalgesia and sensitizing effects on DRG neurons induced by PGE2 (Khasar et al., 1995; Southall and Vasko, 2001).

In addition to the sensitizing effects of over-produced PGE2 on injured axons, the remarkable increase of 4 EP receptor expressing cell profiles in the injured nerve also suggests that over-produced PGE2 may affect the functions of invading macrophages and other inflammatory cells via its EP receptors, through both autocrine and paracrine mechanisms. The increase of EP4-IR cells was overwhelming in abundance and extent, while the increase of other 3 EP receptors is relatively limited, only found in injury site. This observation suggests that PGE2 is one of the PGs over-produced in the injured nerve following nerve injury and its effect on macrophage function might be primarily mediated through EP4 receptors. Indeed, we observed that EP4 receptors, but not other EP receptors, is responsible for the increased IL-6 production in macrophage culture derived from injured nerve segments. Although EP1 receptor expressing cells are never as abundant as EP4 expressing cells, majority of EP1-IR cells were identified as infiltrating macrophages, indicating that PGE2 may also affect macrophage functions through EP1 receptors. The co-expression of EP2- or EP3-IR cells with the macrophage marker ED1 was only detected in a small fraction of cells, indicating that EP2 and EP3 expressing cells are other types of inflammatory cells than macrophages. Further experiments are needed to identify these EP2 and EP3 expressing cells. However, based on available literature, mast cells in injured nerve are one of the possible candidate cells producing PGE2 and expressing EP receptors. Mast cells are known to synthesize and release PGE2 (Chock and Schmauder-Chock, 1988) and express EP receptors, particularly EP3 (Gomi et al., 2000; Nguyen et al., 2002). Through EP3 receptors, PGE2 mediates the production of IL6 and degranulation of activated mast cells (Gomi et al., 2000; Nguyen et al., 2002). Interestingly, mast cells are also increased in injured nerve following nerve injury (Zochodne et al., 1994).

Modulation of the functions of macrophages by over-produced PGE2 may serve as one of contributing events leading to the pathogenesis of neuropathic pain. *In vitro* study showed that EP2, EP3 and EP4 receptors are constitutively expressed in macrophages and differentially modulated by bacterial LPS and interferon-γ (Hubbard et al., 2001). Released PGE2 may act on macrophages, thus forming a negative feedback loop in macrophage activation. PGE2 inhibits the production of various cytokines, including TNFα, IL-1β and IL-12 by macrophages (Zhong et al., 1995; Yamane et al., 2000; Shinomiya et al., 2001), but increases the production of IL-6 (Yamane et al., 2000; Repovic and Benveniste, 2002) and IL-10 (Shinomiya et al., 2001). These effects on cytokines are mediated through EP4 and EP2 receptors (Katsuyama et al., 1998; Yamane et al., 2000), which are also increased in macrophages stimulated by inflammatory agents (Katsuyama et al., 1998; Kurihara et al., 2001). Overall, these lines of evidence suggest that PGE2 plays both pro- and anti-inflammatory roles during inflammation.

However, a recent report clearly supports a pro-inflammatory role of the EP4 receptor in the pathogenesis of rheumatoid arthritis. McCoy et al. showed decreased incidence and severity of the disease in EP4 knockout mice and reduced inflammation as assessed by circulating IL-6 and serum amyloid A level (McCoy et al., 2002). In our study, EP4 up-regulation is the most dramatic among EP receptor subtypes, suggesting that the role of EP4 in the effects of PGE2 on macrophage activity should be more important than other EP receptors. Therefore, further experiments are warranted to address whether up-regulated EP4 contributes to the development of neuropathic pain.

Interestingly, the immunoreactivities of all 4 EP receptors are localized in the nuclei of these cell profiles. Although EP receptors belong to G-protein coupled receptors, they also localize in the nucleus of various types of cells and nuclear EP receptors are functional (Bhattacharya et al., 1998). It is likely that PGE2 derived from up-regulated COX2 in macrophages acts on the EP4 receptors to increase the production of IL6 from macrophages. IL6 is involved in neuropathic pain following SNL (Murphy et al., 1999) and is up-regulated in injured nerve of various neuropathic rats (Cui et al., 2000).

There is evidence for molecular cross talk between inflammatory mediators such as nitric oxide (NO) and PGs. NO is an important pain mediator and is derived from L-arginine by isoforms of nitric oxide synthase (NOS). The inducible isoform iNOS is dramatically increased in injured nerve of rats with CCI, and NO is involved in neuropathic pain (Levy and Zochodne, 1998; Levy et al., 1999; Levy et al., 2001). *In vitro* studies showed that COX2-synthesized PGE2 from macrophages up-regulates iNOS (Chang et al., 2001; Panaro et al., 2001) and indomethacin inhibits iNOS expression in macrophages (Hrabak et al., 2001). Via EP4 receptor and cAMP pathway, PGE2 is involved in the control of NO synthesis by LPS in RAW 264.7 macrophage cultures (Vivancos and Moreno, 2002). Thus, it is highly possible that over-produced PGE2 in macrophages acts on the up-regulated EP4 receptors in the nuclei of macrophages and up-regulates the expression of iNOS.

PGE2 was shown to up-regulate COX2 expression concentration-dependently in LPS stimulated RAW 264.7 macrophages via EP2/EP4 receptors and an adenylyl cyclase/cAMP dependent mechanism (Hinz et al., 2000). PGE2 over-produced by infiltrating macrophages in injured nerve may also behave in the same way via an autocrine feed-forward loop to facilitate the expression of COX2 in macrophages.

4.5. Peripherally Over-Produced PGs Possibly Contribute to the Production of SP and CGRP in the Primary Sensory Neurons, to the Increased Phosphorylation of CREB and to the Up-Regulation of Dynorphin in the Dorsal Horn

Two weeks following partial sciatic nerve injury, SP mRNA and protein are decreased in injured DRG neurons but increased in spared DRG neurons (Ma and Bisby, 1998b), thereby resulting in no obvious decrease in SP expressing cells in L4 to L6 DRG. Similarly, no obvious reduction in CGRP-IR axons was observed between the ipsilateral and contralateral dorsal horn following CCI and PSNL (Ma and Bisby, 1998a). In the current study we observed that 4 weeks after PSNL, SP- and CGRP-IR axons are not significantly different from the contralateral side, confirming our previous observations. Although there is no available literature showing that the release of SP and CGRP in the dorsal horn is altered following PSNL, it has been well documented in both *in vitro* and *in vivo* studies that, PGE2 facilitates the release of SP and CGRP from primary sensory neurons through both direct and indirect mechanisms (Vanegas and Schaible, 2001). Over-produced PGE2 in injured nerve may increase the release of these two peptides from primary sensory afferents in the dorsal horn. Therefore, we expected that local injection of ketorolac would inhibit the peripheral over-production of PGE2, thus reducing the release of SP and CGRP from primary sensory afferents in the dorsal horn. If the release of SP and CGRP in the dorsal horn was reduced by this mechanism, we would have expected that SP- and CGRP-IR axonal terminals in the dorsal horn would increase following intraplantar injection of ketorolac. In contrast to this expectation, intraplantar ketorolac caused a dramatic reduction in SP- and CGRP-IR axons in the contralateral and ipsilateral dorsal horn. Increased release of CGRP in the dorsal horn evoked by electrical stimulation results in a decreased content of CGRP-IR in the dorsal horn (Klein et al., 1990).

It has been well established that nerve growth factor (NGF) up-regulates SP and CGRP in primary sensory neurons (Lindsay et al., 1989; Lindsay and Harmar, 1989). Based on available evidence, we postulate that over-produced PGE2 in injured nerve and target tissue is likely involved in the production of these two peptides in DRG neurons. For example, PG analogs facilitate the promoting effects of NGF on neurite outgrowth of PC12 cells and DRG explants (Satoh et al., 2000; Satoh et al., 2001). In primary hippocampal cell cultures, PGE2 directly increases NGF mRNA and protein in both neurons and glia (Friedman et al., 1990). Interestingly, NGF also increases PGE2 production in cultured mast cells (Marshall et al., 1999). Thus, we hypothesize that peripherally over-produced PGE2 during neuropathic pain possibly facilitates NGF-induced up-regulation of CGRP and SP in spared DRG neurons.

However, the possibility cannot be excluded that ketorolac has a direct effect on the expression of SP and CGRP in the dorsal horn, since it has been reported that some COX inhibitors directly act on DRG neurons to block mRNA expression of acid-sensing ion channels that are up-regulated during inflammation (Voilley et al., 2001). Further experiments using DRG cell culture exposing to PGs and ketorolac are warranted to clarify this issue.

SP and CGRP released from primary sensory afferents in the dorsal horn may contribute to hyperalgesia and allodynia by facilitating the release of excitatory glutamate and aspartate from primary afferents (Kangrga and Randic, 1990; Kangrga et al., 1990) and by increasing the firing of the dorsal horn neurons in response to stimulation (Murase et al., 1989). Thus, increased synthesis and release of SP and CGRP in DRG neurons might be one of the underlying mechanisms for the pro-nociceptive effects exerted by peripherally over-produced PGE2 in injured nerve and target tissue following nerve injury.

cAMP responsive element binding protein (CREB) is a constitutively expressed transcription factor. When phosphorylated or activated it binds to cAMP response element and modulates the transcription of both immediate early genes, including c-fos and c-jun (Sheng et al., 1990; Lamph et al., 1990), and some late effect genes (Tsukada et al., 1987) which are implicated in nociception(White et al., 2000). Three weeks after PSNL, the phosphorylation of CREB in the ipsilateral dorsal horn neurons was increased (Ma and Quirion, 2001). In the present study, both intraplantar and perineural injection of ketorolac not only reversed tactile allodynia but also suppressed the increased phosphorylation of

CREB in the dorsal horn neurons. This observation suggests that the phosphorylation of CREB is possibly involved in the maintenance of neuropathic pain, and that PGs produced in injured nerve or the ipsilateral plantar skin contribute to the increased phosphorylation of CREB in the ipsilateral dorsal horn neurons. Interestingly, locally administered ketorolac not only suppressed pCREB expression in the ipsilateral dorsal horn but also in the contralateral dorsal horn. The reason is currently unknown. As described in the original paper (Seltzer et al., 1990) and also observed by us, PSNL also reduced the paw withdrawal threshold in the contralateral hindpaw. Whether tactile allodynia in the contralateral hindpaw occurs through either central or peripheral mechanisms, our finding indicates that PSNL induced PG up-regulation in the periphery is involved in the maintenance of tactile allodynia in the contralateral paw as well.

Dynorphin is an endogenous ligand of the κ-opioid receptor. Under normal physiological conditions, it exerts an antinociceptive effect via opioid receptor agonism (Przewlocki et al., 1983; Stevens and Yaksh, 1986) while in pathological circumstances, it induces pronociceptive effects through a non-opioid mechanism, in part by activation of glutamate receptors (Vanderah et al., 1996; Laughlin et al., 1997). Dynorphin plays a facilitating role in abnormal pain and neuropathic pain (Vanderah et al., 2000; Caudle and Mannes, 2000; Wang et al., 2001). Dynorphin pervades in the dorsal horn and is up-regulated during inflammation (Ruda et al., 1988; Nahin et al., 1989) and peripheral nerve injury (Kajander et al., 1990). In the current study, we observed that dynorphin-IR cells and axons in the dorsal horn were increased following PSNL, consistent with these previous reports. Moreover, we observed that intraplantar injection of ketorolac markedly suppressed this increase in dynorphin-IR in the dorsal horn following PSNL. This finding is within our expectations, since intraplantar ketorolac suppresses the phosphorylation of CREB in the dorsal horn of PSNL rats. Phosphorylated CREB is involved in regulating the transcription of prodynorphin mRNA into dynorphin (Messersmith et al., 1998). Hence, it is highly possible that suppression of phosphorylated CREB also leads to the suppression of dynorphin content in the dorsal horn following PSNL.

Similar to phosphorylated CREB, we observed that the suppressive effect of intraplantar ketorolac on neuropeptide content in the dorsal horn is bilateral. The reason for this bilateral effect is unclear. Intraplantar injection of ketorolac into the contralateral hindpaw did not relieve tactile allodynia in the ipsilateral hindpaw, suggesting that a local effect prevails. However, the possibility cannot be ignored that local ketorolac may enter the blood stream and inhibit COX1 and COX2 expressing cells in injured nerve, DRG and the dorsal horn, thus causing a global effect.

4.6. Perspective Roles of Macrophage Derived PGE2 in the Underlying Mechanisms of Neuropathic Pain

4.6.1. Role of Over-Produced PGE2 on the Induction of IL6, NGF, Inos Produced by Invading Macrophages

Nerve injury induces dramatic increase in IL-6 (Bourde et al., 1996; Cui et al., 2000) and NGF (Lindholm et al., 1987) in injured nerve. Macrophages are the major producer of IL-6

(Reichert et al., 1996; Cui et al., 2000) and endogenous IL-6 contribues to neuropathic pain (Murphy et al., 1999). In this chapter, we demonstrated that widespread co-localization of IL-6 and COX2 in infiltrating macrophages in injured nerve. In various cell types, PGE2 was shown to up-regulate IL-6 (Williams and Shacter, 1997; Kozawa et al., 1998; Yamane et al., 2000) through specific EP receptor subtypes. Our data revealed that the release of IL6 was significantly increased from cultured cells derived from injured sciatic nerve segments. This increase is further enhanced by PGE2 treatment and inhibited by both non-selective and selective COX2 inhibitors.

It has been shown that NGF is produced by macrophages in injured nerve (Mallat et al., 1989; Liu et al., 1995; Marcinkiewicz et al., 1999). In hippocampal culture, PGE2 increases NGF production in both neurons and glia (Friedman et al., 1990). In injured nerve, PGE2 increases NGF production in non-neuronal cells (Lindholm et al., 1987).

Nerve injury also induces dramatic increase in iNOS in macrophages in injured nerve and its product NO contributes to the development of neuropathic pain (Levy and Zochodne, 1998; Levy et al., 1999; Levy et al., 2001). *In vitro*, PGE2 produced by macrophages up-regulates iNOS (Chang et al., 2001; Panaro et al., 2001) and indomethacin inhibits iNOS expression in macrophages (Hrabak et al., 2001).

Our current data showed that about 50% macrophages up-regulates PGE2 receptor EP4 expression. *Therefore, we hypothesize that, through autocrine or paracrine mechanisms, over-produced PGE2 also induces the up-regulation of NGF and iNOS in macrophages through EP4 receptor.*

4.6.2. Role of Over-Produced PGE2 in the Induction of Bfgf and VEGF and in the Stimulation of Angiogenesis in the Injured Nerve

PGE2 was shown to induce angiogenesis through up-regulating basic fibroblast growth factor (bFGF) (Dormond et al., 2001) and vascular endothelia growth factor (VEGF) (Ben Av et al., 1995), two important growth factors in angiogenesis during development and in various diseases. PGE2 induces increase in VEGF (Mukutmoni et al., 2001) in murine macrophages and bFGF in fibroblasts (Sakai et al., 2001). Nerve injury is followed by angiogenesis and increase in VEGF in injured nerve (Zochodne and Nguyen, 1997; Hoke et al., 2001). VEGF increases the formation of neovasculatures in injured nerve (Sondell et al., 1999). Our preliminary data showed that von-Willebrand factor-IR blood vessel profiles were markedly increased in injured nerve 1 and 2 weeks after PSNL (Ma, unpublished data), suggesting that nerve injury enhances angiogenesis in injured nerve. *We thus hypothesize that over-produced PGE2 up-regulates bFGF and VEGF in macrophages, leading to the increase in microvasculatures in injured nerve.*

4.6.3. Role of Over-Produced PGE2 in the Survival of Infiltrating Macrophages

Macrophage migration inhibitory factor prevents macrophages from apoptosis by inhibiting P53, this process requires the induction of COX2 and involvement of PGE2 (Mitchell et al., 2002). Increased PGE2 synthesis in macrophages protects macrophages against the cytotoxic effects of NO (Zamora et al., 1998). However, invading macrophages in degenerating nerve will be eventually eliminated by apoptosis. Our data showed that COX2-

IR macrophages are dramatically increased during initial 4 weeks after nerve injury, but decline thereafter and finally disappear by 6 months post-lesion. The time course of COX2 correlates well with the evolution of macrophage recruitment in injured nerve. It is possible that increased PGE2 sustains the survival of macrophages during the initial several months after nerve injury. Indeed, partial sciatic nerve injury induces a dramatic increase in the expression of apoptotic marker caspase-3 in Schwann cells, fibroblasts and endothelia in injured nerve, but infiltrating macrophages are rarely caspase-3 positive (Ma, unpublished data). *We therefore hypothesize that over-produced PGE2 by invading macrophages is involved in the survival of macrophages in injured nerve.*

4.6.4. Role of PGE2 in Direct or Indirect Induction of SP and CGRP in DRG Neurons

Substance P and CGRP are two pain-inducing neuropeptides up-regulated in DRG neurons during tissue inflammation. NGF is a stronger inducer of SP and CGRP production (Lindsay and Harmar, 1989; Ma et al., 1995). mRNA of EP1, EP3 and EP4 receptors are present in DRG neurons (Oida et al., 1995). Consistently, we also observed that EP1- and EP4-IR neurons are present in DRG (Ma, unpublished data). PGE2 directly and indirectly facilitates the release of SP and CGRP from primary sensory afferents (Vasko et al., 1994; Vasko, 1995). We showed previously that following PSNL, SP and CGRP mRNA and protein are up-regulated in spared DRG neurons whereas decreased in injured neurons (Ma and Bisby, 1998b; Ma et al., 1999). Our current data also reveal that peripheral injection of ketorolac, which decreases peripherally over-produced PGs, markedly reduces SP and CGRP contents in the dorsal horn. This observation is contrary to expectation that reducing peripheral PG results in the decrease in the release of two peptides from primary sensory afferents in the dorsal horn, thus causing an increase in content. The explanation to our unexpected data is that peripherally derived PG may contribute to the production of SP and CGRP in DRG neurons. *Thus, we hypothesize that peripheral PGE2 is involved in the production of SP and CGRP.* Since PGE2 is possibly involved in the production of NGF, we also wish to determine whether PGE2 directly induces SP and CGRP production or indirectly through induction of NGF.

4.6.5. Role of PGE2 in the Regeneration and Sprouting of DRG Neurons

In ostoblast-like cell culture, PGE2 increases the elongation of cultured cells and sprouting of slend cytoplasmic processes (Conconi et al., 2002). In DRG cultures, PGE2 directly increases neuritogenesis in cultured DRG neurons (Hiruma et al., 2000). Cultured DRG neurons which were pre-axotomized display much more vigorous sprouting than intact DRG neurons (Smith and Skene, 1997). Our preliminary data showed that injured DRG neurons from PSNL rats exhibit more abundant CGRP expressing arborizations than intact neurons 5 days after seeding (Ma, unpublished data). *We hypothesize that PGE2 contributes to vigorous sprouting of pre-axotomized DRG neurons and suppressing PGE2 produced by infiltrating macrophages in vivo affect the sprouting of pre-axotomized DRG neurons.*

4.6.6. Conclusions

Following various types of peripheral nerve injury, COX2, PGE2 and 4 EP receptors are universally up-regulated in invading macrophages in injured nerve. Over-produced PGE2 may directly sensitize both injured and uninjured axons, may exert effect on pain-related neuropeptide production and on the sprouting and regeneration of injured DRG neurons, and may influence the functions of invading macrophages and other inflammatory cells. Through these mechanisms, macrophage derived PGE2 may finally contribute to the pathogenesis of neuropathic pain caused by nerve injury.

References

Ben Av P, Crofford LJ, Wilder RL, Hla T (1995) Induction of vascular endothelial growth factor expression in synovial fibroblasts by prostaglandin E and interleukin-1: a potential mechanism for inflammatory angiogenesis. *FEBS Lett* 372: 83-87.

Bennett GJ, Xie YK (1988) A peripheral mononeuropathy in rat that produces disorders of pain sensation like those seen in man. *Pain* 33: 87-107.

Bhattacharya M, Peri KG, Almazan G, Ribeiro-da-silva A, Shichi H, Durocher Y, Abramovitz M, Hou X, Varma DR, Chemtob S (1998) Nuclear localization of prostaglandin E2 receptors. *Proc Natl Acad Sci* U S A 95: 15792-15797.

Bourde O, Kiefer R, Toyka KV, Hartung HP (1996) Quantification of interleukin-6 mRNA in wallerian degeneration by competitive reverse transcription polymerase chain reaction. *J Neuroimmunol* 69: 135-140.

Brown MC, Perry VH, Lunn ER, Gordon S, Heumann R (1991) Macrophage dependence of peripheral nerve regeneration: possible involvement of nerve growth factor. *Neuron* 6: 359-370.

Caudle RM, Mannes AJ (2000) Dynorphin: friend or foe? *Pain* 87: 235-239.

Chang YH, Lee ST, Lin WW (2001) Effects of cannabinoids on LPS-stimulated inflammatory mediator release from macrophages: involvement of eicosanoids. *J Cell Biochem* 81: 715-723.

Chaplan SR, Bach FW, Pogrel JW, Chung JM, Yaksh TL (1994) Quantitative assessment of tactile allodynia in the rat paw. *J Neurosci Methods* 53: 55-63.

Chock SP, Schmauder-Chock EA (1988) Synthesis of prostaglandins and eicosanoids by the mast cell secretory granule. *Biochem Biophys Res Commun* 156: 1308-1315.

Chouaib S, Welte K, Mertelsmann R, Dupont B (1985) Prostaglandin E2 acts at two distinct pathways of T lymphocyte activation: inhibition of interleukin 2 production and down-regulation of transferrin receptor expression. *J Immunol* 135: 1172-1179.

Clatworthy AL, Illich PA, Castro GA, Walters ET (1995) Role of peri-axonal inflammation in the development of thermal hyperalgesia and guarding behavior in a rat model of neuropathic pain. *Neurosci Lett* 184: 5-8.

Coleman RA, Smith WL, Narumiya S (1994) International Union of Pharmacology classification of prostanoid receptors: properties, distribution, and structure of the receptors and their subtypes. *Pharmacol Rev* 46: 205-229.

Conconi MT, Tommasini M, Baiguera S, De Coppi P, Parnigotto PP, Nussdorfer GG (2002) Effects of prostaglandins E1 and E2 on the growth and differentiation of osteoblast-like cells cultured in vitro. *Int J Mol Med* 10: 451-456.

Cui JG, Holmin S, Mathiesen T, Meyerson BA, Linderoth B (2000) Possible role of inflammatory mediators in tactile hypersensitivity in rat models of mononeuropathy. *Pain* 88: 239-248.

Davies P, MacIntyre DE (1992) Prostaglandins and inflammation. In: Inflammation: basic principles and clinical correlates (Gallin JI, Goldstein IM, Snyderman R, eds), pp 123-138. New York: *Raven Press,*Ltd.

Deleo JA, Colburn RW, Nlichois M, MALHOTRA A (1996) Interleukin-6-mediated hyperalgesia/allodynia and increased spinal IL-6 expression in a rat mononeuropathy model. *J Interferon Cytokine Res* 16: 695-700.

Dormond O, Foletti A, Paroz C, Ruegg C (2001) NSAIDs inhibit alpha V beta 3 integrin-mediated and Cdc42/Rac-dependent endothelial-cell spreading, migration and angiogenesis. *Nat Med* 7: 1041-1047.

Dray A, Perkins M (1993) Bradykinin and inflammatory pain. *Trends Neurosci* 16: 99-104.

Fadok VA, Bratton DL, Konowal A, Freed PW, Westcott JY, Henson PM (1998) Macrophages that have ingested apoptotic cells in vitro inhibit proinflammatory cytokine production through autocrine/paracrine mechanisms involving TGF-beta, PGE2, and PAF. *J Clin Invest* 101: 890-898.

Friedman WJ, Larkfors L, Ayer-LeLievre C, Ebendal T, Olson L, Persson H (1990) Regulation of beta-nerve growth factor expression by inflammatory mediators in hippocampal cultures. *J Neurosci Res* 27: 374-382.

Frisen J, Risling M, Fried K (1993) Distribution and axonal relations of macrophages in a neuroma. *Neuroscience* 55: 1003-1013.

Fukuoka H, Kawatani M, Hisamitsu T, Takeshige C (1994) Cutaneous hyperalgesia induced by peripheral injection of interleukin-1 beta in the rat. *Brain Res* 657: 133-140.

Gomi K, Zhu FG, Marshall JS (2000) Prostaglandin E2 selectively enhances the IgE-mediated production of IL-6 and granulocyte-macrophage colony-stimulating factor by mast cells through an EP1/EP3-dependent mechanism. *J Immunol* 165: 6545-6552.

Hinz B, Brune K, Pahl A (2000) Prostaglandin E(2) upregulates cyclooxygenase-2 expression in lipopolysaccharide-stimulated RAW 264.7 macrophages. *Biochem Biophys Res Commun* 272: 744-748.

Hiruma H, Ichikawa T, Kobayashi H, Hoka S, Takenaka T, Kawakami T (2000) Prostaglandin E(2) enhances axonal transport and neuritogenesis in cultured mouse dorsal root ganglion neurons. *Neuroscience* 100: 885-891.

Hoke A, Sun HS, Gordon T, Zochodne DW (2001) Do denervated peripheral nerve trunks become ischemic? The impact of chronic denervation on vasa nervorum. *Exp Neurol* 172: 398-406.

Hrabak A, Vercruysse V, Kahan IL, Vray B (2001) Indomethacin prevents the induction of inducible nitric oxide synthase in murine peritoneal macrophages and decreases their nitric oxide production. *Life Sci* 68: 1923-1930.

Hubbard NE, Lee S, Lim D, Erickson KL (2001) Differential mRNA expression of prostaglandin receptor subtypes in macrophage activation. *Prostaglandins Leukot Essent Fatty Acids* 65: 287-294.

Ichikawa A, Sugimoto Y, Negishi M (1996) Molecular aspects of the structures and functions of the prostaglandin E receptors. *J Lipid Mediat Cell Signal* 14: 83-87.

Kajander KC, Sahara Y, Iadarola MJ, Bennett GJ (1990) Dynorphin increases in the dorsal spinal cord in rats with a painful peripheral neuropathy. *Peptides* 11: 719-728.

Kangrga I, Larew JS, Randic M (1990) The effects of substance P and calcitonin gene-related peptide on the efflux of endogenous glutamate and aspartate from the rat spinal dorsal horn in vitro. *NEUROSCI LETT* 108: 155-60X.

Kangrga I, Randic M (1990) Tachykinins and calcitonin gene-related peptide enhance release off endogenous glutamate and aspartate from the rat spinal dorsal horn slice. *J NEUROSCI* 10: 2026-238X.

Katsuyama M, Ikegami R, Karahashi H, Amano F, Sugimoto Y, Ichikawa A (1998) Characterization of the LPS-stimulated expression of EP2 and EP4 prostaglandin E receptors in mouse macrophage-like cell line, J774.1. *Biochem Biophys Res Commun* 251: 727-731.

Kawahara H, Sakamoto A, Takeda S, Onodera H, Imaki J, Ogawa R (2001) A prostaglandin E2 receptor subtype EP1 receptor antagonist (ONO-8711) reduces hyperalgesia, allodynia, and c-fos gene expression in rats with chronic nerve constriction. *Anesth Analg* 93: 1012-1017.

Khasar SG, Ouseph AK, Chou B, Ho T, Green PG, Levine JD (1995) Is there more than one prostaglandin E receptor subtype mediating hyperalgesia in the rat hindpaw? Neuroscience 64: 1161-1165.

Kiefer R, Kieseier BC, Stoll G, Hartung HP (2001) The role of macrophages in immune-mediated damage to the peripheral nervous system. *Prog Neurobiol* 64: 109-127.

Kim SH, Chung JM (1992) An experimental model for peripheral neuropathy produced by segmental spinal nerve ligation in the rat. *Pain* 50: 355-363.

Klein CM, Coggeshall RE, Carlton SM, Westlund KN, Sorkin LS (1990) Changes in calcitonin gene-related peptide immunoreactivity in the rat dorsal horn following electrical stimulation of the sciatic nerve. *Neurosci Lett* 115: 149-154.

Kozawa O, Suzuki A, Tokuda H, Kaida T, Uematsu T (1998) Interleukin-6 synthesis induced by prostaglandin E2: cross-talk regulation by protein kinase C. *Bone* 22: 355-360.

Kurihara Y, Endo H, Akahoshi T, Kondo H (2001) Up-regulation of prostaglandin E receptor EP2 and EP4 subtypes in rat synovial tissues with adjuvant arthritis. *Clin Exp Immunol* 123: 323-330.

Lamph WW, Dwarki vJ, Ofir R, Montminy M, Verma IM (1990) Negative and positive regulation by transcription factor cAMP response element-binding protein is modulated by phosphorylation. *Proc Natl Acad Sci* USA 87: 4320-4324.

Laughlin TM, Vanderah TW, Lashbrook J, Nichols ML, Ossipov M, Porreca F, Wilcox GL (1997) Spinally administered dynorphin A produces long-lasting allodynia: involvement of NMDA but not opioid receptors. *Pain* 72: 253-260.

Lee SH, Soyoola E, Chanmugam P, Hart S, Sun W, Zhong H, Liou S, Simmons D, Hwang D (1992) Selective expression of mitogen-inducible cyclooxygenase in macrophages stimulated with lipopolysaccharide. *J Biol Chem* 267: 25934-25938.

Levi G, Minghetti L, Aloisi F (1998) Regulation of prostanoid synthesis in microglial cells and effects of prostaglandin E2 on microglial functions. *BIOCHIMIE* 80: 899-904.

Levine JD, Coderre TJ, White DM, Finkbeiner WE, Basbaum AI (1990) Denervation-induced inflammation in the rat. *Neurosci Lett* 119: 37-40.

Levine JD, Reichling DB (1999) Peripheral mechanisms of inflammatory pain. In: Textbood of Pain (Wall PD, Melzack R, eds), pp 59-84. London: *Churchill Livingston.*

Levy D, Hoke A, Zochodne DW (1999) Local expression of inducible nitric oxide synthase in an animal model of neuropathic pain. *Neurosci Lett* 260: 207-209.

Levy D, Kubes P, Zochodne DW (2001) Delayed peripheral nerve degeneration, regeneration, and pain in mice lacking inducible nitric oxide synthase. *J Neuropathol Exp Neurol* 60: 411-421.

Levy D, Zochodne DW (1998) Local nitric oxide synthase activity in a model of neuropathic pain. *Eur J Neurosci* 10: 1846-1855.

Lindholm D, Heumann R, Meyer M, Thoenen H (1987) Interleukin-1 regulates synthesis of nerve growth factor in non- neuronal cells of the rat sciatic nerve. *Nature* 330: 658-659.

Lindsay RM, Harmar AJ (1989) Nerve growth factor regulates expression of neuropeptide genes in adult sensory neurons. *Nature* 337: 362-34.

Lindsay RM, Lockett C, Sternberg J, Winter J (1989) Neuropeptide expression in cultures of adult sensory neurons - modulation of substance-P and calcitonin gene- related peptide levels by nerve growth factor. *Neuroscience* 33: 53-65.

Liu HM, Lei HY, Kao KP (1995) Correlation between NGF levels in wound chamber fluid and cytological localization of NGF and NGF receptor in axotomized rat sciatic nerve. *Exp Neurol* 132: 24-32.

Liu T, van Rooijen N, Tracey DJ (2000) Depletion of macrophages reduces axonal degeneration and hyperalgesia following nerve injury. *Pain* 86: 25-32.

Ma W, Bisby MA (1998a) Increase of calcitonin gene-related peptide immunoreactivity in the axonal fibers of the gracile nuclei of adult and aged rats after complete and partial sciatic nerve injuries. *Exp Neurol* 152: 137-149.

Ma W, Bisby MA (1998b) Increase of preprotachykinin mRNA and substance P immunoreactivity in spared primary sensory neurons following partial sciatic nerve injuries. *Eur J Neurosci* 10: 2388-2399.

Ma W, Eisenach JC (2002) Morphological and pharmacological evidence for the role of peripheral prostaglandins in the pathogenesis of neuropathic pain. *Eur J Neurosci* 15: 1037-1047.

Ma W, Eisenach JC (2003a) Cyclooxygenase 2 in infiltrating inflammatory cells in injured nerve is universally up-regulated following various types of nerve injury. *Neuroscience* 121: 691-704.

Ma W, Eisenach JC (2003b) Four EP receptors are up-regulated in injured nerve following partial sciatic nerve ligation. *Exp Neurol* 183: 581-592.

Ma W, Eisenach JC (2003c) Intraplantar injection of the cyclooxygenase inhibitor ketorolac reduces immunoreactivities of substance P, calcitonin gene-related peptide, and dynorphin in the dorsal horn of rats with nerve injury or inflammation. *Neuroscience* 121: 681-690.

Ma W, Hatzis C, Eisenach JC (2003) Intrathecal injection of cAMP response element binding protein (CREB) antisense oligonucleotide attenuates tactile allodynia caused by partial sciatic nerve ligation. *Brain Res* 988: 97-104.

Ma W, Quirion R (2001) Increased phosphorylation of cyclic AMP responsive binding protein (CREB) in the superficial dorsal horn neurons following partial sciatic nerve ligation. *Pain* 93: 295-301.

Ma W, Quirion R (2005) Up-regulation of interleukin 6 induced by prostaglandin 2 from invading macrophages following nerve injury: an *in vivo* and *in vitro* study. *J Neurochem in press.*

Ma W, Ramer MS, Bisby MA (1999) Increased calcitonin gene related peptide immunoreactivity in gracile nucleus after partial sciatic nerve injury: age-dependent and originating from spared sensory neurons. *Exp Neurol* 159: 459-473.

Ma W, Ribeiro-da-silva A, Noel G, Julien JP, Cuello AC (1995) Ectopic substance P and calcitonin gene-related peptide immunoreactive fibers in the spinal cord of transgenic mice overexpressing nerve growth factor. *Eur J Neurosci* 7: 2021-2035.

Mallat M, Houlgatte R, Brachet P, Prochiantz A (1989) Lipopolysaccharide-stimulated rat brain macrophages release NGF in vitro. *Dev Biol* 133: 309-311.

Marcinkiewicz M, Marcinkiewicz J, Chen A, Leclaire F, Chretien M, Richardson P (1999) Nerve growth factor and proprotein convertases furin and PC7 in transected sciatic nerves and in nerve segments cultured in conditioned media: their presence in Schwann cells, macrophages, and smooth muscle cells. *J Comp Neurol* 403: 471-485.

Marshall JS, Gomi K, Blennerhassett MG, Bienenstock J (1999) Nerve growth factor modifies the expression of inflammatory cytokines by mast cells via a prostanoid-dependent mechanism. *J Immunol* 162: 4271-4276.

McCoy JM, Wicks JR, Audoly LP (2002) The role of prostaglandin E2 receptors in the pathogenesis of rheumatoid arthritis. *J Clin Invest* 110: 651-658.

Messersmith DJ, Kim DJ, Iadarola MJ (1998) Transcription factor regulation of prodynorphin gene expression following rat hindpaw inflammation. *Mol Brain Res* 53: 260-269.

Michaelis M, Vogel C, Blenk KH, Arnarson A, Janig W (1998) Inflammatory mediators sensitize acutely axotomized nerve fibers to mechanical stimulation in the rat. *J Neurosci* 18: 7581-7587.

Millan MJ (1999) The induction of pain: an integrative review. *Prog Neurobiol* 57: 1-164.

Mitchell RA, Liao H, Chesney J, Fingerle-Rowson G, Baugh J, David J, Bucala R (2002) Macrophage migration inhibitory factor (MIF) sustains macrophage proinflammatory function by inhibiting p53: regulatory role in the innate immune response. *Proc Natl Acad Sci* U S A 99: 345-350.

Mukutmoni M, Hubbard NE, Erickson KL (2001) Prostaglandin E(2) modulation of vascular endothelial growth factor production in murine macrophages. *Prostaglandins Leukot Essent Fatty Acids* 65: 123-131.

Murase K, Ryu PD, Randic M (1989) Excitatory and inhibitory amino acids and peptide-induced responses in acutely isolated rat spinal dorsal horn neurons. *Neurosci Lett* 103: 56-63.

Murphy PG, Ramer MS, Borthwick L, Gauldie J, Richardson PM, Bisby MA (1999) Endogenous interleukin-6 contributes to peripheral neurophathic pain. *Eur J Neurosci* 11: 2243-2253.

Nahin RL, Hylden JL, Iadarola MJ, Dubner R (1989) Peripheral inflammation is associated with increased dynorphin immunoreactivity in both projection and local circuit neurons in the superficial dorsal horn of the rat lumbar spinal cord. *Neurosci Lett* 96: 247-252.

Nguyen M, Solle M, Audoly LP, Tilley SL, Stock JL, McNeish JD, Coffman TM, Dombrowicz D, Koller BH (2002) Receptors and signaling mechanisms required for prostaglandin E2-mediated regulation of mast cell degranulation and IL-6 production. *J Immunol* 169: 4586-4593.

Oida H, Namba T, Sugimoto Y, Ushikubi F, Ohishi H, Ichikawa A, Narumiya S (1995) In situ hybridization studies of prostacyclin receptor mRNA expression in various mouse organs. *Br J Pharmacol* 116: 2828-2837.

Omana-Zapata I, Bley KR (2001) A stable prostacyclin analog enhances ectopic activity in rat sensory neurons following neuropathic injury. *Brain Res* 904: 85-92.

Panaro MA, Brandonisio O, Sisto M, Acquafredda A, Leogrande D, Fumarola L, Mitolo V (2001) Nitric oxide production by Leishmania-infected macrophages and modulation by prostaglandin E2. *Clin Exp Med* 1: 137-143.

Perkins NM, Tracey DJ (2000) Hyperalgesia due to nerve injury: role of neutrophils. *Neuroscience* 101: 745-757.

Przewlocki R, Stala L, Greczek M, Shearman GT, Przewlocka B, Herz A (1983) Analgesic effects of mu-, delta- and kappa-opiate agonists and, in particular, dynorphin at the spinal level. Life Sci 33 *Suppl* 1: 649-652.

Rakovska A, Milenov K (1984) Antagonistic effect of SC-19220 on the responses of guinea-pig gastric muscles to prostaglandins E1, E2 and F2 alpha. *Arch Int Pharmacodyn Ther* 268: 59-69.

Ramer MS, Murphy PG, Richardson PM, Bisby MA (1998) Spinal nerve lesion-induced mechanoallodnia and adrenergic sprouting in sensory ganglia are attenuated in interleukin-6 knockout mice. *Pain* 78: 115-121.

Reddy ST, Herschman HR (1994) Ligand-induced prostaglandin synthesis requires expression of the TIS10/PGS-2 prostaglandin synthase gene in murine fibroblasts and macrophages. *J Biol Chem* 269: 15473-15480.

Reddy ST, Winstead MV, Tischfield JA, Herschman HR (1997) Analysis of the secretory phospholipase A2 that mediates prostaglandin production in mast cells. *J Biol Chem* 272: 13591-13596.

Reichert F, Levitzky R, Rotshenker S (1996) Interleukin 6 in intact and injured mouse peripheral nerves. *Eur J Neurosci* 8: 530-535.

Repovic P, Benveniste EN (2002) Prostaglandin E2 is a novel inducer of oncostatin-M expression in macrophages and microglia. *J Neurosci* 22: 5334-5343.

Ruda MA, Iadarola MJ, Cohen LV, Young WS, III (1988) In situ hybridization histochemistry and immunocytochemistry reveal an increase in spinal dynorphin biosynthesis in a rat model of peripheral inflammation and hyperalgesia. *Proc Natl Acad Sci* U S A 85: 622-626.

Sakai Y, Fujita K, Sakai H, Mizuno K (2001) Prostaglandin E2 regulates the expression of basic fibroblast growth factor messenger RNA in normal human fibroblasts. *Kobe J Med Sci* 47: 35-45.

Satoh T, Furuta K, Tomokiyo K, Nakatsuka D, Tanikawa M, Nakanishi M, Miura M, Tanaka S, Koike T, Hatanaka H, Ikuta K, Suzuki M, Watanabe Y (2000) Facilitatory roles of novel compounds designed from cyclopentenone prostaglandins on neurite outgrowth-promoting activities of nerve growth factor. *J Neurochem* 75: 1092-1102.

Satoh T, Furuta K, Tomokiyo K, Namura S, Nakatsuka D, Sugie Y, Ishikawa Y, Hatanaka H, Suzuki M, Watanabe Y (2001) Neurotrophic actions of novel compounds designed from cyclopentenone prostaglandins. *J Neurochem* 77: 50-62.

Schafers M, Marziniak M, Sorkin LS, Yaksh TL, Sommer C (2004) Cyclooxygenase inhibition in nerve-injury- and TNF-induced hyperalgesia in the rat. *Exp Neurol* 185: 160-168.

Schiltz JC, Sawchenko PE (2002) Distinct brain vascular cell types manifest inducible cyclooxygenase expression as a function of the strength and nature of immune insults. *J Neurosci* 22: 5606-5618.

Schmauder-Chock EA, Chock SP (1989) Localization of cyclo-oxygenase and prostaglandin E2 in the secretory granule of the mast cell. *J Histochem Cytochem* 37: 1319-1328.

Seltzer Z, Dubner R, Shir Y (1990) A novel behavioral model of neuropathic pain disorders produced in rats by partial sciatic nerve injury. *Pain* 43: 205-218.

Sheng M, Mcfadden G, Greenberg ME (1990) Membrane depolarization and calcium induce c-Fos transcription via phosphorylation of transcription factor CREB. Neuron 4: 571-582.

Shinomiya S, Naraba H, Ueno A, Utsunomiya I, Maruyama T, Ohuchida S, Ushikubi F, Yuki K, Narumiya S, Sugimoto Y, Ichikawa A, Oh-ishi S (2001) Regulation of TNFalpha and interleukin-10 production by prostaglandins I(2) and E(2): studies with prostaglandin receptor-deficient mice and prostaglandin E-receptor subtype-selective synthetic agonists. *Biochem Pharmacol* 61: 1153-1160.

Shu S, Ju G, Fan L (1988) The glucose oxidase-DAB-nickel method in peroxidase histochemistry of the nervous system. *Neurosci Lett* 85: 169-171.

Simkin NJ, Jelinek DF, Lipsky PE (1987) Inhibition of human B cell responsiveness by prostaglandin E2. *J Immunol* 138: 1074-1081.

Smith DS, Skene JH (1997) A transcription-dependent switch controls competence of adult neurons for distinct modes of axon growth. *J Neurosci* 17: 646-658.

Sondell M, Lundborg G, Kanje M (1999) Vascular endothelial growth factor stimulates Schwann cell invasion and neovascularization of acellular nerve grafts. *Brain Res* 846: 219-228.

Sotgiu ML, Biella G, Formaglio F, Marchettini P (1998) Central effect of ketorolac involving NMDA receptors activity. *Brain Res* 813: 223-226.

Southall MD, Vasko MR (2001) Prostaglandin receptor subtypes, EP3C and EP4, mediate the prostaglandin E2-induced cAMP production and sensitization of sensory neurons. *J Biol Chem* 276: 16083-16091.

Stevens CW, Yaksh TL (1986) Dynorphin A and related peptides administered intrathecally in the rat: a search for putative kappa opiate receptor activity. *J Pharmacol Exp Ther* 238: 833-838.

Syriatowicz JP, Hu D, Walker JS, Tracey DJ (1999) Hyperalgesia due to nerve injury: role of prostaglandins. *Neuroscience* 94: 587-594.

Taffet SM, Russell SW (1981) Macrophage-mediated tumor cell killing: regulation of expression of cytolytic activity by prostaglandin E. *J Immunol* 126: 424-427.

Takayama K, Garcia-Cardena G, Sukhova GK, Comander J, Gimbrone MA, Jr., Libby P (2002) Prostaglandin E2 suppresses chemokine production in human macrophages through the EP4 receptor. *J Biol Chem* 277: 44147-44154.

Thalhammer JG, Vladimirova M, Bershadsky B, Strichartz GR (1995) Neurologic evaluation of the rat during sciatic nerve block with lidocaine. *Anesthesiology* 82: 1013-1025.

Tracey DJ, Walker JS (1995) Pain due to nerve damage - are inflammatory mediators involved. *Inflamm Res* 44: 407-411.

Tsukada T, Fink JS, Mandel G, Goodman RM (1987) Identification of a region in the human vasoactive intestinal polypeptide gene responsible for regulation by cyclic AMP. *J Biol Chem* 262: 8743-8747.

Vanderah TW, Gardell LR, Burgess SE, Ibrahim M, Dogrul A, Zhong CM, Zhang ET, Malan TP, Jr., Ossipov MH, Lai J, Porreca F (2000) Dynorphin promotes abnormal pain and spinal opioid antinociceptive tolerance. *J Neurosci* 20: 7074-7079.

Vanderah TW, Laughlin T, Lashbrook JM, Nichols ML, Wilcox GL, Ossipov MH, Malan TP, Jr., Porreca F (1996) Single intrathecal injections of dynorphin A or des-Tyr-dynorphins produce long-lasting allodynia in rats: blockade by MK-801 but not naloxone. *Pain* 68: 275-281.

Vanegas H, Schaible HG (2001) Prostaglandins and cycloxygenases in the spinal cord. *Prog Neurobiol* 64: 327-363.

Vasko MR (1995) Prostaglandin-induced neuropeptide release from spinal cord. *Prog Brain Res* 104: 367-380.

Vasko MR, Campbell WB, Waite KJ (1994) Prostaglandin E2 enhances bradykinin-stimulated release of neuropeptides from rat sensory neurons in culture. *J Neurosci* 14: 4987-4997.

Vivancos M, Moreno JJ (2002) Role of Ca(2+)-independent phospholipase A(2) and cyclooxygenase/lipoxygenase pathways in the nitric oxide production by murine macrophages stimulated by lipopolysaccharides. *Nitric Oxide* 6: 255-262.

Voilley N, de Weille J, Mamet J, Lazdunski M (2001) Nonsteroid anti-inflammatory drugs inhibit both the activity and the inflammation-induced expression of acid-sensing ion channels in nociceptors. *J Neurosci* 21: 8026-8033.

Wagner R, Janjigian M, Myers RR (1998) Anti-inflammatory interleukin-10 therapy in CCI neuropathy decreases thermal hyperalgesia, macrophage recruitment, and endoneurial TNF-alpha expression. *Pain* 74: 35-42.

Wagner R, Myers RR (1996a) Endoneurial injection of TNF-alpha produces neuropathic pain behaviors. *Neuroreport* 7: 2897-2901.

Wagner R, Myers RR (1996b) Schwann cells produce tumor necrosis factor alpha: expression in injured and non-injured nerves. *Neuroscience* 73: 625-629.

Wang Z, Gardell LR, Ossipov MH, Vanderah TW, Brennan MB, Hochgeschwender U, Hruby VJ, Malan TP, Lai J, Porreca F (2001) Pronociceptive actions of dynorphin maintain chronic neuropathic pain. *J Neurosci* 21: 1779-1786.

White DM, Walker S, Brenneman DE, Gozes I (2000) CREB contributes to the increased neurite outgrowth of sensory neurons induced by vasoactive intestinal polypeptide and activity-dependent neurotrophic factor. *Brain Res* 868: 31-38.

Williams JA, Shacter E (1997) Regulation of macrophage cytokine production by prostaglandin E2. Distinct roles of cyclooxygenase-1 and -2. *J Biol Chem* 272: 25693-25699.

Yamane H, Sugimoto Y, Tanaka S, Ichikawa A (2000) Prostaglandin E(2) receptors, EP2 and EP4, differentially modulate TNF-alpha and IL-6 production induced by lipopolysaccharide in mouse peritoneal neutrophils. *Biochem Biophys Res Commun* 278: 224-228.

Zamora R, Bult H, Herman AG (1998) The role of prostaglandin E2 and nitric oxide in cell death in J774 murine macrophages. *Eur J Pharmacol* 349: 307-315.

Zhong WW, Burke PA, Drotar ME, Chavali SR, Forse RA (1995) Effects of prostaglandin E2, cholera toxin and 8-bromo-cyclic AMP on lipopolysaccharide-induced gene expression of cytokines in human macrophages. *Immunology* 84: 446-452.

Zochodne DW, Nguyen C (1997) Angiogenesis at the site of neuroma formation in transected peripheral nerve. *J Anat* 191 (Pt 1): 23-30.

Zochodne DW, Nguyen C, Sharkey KA (1994) Accumulation and degranulation of mast cells in experimental neuromas. *Neurosci Lett* 182: 3-6.

In: Progress in Inflammation Research
Editor: James A. Pitzer, pp. 95-145
ISBN 1-59454-277-5

Chapter III

The Acute Phase Inflammatory Response in Stroke: Systemic Inflammation and Neuroinflammation

Mario Di Napoli, Arsen Arakelyan†, Anna Boyajyan,† Daniel Godoy‡ and Francesca Papa**

*Neurological Section, SMDN – Center for Cardiovascular Medicine and Cerebrovascular Disease Prevention, Sulmona (L'Aquila), Italy.

† Laboratory of Macromolecular Complexes, Institute of Molecular Biology of Armenian National Academy of Sciences, Yerenav, Republic of Armenia.

‡ Neurointensive Care Unit, Community Medical Institute, Junin Hospital, Junin, Buenos Aires, Argentina.

Abstract

Stroke is among the most common diseases of advanced age becoming a steadily increasing financial healthcare problem in the industrialized world with the increasing longevity and aging of the population. To-date there are not effective therapeutics. However, during the last years promising findings suggest that systemic inflammation and neuroinflammation are central features in cerebrovascular disease. Atherosclerosis, the pathologic process underlying most coronary artery disease and the majority of ischemic stroke (IS) in humans, is an inflammatory process. Complex interactions occur between the classic risk factors for atherosclerosis and its clinical consequences. These interactions appear to involve inflammatory mechanisms both in the periphery and in the central nervous system (CNS). Inflammation in the CNS or in the periphery may be a risk factor for the initial development of cerebral ischemia. Peripheral infection and inflammatory processes are likely to be important in this respect. CNS inflammation is

* Address for correspondence: Dr. Mario Di Napoli, MD; SMDN – Center for Cardiovascular Medicine and Cerebrovascular Disease Prevention, Neurological Section, Via Trento, 41 I-67039 – Sulmona (AQ) Italy. Phone +39 (0)864 52716; Fax. +39 (0)864 52716; Email: mariodinapoli@katamail.com

important in the pathophysiologic processes occurring in IS, subarachnoid hemorrhage and following hemorrhagic stroke. Stroke elicits an inflammatory response in the injured brain that is mediated by various factors, leading to the accumulation of inflammatory cells. The inflammatory reaction, which has a rapid onset and continues after the stroke, is thought to acutely contribute to the evolution of tissue injury. It appears that inflammation may be important both before, in predisposing to a stroke, and afterwards, where it is important in the mechanisms of cerebral injury and repair. Many compounds have been identified in stroke, which are known to promote and sustain inflammatory responses at local and systemic level, producing a neuroinflammatory response and a systemic acute phase response. The acute phase inflammatory response after stroke is a reflection of an unspecific Systemic Inflammatory Response Syndrome. Classic acute-phase reactants and body temperature are also modified in stroke, and may be useful in the prediction of events, outcome, and as therapeutic targets. The pentraxin C-reactive protein is found as a stronger and independent predictor of stroke risk and of prognosis in stroke patients when compared to other prothrombotic and inflammatory markers. Its synthesis is markedly upregulated in stroke. Since it as known to activate the complement cascade in an antibody-independent fashion and chronic activation can cause destruction of host tissue, this pentraxin may be important initiators of an autodestructive process influencing short-term and long-term prognosis of stroke patients. Considerable opportunities therefore exist for the development of novel therapies. Whether these targets will be useful in the development of therapies for the treatment of stroke in humans is far from clear, they provide fertile ground for scientific investigation. At the moment, beyond the traditional anti-thrombotic agents, statins and angiotensin-converting enzyme inhibitors may prove to be important additions to our armamentarium for stroke prevention and treatment acting partly via anti-inflammatory mechanisms.

Keywords Cerebrovascular disease, stroke, erebral ischemia, prognosis, cytokines, chemokines, complement, atherosclerosis, inflammation, C-reactive protein.

Introduction

The last decade has witnessed a major reassessment of our perceptions about the acute stroke. A consensus has emerged that inflammation plays a decisive role in the pathophysiology of these acute cerebrovascular events. Stroke triggers an inflammatory reaction that causes injury to the brain and progresses for several days. Data are accumulating which demonstrate that inflammation plays an important role in the development of secondary brain damage following stroke, and is associated with increased infarct size, neuronal loss and impaired clinical outcome. [1-3] Ischemia is accompanied by increased free radical generation, which induces expression of inflammatory cytokines and chemokines. Cytokines upregulate the expression of adhesion molecules on endothelial cells, leukocytes and platelets, and mediate the interaction between endothelial cells and leukocytes, leading to infiltration of leukocytes into the brain parenchyma. Cytokines activate also resident microglia, whereas chemokines direct blood-borne cells toward their targets. Inflammatory cells contribute to brain damage by producing free radicals and other inflammation-related products that are toxic and lead to blood-brain barrier (BBB) dysfunction, edema and cell death. Together with local effects, cytokines cause systemic actions such as activation of the hypothalamus-hypophysic-adrenal axis, hepatic synthesis of the acute phase reactants, marrow stimulation, etc. Usually, both the production and the action of the cytokines are regulated by a net of endogen mediators. However, sometimes the balance is broken producing a massive and self-destroying inflammatory reaction.

Clinical trials that are aimed at limiting the post-ischemic inflammatory response, however, have thus far yielded disappointing results. These clinical failures probably reflect insufficient preclinical data and inadequate trial design, and therefore do not exclude a role for inflammation in ischemic brain injury. [3] Although each element of the inflammatory response can contribute to post-ischemic brain injury, the most deleterious aspect of the response and the most appropriate target for intervention is unclear. To improve the therapeutic outcome, the significance of brain inflammation and its contribution to ischemic brain injury must be clearly understood.

Inflammation as Precipitating Event in Cerebrovascular Disease

The most common variety of complete stroke is atherothrombotic brain infarction, which is related closely to cerebral thrombosis. [4] It accounts for ≈60% of all strokes (excluding transient ischemic attacks or TIAs). The next most common is cerebral embolus (≈25%). Of all strokes, ≈88% are ischemic (IS), ≈9% are intracerebral hemorrhage (ICH), and ≈3% are subarachnoid hemorrhage (SAH). The pathogenic process leading from cerebrovascular or extra cranial atherosclerosis to acute IS and eventual cell death is complex and not completely understood. ICH and SAH are more likely to involve extremes of blood pressure and/or structural anomalies (e.g. Berry aneurysm) but atherosclerosis may also play a role. [4]

IS can originate from atherosclerotic large cerebral arteries (e.g. carotid, middle cerebral, and basilar arteries) or atherosclerotic small cerebral arteries (e.g. lenticulostriate, basilar penetrating, and medullary arteries). [4] IS can also come from a cardioembolic source. While most studies of atherogenesis have concentrated on the coronary arteries similar but not identical processes occur in the cerebral circulation. [5] In the brain, this process is better understood in the larger arteries than in small arteries that supply deep cerebral white matter. Some studies suggest that the underlying pathogenesis in small arteries may differ from that of larger arteries. More research is needed to define these differences.

Atherogenesis is a decades-long process where the lumen (diameter) of a blood vessel narrows through a combination of cellular (e.g. lipid-laden macrophages) and extracellular interactions making it more vulnerable to blockage from unstable thrombotic plaque. [6,7] Autopsy studies of blood vessels in fetuses, children and young adults have found that the earliest lesion of atherosclerosis is the fatty streak. [6,7] Nearly 70% of children between ages 12 and 14 years had evidence of these lesions. These are grossly visible as areas of yellowish discoloration on the surface of the intimal layer of the vessel wall, and are apparent throughout the arterial vasculature. These lesions consist mainly of lipid-filled macrophages, called *foam cells*. More advanced focal lesions occur in areas of eccentric thickening (i.e. at branch points of the arterial vessel) where turbulent flow is high and involve large amounts of extra-cellular lipids that displace normal cells and matrix. As early as one's thirties, some atheromatous lesions evolve into complicated fibrous plaques, which consist of a central acellular area of oxidized lipid covered by a cap of smooth muscle cells and collagen. The caps grow usually slowly, but with deposition of platelets and fibrin on the surface—which may be due to endothelial injury—the caps can thicken quickly, possibly secondary to thrombosis-dependent fibrotic organization. These lesions can then be calcified. The progression of early atherosclerotic lesions to clinically relevant advanced atherosclerotic lesions occurs with remarkable plasticity over the lifespan—from the thirties to the nineties in some cases. [8] Risk factors for atherosclerotic disease [e.g. hypercholesterolemia, hypertension, cigarette smoking, inflammatory markers such as C-reactive protein (CRP)] can accelerate the process markedly. [9]

Atherogenesis and Inflammation as Pathogenic Mediators

Immunological and inflammatory mechanisms are active early in the atherosclerotic process. [9,10] Known long-term risk factors for human stroke (e.g. arterial hypertension, hyperlipidemia, diabetes mellitus, obesity, smoking, etc.) act also stimulating inflammatory cells to release markers of inflammation. [5,11-13] Early atherosclerosis is preceded by inflammatory cell deposition (e.g. macrophages, T lymphocytes) into the subendothelial layer of large cerebral arteries and its major branches and into the intima and media of small brain vessels. Inflammatory cell infiltrates clearly lodge within vascular walls of human arteries. Most atherothrombotic strokes result also from a fracture in the protective fibrous cap of the plaque on carotid arteries. Ample evidence now supports the concept that the protective fibrous cap, far from being fixed and static, actually can undergo continuous and dynamic remodeling and displays considerable metabolic activity. [14-17] Fibrils of interstitial collagen confer biomechanical strength on the fibrous cap. The balance between synthetic and degradative processes closely controlled by inflammatory mediators regulates the level of collagen in this structures. This ongoing process is reinforced by the progressive deposition of oxidized lipids in the subendothelial layers and can be stimulated by many means but infections, which has been detected in coronary, [18-21] carotid [22] and cerebral [23-25] arterial plaques. It appears to activate and accelerate the atherosclerotic process in larger arteries and contribute to maturation and instability of atherosclerotic plaques. However, well-controlled prospective data are lacking. [26] These plaques inevitably contain inflammatory cells and release proteases and procoagulant factors in response to further systemic stimuli. [5,11-13] These factors include clotting factors and fibrinogen, which can trigger plaque rupture and thromboembolism.

The actual mechanism that leads to plaque rupture and thromboembolism is not completely understood. Proinflammatory cytokines induce the expression of enzymes capable of breaking down constituents of the arterial extracellular matrix. In particular, matrix metalloproteinases (MMPs), including interstitial collagenases and gelatinases, can degrade the collagen fibrils that lend strength to the plaque's fibrous cap. [27-29] Inflammatory stimuli such as cytokines and *fas* ligand, factors overexpressed in atherosclerotic plaques, can trigger the complex mechanisms of apoptosis in both smooth muscle cells and endothelia cells reducing the integrity of the fibrous cap and uncovering the thrombogenic subendothelial matrix. [30-32] Endothelial cells can also express proteinases regulated by inflammatory cytokines and oxidized lipoproteins. [33] Activation of proteases in response to inflammatory stimuli can sever the tethers that hold the endothelial cell to its underlying matrix, promoting desquamative injury to the intima, a possible prelude to local thrombosis resulting from superficial erosion.

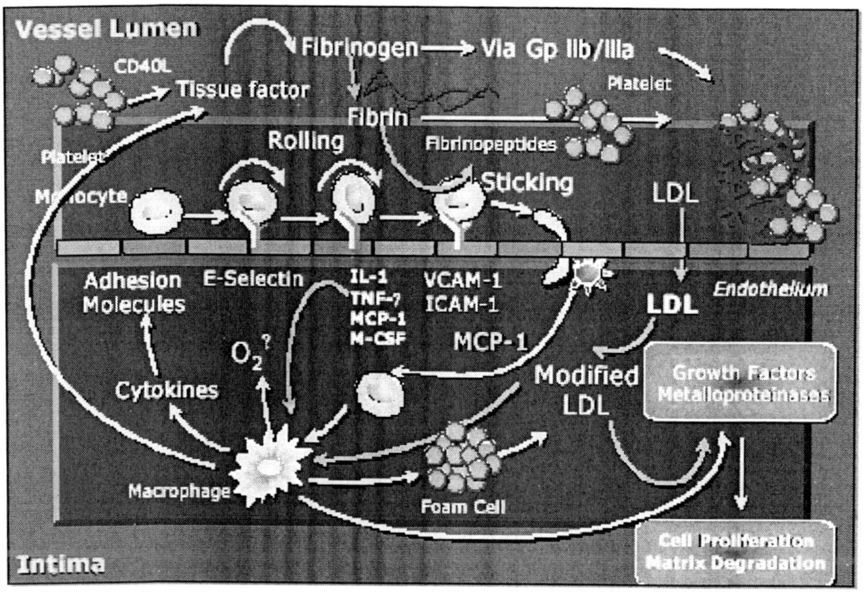

Figure 1. The central role of inflammation as a determinant of the biology underlying the acute thrombotic complications of atherosclerosis. The figure depicts the current complex understanding of the interelationship between inflammation and thrombogenicity. See text for details.

Inflammation may play a role possibly through stimulating activation of the coagulation/fibrinolysis system and stimulating platelet function from a superficial erosion of the intima without a frank rupture through the plaque fibrous cap. Endothelial cells express tissue factor procoagulant in response to inflammatory mediators and bacterial products such as endotoxin. [34] The fibrinolytic pathway also fluctuates, depending on the inflammatory status. [35-37] For example, increases in CRP have been associated with increased thrombin-antithrombin complex concentrations in acute thrombotic stroke patients. [38-40] Activated generation of thrombin, which acts as the terminal enzyme of the coagulation cascade, stimulates platelet release and aggregation. Platelets may further activate the coagulation system through coagulant proteins such as fibrinogen, factors V, VIII, IX, and XIII, and plasminogen activator inhibitor 1 (PAI-1). [35,41-43] The expression of PAI-1 can vary in the presence of inflammatory mediators. [44-47] CRP itself can also directly induce complement activation, thereby contributing to inflammation and thromboembolism in cerebral vessels and brain injury. [48,49] The CRP concentration might be related to the composition of the carotid atherosclerotic plaque, such that higher CRP is associated with a more active or unstable plaque, with greater propensity to stroke. Therefore, CRP-associated stroke risk is more significant when there is greater measurable plaque burden that is subject to rupture. [15,50,51] Potential biological activities of CRP within plaques, such as complement activation, induction of leukocyte chemotaxis and adhesion molecules, opsonization of LDL, and induction of monocyte tissue factor production, add support to these hypotheses. [48,49]

Endothelial cells in atherosclerotic arteries show impaired vasodilator function. [52] This may result in part from decreased production of nitric oxide (NO). [53] Also, augmented release of superoxide anion ($O_2^{\bullet -}$) may annihilate NO radical, neutralizing its vasodilator capacity. [54] In addition to producing vasodilatation, NO can impair platelet aggregation. NO also has a direct anti-inflammatory effect, augmenting production of the inhibitor of nuclear factor kappa B (NF-κB), a transcription factor involved in the expression of the genes encoding many proinflammatory functions of vascular wall cells and infiltrating leukocytes. [55-57] These various findings all highlight the central role of inflammation as a determinant of the biology underlying the acute thrombotic complications of atherosclerosis (**Figure 1**).

The Inflammatory Response in the Brain: Neuroinflammation in Cerebral Ischemia

The disruption of blood flow to a portion of the brain unleashes an ischemic cascade, leading to the death of neurons and cerebral infarction (**Figure 2**). Within minutes of a stroke, the zone of initial cell death (necrosis) is surrounded by additional damaged and dying brain cells (apoptosis). This process can continue for hours, leading to brain damage, perhaps irreversible. [57-61] Numerous studies indicate that local inflammatory response plays an important role in the pathogenesis of IS and delayed ischemic cell death. On the one hand the response is pointed toward the removal of damaged tissue from the ischemic area; while on the other hand it enlarges the ischemic area, and the severity of disease. [62-65]

Inflammatory Cells

Inflammation is characterized by an accumulation of inflammatory cells and mediators in the ischemic brain. Data have accumulated that have led to the notion that peripheral inflammatory cells play a prominent role in the pathogenesis of cerebral ischemia. This hypothesis was derived from pharmacological studies in animals, which led to several observations: (*i*) leukocytes are present in ischemic tissue after ischemia; [66-68] (*ii*) neutropenia is associated with reduced ischemic damage; [69-71] (*iii*) treatments that prevent leukocyte vascular adhesion and extravasation into the brain parenchyma, eg, using anti-intercellular adhesion molecule (ICAM)-1 [72,73] and anti-CD11/CD18 antibodies, can be neuroprotective; [29,72-76] and (*iv*) studies using ICAM-1 knockout animals have

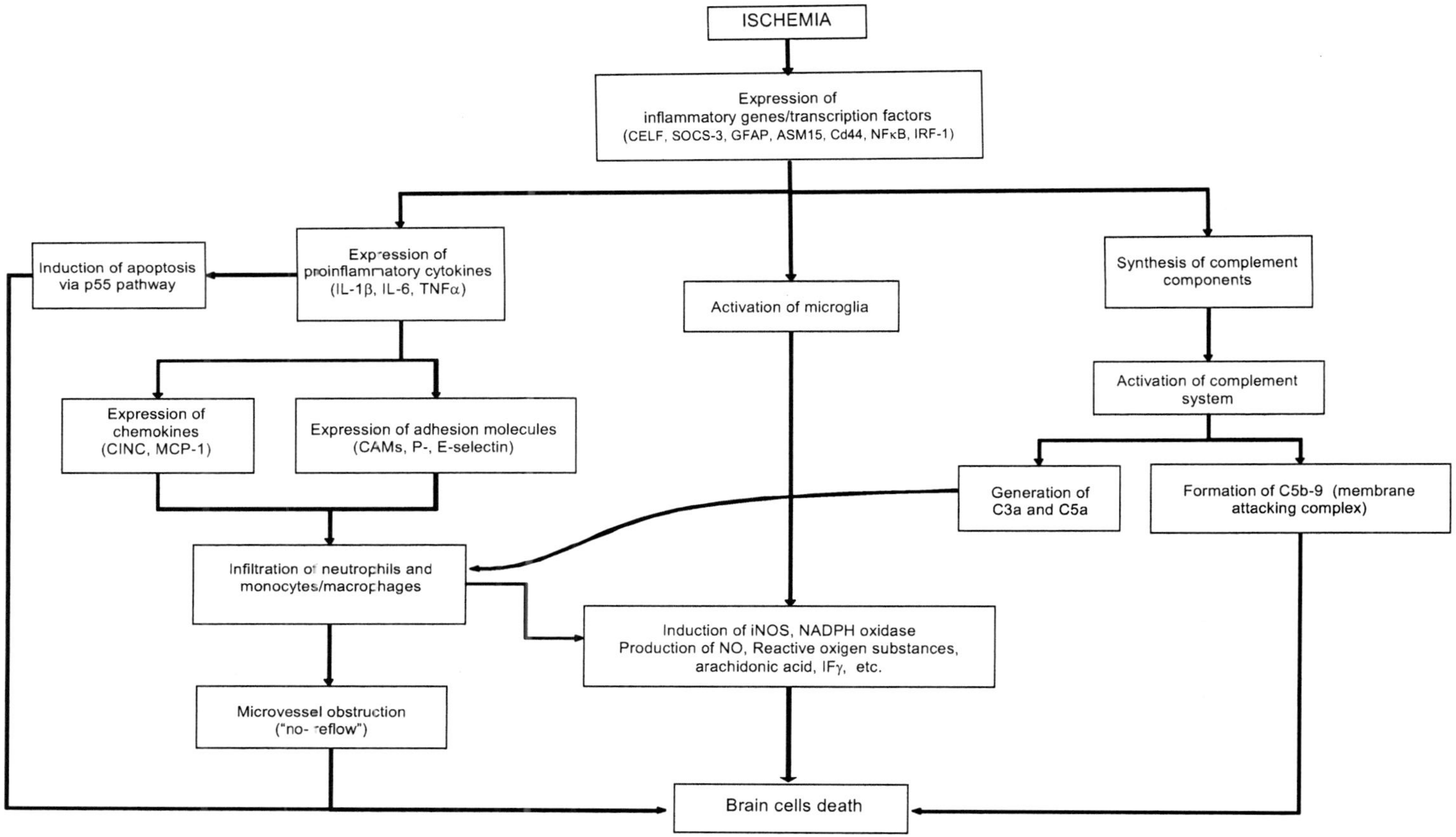

Figure 2. Development of local inflammatory response in brain after cerebral ischemia. The figure summarizes the possible mechanisms of development and interaction between cellular and humoral inflammatory mediators as well as their role in ischemic cell death.

demonstrated significant reduction in ischemic infarct size, relative to that of wild-type animals. [77-79] Both models of permanent and transient focal ischemia are characterized by massive infiltration of hematogenous immunocompetent cells. Despite this similarity in general, the temporal profiles of this process are quite different. After permanent middle cerebral artery occlusion (MCAo), neutrophils start to accumulate in vessels within few hours and infiltrate into the infarct zone after 12 hours. This process peak at 24 hours and then number of neutrophils significantly decrease. [80,81]

Monocytes/macrophages start to infiltrate the parenchyma at 12 hours and further increase in numbers up to day 14. [82,83] The entire infarct area is covered by macrophages at 3 days after MCAo. [83] In transient MCAo these processes seem to evolve more rapidly than after permanent MCAo. Despite the same temporal profile of neutrophil accumulation in the vessels, significant infiltration in parenchyma appears within 6 hours. [84,85] Accumulation of monocytes is observed during first 7 days and their number is already decreased after 14 days. [86] The accumulation of the neutrophils can lead to obstruction of microvessels (*no-reflow* phenomenon) and exacerbate the area of ischemia. [87] This was proven by observations that blocking neutrophil accumulation after transient MCAo significantly reduced infarct size, [87,88] but was ineffective after permanent MCAo. [72,86,89] Blood-derived macrophages and activated microglial cells are able to contribute the post-ischemic brain damage by expressing iNOS, production cytotoxic agents, free radicals. [90] Accumulation and infiltration of hematogenous cells in brain is complex process that requires the interaction between several cell adhesion molecules and chemokines. Number of animal studies showed that after transient or permanent focal ischemia the up-regulation of adhesion molecules, especially ICAM-1, P- and E-selectin, preceded the invasion of neutrophils into brain. [73,91,92] Also, it has been shown that treatment with anti-ICAM antibodies significantly reduced the infarct size after transient MCAo. [87,88] This process is accompanied by expression of chemokines at the site of damage. After MCAo the levels of cytokine-induced neutrophil chemoattractant (CINC) mRNA elevated after 6 hours, this process peaks at 12 hours and rapidly decreases at 24 hours. [93,94] It is known that CINC acting mainly as neutrophil chemoattractant. [93,94] The temporal expression of Monocyte Chemoattractant Protein-1 (MCP-1) follows that of CINC. [95] High levels of MCP-1 mRNA have been found at 6 hours. The maximal expression of this chemokine is observed between 12 hours and 2 days. [96,97]

Microglia/Macrophages

Resident brain cells are also involved in the inflammatory response. It is known that microglial cells respond to any pathological event in the brain, and after activation they become undistinguishable from blood derived macrophages. The study performed by Schroeter et al. [83] has shown that at the initial days after photochemically induced ischemia macrophages in the brain was mainly derived from microglial cells. Macrophages in ischemic brain lesions derive from distinct sources, including perivascular monocytes, infiltrating macrophages derived from blood monocytes, and parenchymal microglial cells. As a major glial component of the CNS, microglia plays a critical role as resident immunocompetent and phagocytic cells in the CNS, [98] and serve as scavenger cells in the event of infection, inflammation, trauma, ischemia and neurodegeneration in the CNS. [98] Upon activation as part of the inflammatory response, microglia are transformed into phagocytes, which are capable of releasing potentially cytotoxic substances such as oxygen radicals, NO, proteases and cytokines, [99] including interleukin (IL)-1, IL-6 and tumor necrosis factor-α (TNFα). [100-102] Following the formation of ischemic brain lesions, endogenous stimulators activate monocytic cells via CD14, a receptor that mediates inflammatory events. [103,104]

Cytokines

Cytokines are upregulated in the brain after a variety of insults, including stroke. As well as being expressed by cells of the immune system, cytokines are also endogenously produced by resident brain cells, including glia and neurons. Cytokines possess both pro- and anti-inflammatory properties, both of which play a role in the progression of stroke. [105-109] Cytokines and their receptors are responsible for initiation and regulation of the inflammatory response and play an important role in leukocyte and monocyte/macrophage infiltration into ischemic regions. The main interest is represented by IL-1β, IL-6, TNFα, MCP-1, and CINC. The last two belong to a superfamily of structurally related small, inducible, secreted, pro-inflammatory cytokines, named chemokines. MCP-1 and CINC-1, potent chemoattractant factors, function as inflammatory mediators and have been implicated in many inflammatory and autoimmune diseases.

IL-1

The IL-1 family comprises the agonistic isoforms IL-1α and IL-1β, and their endogenous inhibitor, the IL-1 receptor antagonist (IL-1ra). [110] The expression of IL-1β mRNA is observed rapidly within 15 min after permanent MCAo and remained persistent up to 4 days. [102,111] The same temporal profile of expression observed for its corresponding receptor, IL-1r. [100] The important role of IL-1β in pathomechanisms of brain injury after stroke is documented by observation that treatment with natural IL-1ra decreases the neuronal cell death in peri-infarct zone and reduces infarct size after permanent focal cerebral ischemia. [112,113] Furthermore, transgenic mice overexpressing IL-1ra showed reduced infarct size after focal ischemia. [114]

TNFα

The expression of TNFα was documented after experimentally induced stroke. [115,116] The initial source of TNFα within the brain appears to be the microglia and macrophages, although it is also found in ischemic neurons. [116-118] TNFα mRNA is upregulated within 20 min after permanent MCAo and is persistent until day 5. [119] The overexpression of TNFα receptors p55 and p75 is observed after 6 and 12 hours respectively. [120] Many reports indicate that TNFα potentiates ischemic injury, however, in some settings it may also be beneficial. Intracerebral administration of TNFα 24 hours before MCAo significantly enlarges lesion size and there is an evidence that infarct size can be reduces with use of anti-TNFα antibodies, [116,117] while, it has been demonstrated that *in vitro* this cytokine shows protective effect on neurons if added before induction of ischemia. [121]

IL-6

IL-6 belongs to a family of factors that includes ciliary neurotrophic factor, leukemia inhibitory factor, oncostatin, IL-11 and cardiotrophin-1. IL-6 mRNA and bioactivity are induced rapidly in experimental focal cerebral ischemia. Elevated levels of IL-6 in CSF of acute stroke patients correlate with infarct volume and with a poorer clinical outcome. [105] The expression of IL-6 mRNA is observed at 3 hours after permanent focal ischemia and peaks at 12 hours [122] The role of IL-6 in stroke, however, is far from clear because multiple regulatory levels are apparent. [125] In one hand, IL-6 regulates synthesis and expression of number acute-phase reactants (CRP, fibrinogen, etc.) [126] in other, IL-6 possess antiinflammatory effects and shown to be protective both *in vitro* and *in vivo*. [124]

Furthermore, IL-6 and TNFα are responsible for activation of iNOS, an enzyme participating in formation of NO, and COX-2, free radical producing enzyme. [127] Another important pathway of exacerbating brain damage induced by IL-6 and TNFα is apoptosis of neuronal and glial cells. It is known that TNFα is an activator of the apoptosis at various target cells via its p55 receptor, which is shown to be overexpressed in ischemic lesions. [31,128,129]

IL-10

IL-10 is an anti-inflammatory cytokine that inhibits both IL-1β and TNFα. [130] It reduces injury from experimentally induced stroke, ICH and in IS. [108,130,131] IL-10 regulates a variety of signaling pathways and promotes neuronal and glial cell survival by blocking the effects of pro-apoptotic cytokines, as well as promoting expression of cell-survival signals. IL-10 also limits inflammation in the brain by suppressing cytokine receptor expression and inhibiting receptor activation. [130-132]

Chemokines

Chemokines are a family of over 40 cytokines that are involved in chemotaxis and include both ligands and receptors. [133] Chemokines mediate both leukocyte migration and microglial activation, and are extensively expressed after cerebral ischemia. [118,133-135] IL-8 (neutrophil activation peptide) is thought to contribute to tissue damage by preventing neutrophil infiltration, and an anti-IL-8 antibody significantly reduced brain edema and infarct size. [133,135] IL-6 and TNFα regulate the expression of MCP-1 and CINC in the brain. [108,133] The increased expression of MCP-1 and CINC was observed in experimental stroke models where infiltrated leukocytes were supposed to induce tissue injury. Animal and cell culture studies have shown that MCP-1 and CINC may play an important role in ischemia-induced inflammatory response and in ischemic brain damage. These studies indicated that MCP-1 in cerebral ischemia actually plays a significant role in the migration of macrophages into the lesion, and CINC precedes neutrophil accumulation. In MCAo the level of CINC mRNA increased after 6 hours, this process peaked at 12 hours and rapidly decreased at 24 hours. [93] It is known that CINC is acting mainly as neutrophil chemoattractant. [94] The temporal expression of MCP-1 follows that of CINC. High levels of MCP-1 mRNA have been found at 6 hours. The maximal expression of this chemokine was observed between 12 hours and 2 days. [96,97] The differential temporal production of MCP-1 and CINC contributes to the regulation of infiltrated white blood cells (WBC) subtypes and the inhibition of MCP-1 and CINC signaling could be a new acute treatment approach to limit infarct size after stroke. [93,96,97,136-139]

The Complement System

The complement system is one of major systems in innate immunity: it consists of more than 20 circulating proteins and a similar number of cell-surface receptor and regulator proteins. The activation of complement by the classical, alternative or lectin pathways generates opsonins, inflammatory mediators and cytolytic protein complexes. [140,141] It provides a first line of defense against infection, and so is a major component of innate immunity. However, undesirable complement activation contributes to the pathology of many human diseases by damaging tissue and promoting inflammation. Activation of complement by the classical, alternative, and the lectin pathways generates opsonins, inflammatory mediators and cytolytic protein complexes that play an essential role in tissue damage. Complement plays a critical role in several stages of the processing of immune complexes. Incorporation of complement proteins into immune complexes modifies the lattice structure. Covalently incorporated cleavage products of complement proteins C3 and C4 then influence the fate of immune complexes by acting as ligands, firstly, for receptors on cells that transport immune complexes through the body and, secondly, for receptors on cells that take up and process circulanting immune complexes (CIC). [140,141]

The overlap of the complement cascade with other biochemical events occurring in stroke is quite complex and is only beginning to be understood. In the animal and cell culture models of stroke it has been shown that complement plays a key role in stroke outcome, and complement depletion improves neurological function after cerebral ischemia. [142-145] However, very little attention has been paid to the activation of the complement system in stroke patients, particularly on brain level. There is only one report on this issue related to human studies, where using postmortem brain slices of patients with acute IS it was shown a deposition of complement membrane attack complex C5b-C9 in infarction zone. [146]

Adhesion Molecules

Leukocytes adhere to the endothelium prior to tissue infiltration via a series of carefully orchestrated steps. [73,91,92] Accumulation and infiltration of the brain by WBC is a complex process that requires the interaction between several cell adhesion molecules and chemokines. Leukocytes roll on the endothelial surface and then adhere to the endothelial cells, which is followed by diapedesis. Three families of leukocyte endothelial adhesion molecules have been identified: the selectins, the immunoglobulin gene superfamily and the integrins. The rolling of leukocytes is mediated by interaction of E- and P-selectin (found on the surface of endothelial cells), and L-selectin (normally found on the surface of leukocytes) with their respective ligands. Firm adhesion and activation of leukocytes is mediated by binding of the CD11/CD18 complex to receptors of the immunoglobulin gene superfamily, such as ICAM-1 and -2, vascular cell adhesion molecule-1 (VCAM-1), platelet-endothelial cell adhesion molecule-1 and the mucosal addressin. Leukocyte integrins [including CD11 (α-chain), CD18 (β2 chain) and CD29 (β1 chain)] are activated by chemokines, chemoattractants and cytokines. Once leukocyte rolling has stopped, an interaction between CD11/CD18 and ICAM-1 causes the leukocytes to shed L-selectin and transmigrate across the vessels to the abluminal side of the target tissue. IL-6 and TNFα also regulates the expression of cell adhesion molecules on the endothelial cells and induce infiltration of the brain by WBC in the site of inflammation. [147,148] Number of animal studies have documented that after transient or permanent focal ischemia the up-regulation of adhesion molecules, especially ICAM-1, P- and E-selectin, preceded the invasion of neutrophils into brain. [[73,91,92] There is ample evidence from animal models of MCAo that expression of CAMs is associated with cerebral infarct size. Thus, absence of CAMs in knockout animals resulted in reduced infarct size. When MCAo in experimental stroke was followed by reperfusion, administration of anti-CAM antibodies decreased infarct size. Thus far, anti-CAM treatment has not been successful in patients with IS. Inflammatory CAM may also play a role in the pathogenesis of delayed cerebral ischemia after SAH. In animal models, increased expression of CAMs has been observed in vasospastic arteries. [87,88,149]

Inflammatory Mediators Generated by Leukocytes and Microglia

Once activated, peripheral inflammatory cells and resident microglia are capable of generating a variety of potentially toxic substances leading to secondary brain injury. These toxic substances include the products of enzyme systems that generate reactive oxygen and nitrogen species, which damage tissues by disrupting cell membranes, altering DNA and activating other oxidant-inducible systems.

Inducible Nitric Oxide Synthase (NOS)

Inducible NOS (iNOS) is not normally found in most cells, however, its expression is induced during development and in pathological states, particularly those associated with inflammation. After an ischemic episode, iNOS is induced almost exclusively in inflammatory cells, including neutrophils infiltrating the injured brain, cerebral blood vessels and activated microglia. [2,150-153] Through conversion of L-arginine, iNOS can generate toxic levels of NO, which may contribute to inflammation-induced cytotoxicity. The mechanisms by which NO exerts its cytotoxic effects include inhibition of ATP-producing enzymes, DNA damage and oxidative damage caused by peroxynitrite. [154] In contrast to neuronal NOS, which generates NO in the early stages of ischemia onset, iNOS appears somewhat later in inflammatory cells. [2,127,155] Consistent with the notion that NO generated in inflammatory cells causes tissue damage, iNOS-null mice have smaller infarcts and improved neurological outcome compared with wild-type littermates, and treatment with antisense oligodeoxynucleotides to iNOS protected against ischemia-induced brain injury. [127]

NADPH Oxidase

Massive increases in oxygen levels during reperfusion result in the overproduction of oxygen free radicals and lead to tissue damage. Such free radicals are generated by a variety of enzyme systems in different cell types. However, one of the major sources of $O_2^{\bullet -}$ is NADPH oxidase, which has been localized to inflammatory cells. [156,157] The essential components of NADPH oxidase include p47phox, p67phox and cytochrome b558 (which consists of two subunits, p22phox and gp91phox). [156] Mice lacking functional NADPH oxidase are significantly protected after cerebral ischemia. [158] Preventing the generation of reactive species by inflammatory cells may therefore be an important therapeutic endpoint for stroke. This may not only limit the extent of ischemic injury, but might also preserve the BBB and prevent edema and ICH.

Intracellular Regulators of Inflammation

Cerebral ischemia also stimulates pathways that produce significant changes in gene expression and enzyme activation, thereby contributing to brain inflammation. Various transcription factors have now been studied in cerebral ischemic models.

Early Gene Expression

Inflammatory/immune reactions are developed as early as in a few hours after the onset of stroke. This is initiating by ischemia-reperfusion induced different transformations occurred in the organism at cellular, molecular and metabolic levels. Ischemia associated hypoxia, Ca^{2+}- activation of metabolic reactions, and increase in free radicals level may stimulate an expression of several genes responsible for initiation of the immune response in ischemia. [159-162] It has been shown the activation of specific genes within hours to days after a stroke, leading to the formation of immune response related factors. [62,64,65,138,163-165] Of the genes induced 24 h after ischemia approximately half were unique for stroke condition. A significant component of the response involves immune-process related genes likely to represent responses to dying neurons, glia and vessels in ischemia. These genes, which are usually induced by all injury conditions, included but were not limited to: CELF, SOCS-3, GFAP, ASM15, CD44, immediate-early serum-responsive JE, Hsp27, heme oxygenase (Hsp32), α_2-globulin-related protein, and TIMP-1. [166] It was also demonstrated that the mRNA encoding for the transcription factor interferon regulatory factor 1 (IRF-1) is markedly upregulated after focal cerebral ischemia. It was shown that IRF-12/2 mice are substantially protected from the brain damage and neurological deficits produced by MCAo. The protection develops 2–3 day after induction of ischemia. The findings suggest that IRF-1–inducible genes contribute to the late stages of tissue damage after cerebral ischemia. IRF-1 is a critical transcription factor in the molecular mechanisms of ischemic brain injury and, as such, might be a target for therapeutic interventions in IS. [167]

Nuclear Factor-κB

The NF-κB appears to be a major mediator of the brain's response to ischemia and reperfusion, playing a complicated set of roles in the pathogenesis of stroke. [56,57,168-170] NF-κB is a key regulator of the inflammatory cascade and many inflammatory mediators such as inflammatory cytokines, adhesion molecules and iNOS have NF-κB binding sequences in their promoters. [165,171] NF-κB is activated by a number of factors that are present in focal ischemia, including activated glutamate receptors, reactive oxygen species, TNFα and IL-1β. [55,57,161,172-175] NF-κB regulates the expression of many genes that encode proteins involved in immunity, inflammation, oxidative damage and apoptosis, [174] and has several different targets and effects in various cell types and tissues, which can appear paradoxical. [55,57,161,172-175] In some studies, preventing NF-κB activation was shown to be protective, whereas in other studies, activation of NF-κB enhanced neuronal survival. [56] These conflicting results may be due to the fact that NF-κB can upregulate both proinflammatory and pro-survival factors and act in a different manner in cellular types. [56]

MAPK

MAPK is one of the most important kinase families in inflammatory cells, [176] which comprises four subfamilies: (*i*) extracellular signal-regulated kinases (ERK)1/2 (or p44/42 MAPK); (*ii*) c-jun *N*-terminal kinases (JNKs) or stress activated protein kinases (SAPKs); (*iii*) ERK5/big MAP kinase 1 (BMK1); and (*iv*) p38 MAPK. The p38 and p44/42 MAPKs most likely play a significant role in initiating and sustaining the inflammatory reaction in the brain. Of the MAPKs, p38 is of particular interest with regard to the inflammatory cascade.

The levels of activated p38 increased in microglial cells in experimental models of ischemia. [176,177] Like NF-κB, p38 is also activated by, and induces the expression of many inflammatory mediators. [176,177]

The Systemic Inflammatory Response

In addition to the development of the local inflammatory processes in the brain, stroke evokes an immune response at the systemic level (Figure 3). The systemic inflammatory response is a well-known phenomenon in various types of insults, infectious and non infectious and it is called Systemic Inflammatory Response Syndrome (SIRS). SIRS includes at least two of the following parameters: (*i*) body temperature of >38°C or <36°C ; (*ii*) heart rate of >90 beats/min ; (*iii*) tachypnea, as manifested by respiratory rate of >20 breaths/min or hyperventilation, as indicated by $paCO_2$ of <32 torr (<4.3kPa); (*iv*) WBC count >12,000/mm^3, <4,000/mm^3 , or the presence of >10% immature neutrophils ("bands"). [178,179] SIRS is evident in both ischemic [39,132,180-182] and hemorrhagic stroke. [183-185]

One among the systemic markers of the SIRS during ischemia is an increased total blood WBC count, which is observed during IS. [186,187] Furthermore, the patterns of increase of neutrophil and monocyte counts correspond to temporal patterns of infiltration and accumulation of these cells in damaged brain area. The latter observation suggests that the WBC count increases in response to inflammatory stimuli in ischemic area in the brain. An increased total WBC count within the first 12 hours of stroke is an independent and strong risk factor for mortality, no neurological improvement, and the need for prolonged hospitalization in the course of acute IS. [186,187] Kostulas *et al.* evaluated numbers of peripheral blood mononuclear cells (PBMC) expressing mRNA for IL-1β, IL-8, and IL-17 and macrophage inflammatory protein-1a (MIP-1a) after IS. [188] This longitudinal study revealed systemic increases of levels of IL-1β, IL-8, and IL-17 that correlated with Scandinavian Stroke Scale scores. [188] Based upon the assessment of the plasma levels of IL-8 in patients on days 1, 3 and 7 after IS it was proposed that elevated IL-8 may contribute to stroke pathophysiology by activating polymorphonuclear leukocyte early after ischemia. [189] Another marker of the immune system activation during ischemia on the systemic level is an increased concentration of CIC in the blood. [190] Significantly, elevated CIC levels within 24 hours and at days 7 and 30 after IS onset are associated with worsening of neurological status and 30-day fatality. [25] CIC can induce severe lesions by the formation of immune complex deposits, which lead to vascular inflammation and pathological tissue injury. CIC may interact with both humoral and cellular immune recognition systems, activate complement cascade and finally significantly affect the development of inflammatory immune response in stroke. [191,192] High levels of CIC in cerebral ischemia may also reflect BBB leakage and the development of autoimmune reactions targeted at brain specific antigens released in circulation from the ischemic brain. [193-197]

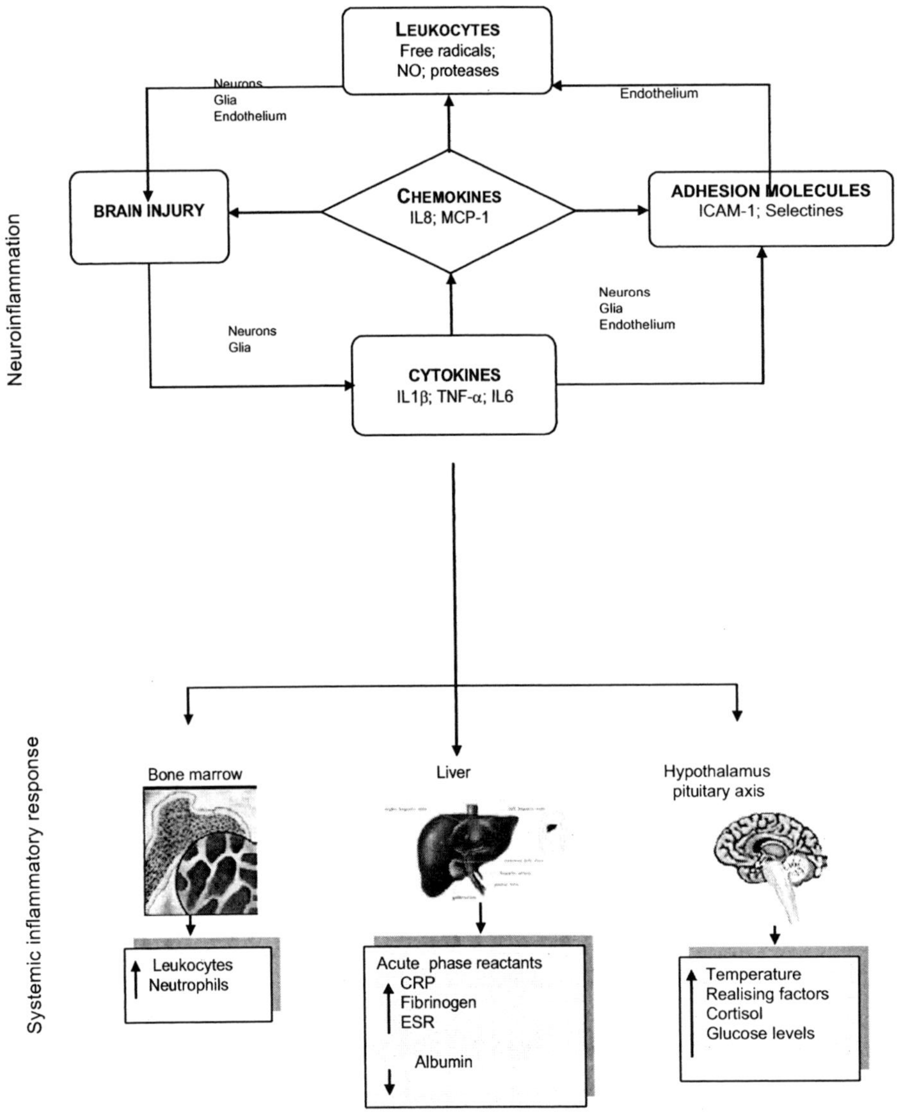

Figure 3. Neuroinflammation and systemic inflammatory response. The figure depicts the known reverberating pathways and feed-back loops acting in neuroinflammation and in the systemic inflammatory response. See text for details.

The Acute-Phase Reactants

Classic acute-phase reactants and body temperature are modified in stroke, and may be useful in the prediction of events, outcome, and as therapeutic targets. [99] However, the relationship between peripheral inflammatory markers and outcome in stroke patients remains poorly understood such as the relationship between peripheral mediators and CNS events is uncertain. [198] Peripheral infection, which commonly precedes or complicates stroke, [199] is also a major stimulus for production of cytokines and an acute phase response. Although most cytokines are only present at biologically effective concentrations at the site of inflammation, IL-6 is a major circulating cytokine produced in response to inflammatory insult and infection, and is a potent stimulus for production of hepatic acute phase proteins, [200] induction of fever, [201] and activation of the hypothalamic pituitary-adrenal (HPA) axis. [106] The increased levels of IL-6, TNFα [105,202] and other markers of the acute phase response [203-210] in the blood of patient with IS were observed in a number of studies. It was also shown that IL-6 secretion can be triggered by sympathetic neurons. [211] Peak plasma IL-6 and other peripheral markers of inflammation in the first week of IS correlate with brain infarct volume, stroke severity and long-term outcome. Thus, in patients with acute IS, some studies have reported an association between circulating IL-6 concentration and brain infarct volume, stroke severity, or outcome up to 6 months. [105.107-109.125] Conversely, other studies have reported no association between serum IL-6 concentration and infarct volume or stroke severity at 3 months. [212,213] Recently, Smith *et al.* reported that peak plasma IL-6 concentration in the first week of IS correlated significantly with computer tomography (CT) brain infarct volume at 5 to 7 days, and clinical outcome at 3 months. [214] Secondary analyses also demonstrated strong associations between peak plasma IL-6 and stroke severity, clinical outcome, or mortality at 12 months. In keeping with these findings, other peripheral markers of inflammation, including CRP, serum amyloid A (SAA), WBC count, erythrocyte sedimentation rate (ESR) or plasma cortisol concentration, were associated with severity of stroke, CT brain infarct volume and clinical outcome. [214]

Serum Amyloid A (Saa)

SAA is an acute phase protein complexed to high-density lipoproteins (HDL) as an apoprotein (apo SAA). [215] It is mainly found in HDL_3 fraction, but small amounts can be found in other HDL fractions as well as in low-density lipoproteins (LDL) and very low-density lipoproteins (VLDL). SAA is an impressive of acute-phase proteins, increasing within 24 h by up to 1000-fold, and resulting in displacement of apo A-I, apo A-II and apo A-III proteins from the HDL complex. Six major isoforms of SAA can be extracted from the plasma HDL fraction of patients with inflammatory diseases. The molecular weight of SAA is 11.4-12.5 kDa and the protein has from 104 to 112 amino acids. [215] The function of SAA remains unclear. [215] SAA can influence lymphocytic responses to antigens, plays a role in cholesterol metabolism during the course of acute inflammation, induces the synthesis of collagenase and can inhibit fever induced by IL-1 or TNFα, can suppress thromboxin synthesis and platelet release of serotonin, and inhibit platelet aggregation and endothelial cell proliferation. [215] In IS, SAA levels are a sensitive indicator of clinical severity of IS and an early indicator of possible infectious complications. [216]

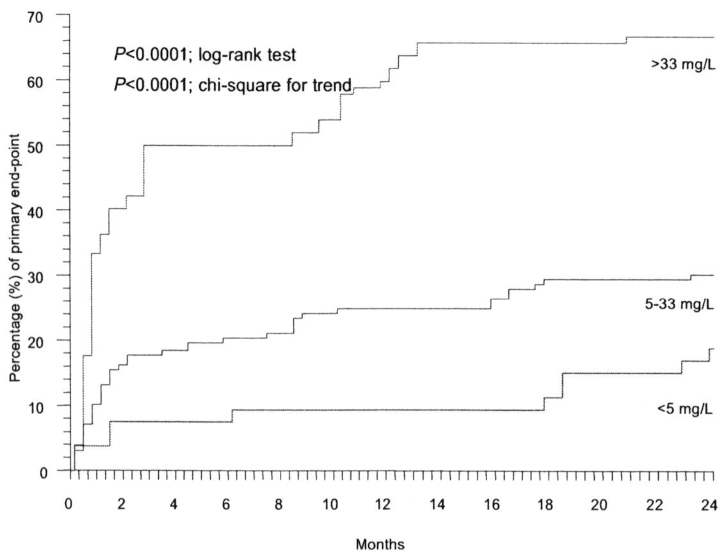

Figure 4. Two-year cumulative probability of fatal or non-fatal cardiovascular events in first-ever ischemic stroke patients according to C-reactive protein levels within 24 hours after stroke onset. Data are shown using tertile cut-points derived from an Italian stroke patients cohort. Adapted from reference 36.

C-Reactive Protein (CRP)

CRP is an indicator of underlying systemic inflammation. CRP together with serum amyloid P protein (SAP), is a member of the family of proteins known as pentraxins. [217] CRP is a ubiquitous protein found in both vertebrates and invertebrates phylogenetically spanning 400 million years of evolution. Originally CRP was defined as a substance, observed in the plasma of patients with acute infections, that reacted with the C polysaccharide of the pneumococcus. [218] It is one of the plasma proteins that are called acute phase reactants because of a pronounced rise in concentration after tissue injury or inflammation; in the case of CRP the rise may be 1000-fold or more. CRP is composed of 5 identical, 21,500-molecular weight subunits. It is detectable on the surface of about 4% of normal peripheral blood lymphocytes. Acute phase reactant CRP is produced in the liver; CRP detectable on lymphocytes is produced by those cells. [219] On the basis of *in vitro* and *in vivo* experiments, it has been proposed that the function of CRP is related to its ability to recognize specifically foreign pathogens and damaged cells of the host and to initiate their elimination by interacting with humoral and cellular effector systems in the blood. Thus, the CRP molecule has both a recognition and an effector function. [218] It has been proposed that one of its major physiologic functions is to act as a scavenger for chromatin released by dead cells during the acute inflammatory process. [220] CRP has a long plasma half-life and is now understood to be a mediator as well as a marker of cerebrovascular disease. [11]

Special attention is paid to the involvement of CRP in pathogenesis of stroke. The association of increased levels of CRP with IS has been reported by several studies. It has been shown that increased levels of CRP are associated with a worse outcome in patients with IS (Figure 4). [208-210] Increased levels of CRP are also associated with increased risk of future stroke in the elderly. [131,221] CRP role in pathogenesis of IS is not completely understood. It is not known whether CRP is just a marker of systemic inflammatory processes or directly involved in mechanisms of brain damage.

The Complement System

The data concerning the involvement of complement system in pathogenesis of IS at the systemic level is rare. However, the study performed by Di Napoli *et al.* [222] suggests that involvement of systemic complement activation is changeable between IS subtypes and mostly could be observed in cardioembolic stroke when comparing with atherothrombotic or lacunar strokes. In addition, in preliminary studies (Boyajyan A, 2004; unpublished results) classical (CCHA) and alternative pathway haemolytic activities (ACHA) of complement were determined in serum of patients with acute IS on days 1, 3, 5 and 7 after onset of stroke. On day 1, no significant changes were found in CCHA in patients compared to healthy subjects, but on day 3 CCHA significantly decreased. On day 5, CCHA increased and returned to normal on day 7. For ACHA no significant difference, compared to healthy subjects, was detected on days 1 and 3, whereas on days 5 and 7 ACHA significantly increased with maximum level on day 7. There was positive correlation between the CCHA and ACHA on days 1, 3, 5 and 7 after the onset of stroke. The results suggest that complement activation by both the classical and the alternative pathway could play an important role in the pathogenesis of IS. ACHA in acute IS may be increased via a compensation mechanism launched by a depletion of components of complement activation by the classical pathway.

The Inflammatory Response in Intracerebral Hemorrhage and Subarachnoid Hemorrhage

Less consistent data are present on the role of inflammatory response following hemorrhagic stroke. However, a consensus has emerged that inflammation plays also a decisive role in the pathophysiology of acute hemorrhagic events (Figure 5). A SIRS is evident in both patients with ICH and SAH and its development is predictive of outcome. [183,184,223] Inflammatory response occurs in and around blood clot and may participate in the absorption of the blood clot and the removal of injured cells and it is also involved in secondary injury following ICH participating to the secondary edema formation. [224] Several mechanisms interact with themselves acting as perpetuators. [185] In experimental models, inflammatory cells are activated within hours, caracterized by adherence of neutrophils to damaged brain endothelia and subsequent brain entry. [224] Macrophages follow neutrophils within hours to days with a peak at 48 hours, lymphocytes becomes apparent within 48 hours and persisted for 1 week while the activation of resident microglia and astrocytes is evident at 4 hours and persists for 4 weeks, accompanied by neuronal and glial death. [225,226] Inflammatory response is maximal at 48–72 hours following ICH and is associated with cells death for a period of at least 4 weeks. [225-227] Several evidences now supports the concept that proinflammatory cytokines induce the expression of enzymes capable of breaking down constituents of the extracellular matrix, apoptosis induction and neurotoxicity. In particular, Powers *et al.* examined MMPs expression in vivo using a collagenase induced rat model of ICH showing that ICH increased MMP-mRNA levels in the vicinity of the hematoma. [228]

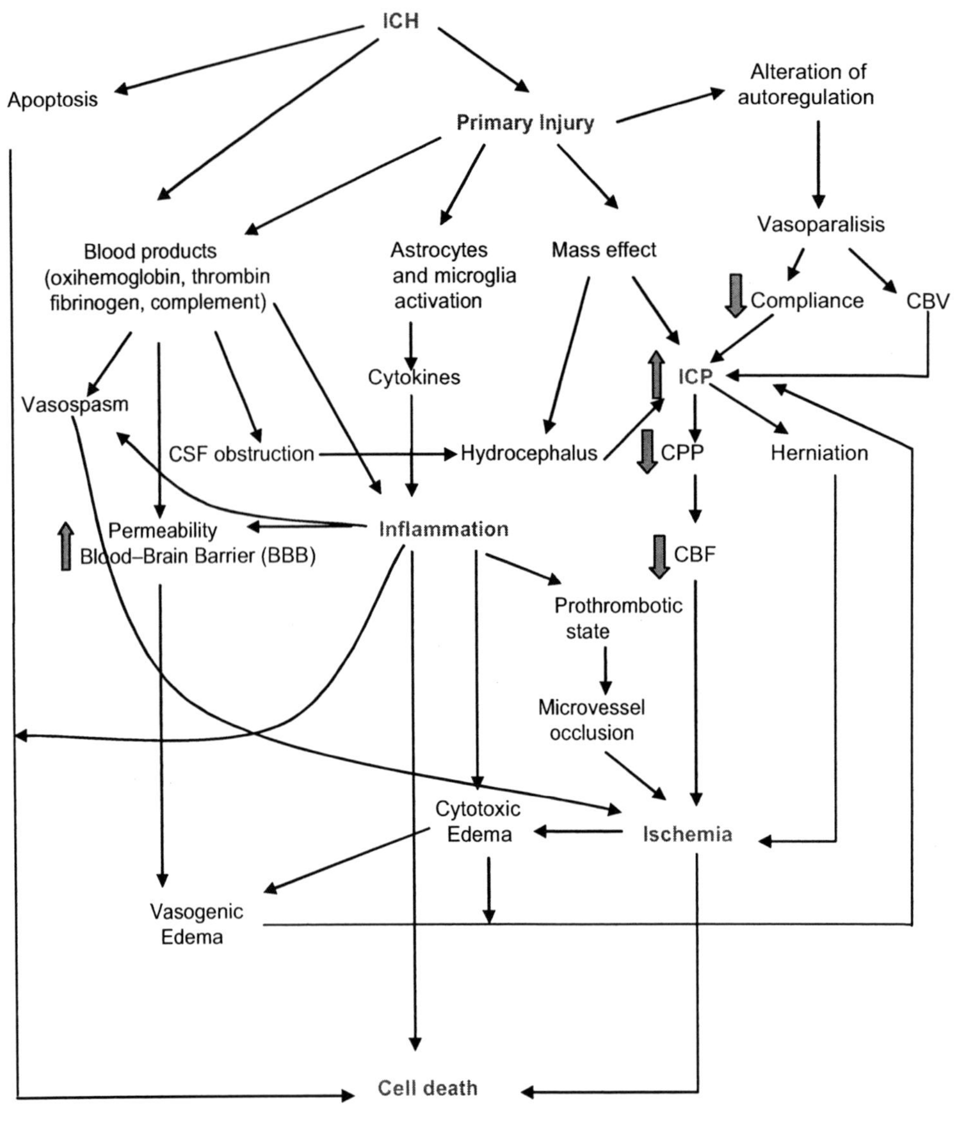

Figure 5. Development of local inflammatory response in brain after intracerebral hemorrhage (ICH). ICP indicates intracranial pressure, CBV cerebral blood volume, CPP cerebral pulse pressure, CBF cerebral blood flow, CSF cerebrospinal fluid.

Inflammation may also contribute to the mechanism of cerebral vasospam in SAH acting on endothelin-1 pathway. [229] Activated mononuclear leukocytes in the CSF of SAH patients synthesize and release endothelin-1 in parallel with known acute-phase reactants. [229]

Clinical Application of Inflammation Markers in Cerebrovascular Disease

Health education and preventive measures to improve health-related behavior by the entire population are fundamental aspects of prevention. Promotion of a healthy lifestyle will not only result in decreased stroke-related mortality and morbidity but also in a reduction in mortality and morbidity due to all cardiovascular (CVD) causes. Clinicians should focus on the identification and treatment of persons who are at increased stroke risk and therapeutic agents should be targeted to those individuals who would benefit most. Risk prediction at the individual level is still not satisfactory and the searching of predictive markers is surely of interest. In an attempt to improve global cerebrovascular risk prediction, considerable interest has focused on inflammatory markers. Several inflammatory markers are been identified. However, CRP has been shown a consistent positive association with incident stroke and CVD events in several prospective studies in initially healthy subjects, [131,221,230-234] in patients with acute IS [36,207-210,235-240] and in patients with severe atherosclerosis. [181,241-243]

These highly consistent clinical data are supported by abundant laboratory and experimental evidence that demonstrate that atherothrombosis also represents a chronic inflammatory process. [244] However, in order to lay the basis for a rational and speedy introduction of the measurement of this novel cerebrovascular risk indicator into routine clinical, it is useful to investigate on the reported predictive role of CRP in primary and secondary prevention, on the assessment of its normal blood levels and of its determinants, on the cost-effectiveness of its measurement, and finally on its possible direct cerebrovascular pathogenetic mechanisms and potential new pharmacological treatments.

Evidence Supporting C-Reactive Protein Use in Primary Prevention of Stroke

Studying the effect that a general inflammatory marker, such as CRP, has on cerebrovascular risk prediction is far from a simple task. Methodological problems are inherent in design, implementation, and analysis of any such study. Actually, on an epidemiological point of view, several prospective studies demonstrate that a single, non-fasting measure of CRP is a strong predictor of future fatal and not fatal cerebrovascular events (Figure 6). [131,221,230,232-234,243,245-248] The relationship between a patient's baseline level of CRP and future vascular risk has been consistent in different studies, and in most cases has proven independent of age, smoking, cholesterol levels, blood pressure, and diabetes, the major risk factors evaluated in daily practice. These effects are present among women, as well as men, among the elderly, as well as, those in middle age, among smokers and non-smokers, and among those with and without diabetes mellitus. Even after correction for these risk factors, high-normal CRP levels still predict an increased risk for development of a cerebrovascular event. The effect of CRP on vascular risk remained highly significant after adjustment for traditional risk factor typically used in global risk-assessment programs. [249] However, while we have abundant data bearing on relative risks, we know little or nothing about predictive values or absolute risk for cerebrovascular risk. [250] Thus, we do not know what the actual risk for cerebrovascular disease is in a given individual with modest CRP elevation. We do not know what the likelihood of a false positive result is, ie, how many individuals are incorrectly identified as being likely to develop cerebrovascular disease. We really need to know this, so that we can arrive at some sort of an estimate of cost--effectiveness, before undertaking large-scale screening or interventions.

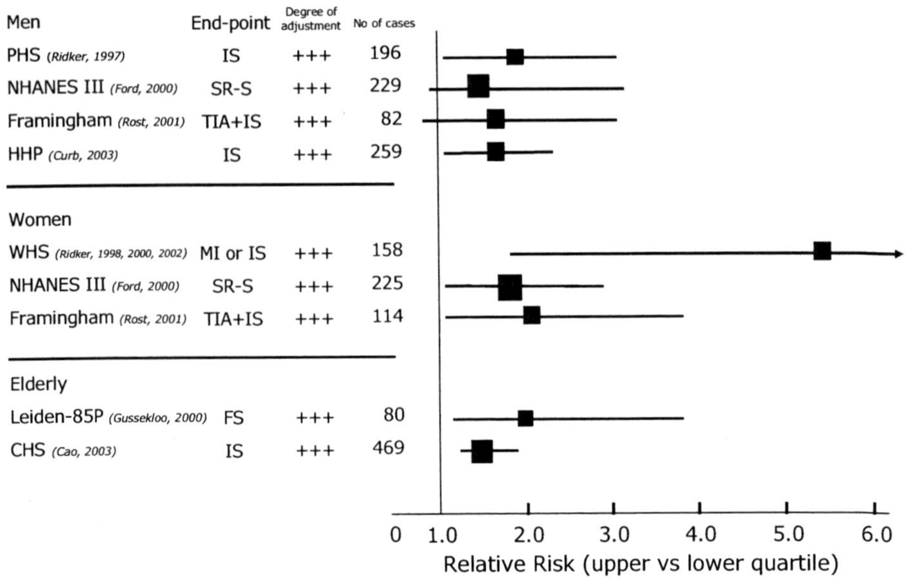

Figure 6. Prospective studies relating baseline C-reactive protein levels to the risk of first cerebrovascular event. Relative risk compare top and bottom quartile of baseline measurements. Black squares indicate the relative risk in each study, with the size of square proportional to number of cases. All studies adjusted for some other standard vascular risk factors. The key observation in all these studies is that the presence of a heightened inflammatory response as determined by a high level of CRP is consistently associated with increased cerebrovascular risk in several different population groups, both at low and at high absolute risk for these events. IS indicates ischemic stroke; SR-S, self-reported stroke; TIA, transient ischemic attack; MI, myocardial infarction; FS fatal stroke; PHS, Physicians' Health Study; NHANES III, 3rd National Health and Nutrition Examination Survey; Framingham, Framingham Heart Study; HHS, Honolulu Heart Study; WHS, Women's Health Study; Leiden-85P, Leiden Heart Study; and CHS, Cardiovascular Health Study.

Furthermore, high sensitivity (hs-) CRP assay is far from a perfect test. Quality control and the relevance of experimental design before ascribing pathophysiological functions, are also often ignored. It is critically important to recognize that the CRP response is nonspecific and is triggered by many disorders unrelated to CVD. Furthermore, the present torrent of studies of CRP in CVD and associated conditions is facilitated by the ready commercial availability of automated CRP assays and of CRP itself as a research reagent. The current enthusiasm over CRP in CVD is widely characterized by failure to recognize appropriately the nonspecific nature of the acute phase response, and by lack of critical biological judgment. Hardly a week passes without report of a new potential association between CRP values and some commonly encountered medical condition, physiologic state, vascular risk factor. Examples include cardiac arrhythmias, [251,252] renal insufficiency, [253,254] diabetes mellitus, [43,255-261] obstructive sleep apnea, [262,263] arterial hypertension, [264-266] obesity, [256,260,267-271] insulin resistance syndrome, [270,272] metabolic syndrome, [272-275] estrogen use, [276-278] frequent physical activity, [279-282] moderate alcohol consumption, [283-285] high protein diet, [269] and depressive symptoms. [286-288] In contrast, the positive association of CRP values with other classical CVD disease risk factors, such as periodontal disease [289-291] and smoking, [269,292] seems more clearly related to local non-arterial inflammation. CRP levels have also been shown to be influenced by genetic factors as well, [293-296] and modest CRP elevation may be a marker of biologic aging [297] and decline of cognitive function. [298,299]

Specificity of CRP for inflammation is clearly not infallible, with non inflammatory states. In addition to indicating that modest CRP elevation does not necessarily bespeak the existence of an inflammatory state, these data pose several problems: just how to intervene? If CRP elevation is due to a noninfectious inflammatory stimulus, which type of anti-inflammatory agent should we use? If, on the other hand, it is due to depression, ingestion of a high protein diet, aging, frequent physical activity, i.e., should we attempt to alter these states? If we understood the mechanisms responsible for the association between modest CRP elevation and future cerebrovascular events, we would know how to intervene when elevated CRP levels are found. At present, however, we do not know what those mechanisms are, neither precisely what to do. Given our current state of knowledge, intervention is even less possible, because this hypothesis should prove correct. The primary goal of stroke screening programs should be the identification of high-risk individuals who can be targeted for smoking cessation, diet, exercise, and blood pressure control. It is well established that compliance with lifestyle recommendations is directly related to the absolute risk perceived by individual patients. In particular, weight loss, diet, exercise, and smoking cessation all lead to both reduced CRP levels and reduced vascular risk. There is not direct evidence that lowering CRP levels will result in reduced risk of cerebrovascular events[11] and it is far from certain that effecting such changes would have a favorable effect on the pathogenesis of atherothrombotic events: [217,218,300] studies addressing this issue are only now being designed. However, many interventions known to reduce CVD risk have been linked to lower CRP levels.

Finally, in using CRP for assessment of cerebrovascular risk, it is also essential to clearly establish true high CRP values that are not distorted by either trivial or serious intercurrent pathologies. When measured with hs-assays, the population distribution of CRP has generally been consistent across sex and ethnic groups, and values of 0.3, 0.6, 1.5, 3.5, and 6.6 mg/L have been reported as estimates of the 10th, 25th, 50th, 75th, and 90th percentile cut-points for middle-aged Americans. [245] Similar results are also found in different European, North American and Japanese cohorts. [301-307] However, levels of CRP can fluctuate substantially from day to day. The within-subject variability in CRP levels in apparently healthy individuals is 4 to 6 times greater than that for cholesterol. The distribution of CRP in apparently healthy individuals is wide and skewed with interquartile values ranging between 150-250% of the median and an estimate of the composite coefficient of variation of ≈120%. [308-310] The CRP mean within-subject variability is of ≈30% for several group and period. [309] This means that it would not be unusual for a subsequent CRP measurement to be ≈60% higher or lower than the initial reading. Although it has suggested that CRP has the same degree of measurement stability as total cholesterol, [305,307,311,312] this conclusion was based on Ridker-Rifai quartile model: [311] classifying CRP into 4 arbitrarily defined categories, of unequal sizes, and cholesterol into quartiles of equal size. Approximately 60% of repeated measurements were found to fall into the same category for CRP or the same quartile for cholesterol. However, such an approach may be misleading because the results will depend greatly on which cutpoints are selected to define the 4 categories and on the relative sizes of the categories. In addition, the high degree of variability in CRP levels means that 2 measurements can be quite far apart and still be in the same quartile. In fact, the within-subject variability easily result from a wide variety of minor inflammatory stimuli but if this effect can be avoided in large observational population studies, in which such effects are diluted out by sheer numbers, this is not possible in a single patient, on a single date. Furthermore, analytical variation and assay imprecision can produce clinically significant variation in risk estimates that only multiple measurements may reduce. [312] At the same time, women taking HRT will have higher levels of CRP [234,306,313,314] and risk estimates for such women may need to be calibrated downward.

Several pharmacological agents proven to reduce vascular risk influencing CRP levels. Of these, the statin drugs are the most important, and studies with pravastatin, lovastatin, cerivastatin, simvastatin, and atorvastatin have all shown that, on average, median CRP levels decline 15% to 25% as early as 6 weeks after initiation of therapy. [315] Although data are less robust, other lipid-lowering agents reported to reduce CRP include niacin, fibrates, and gemfibrozil. Aspirin and clopidrogrel also have an intriguing interaction with CRP. However, these effects are not actually tested in the primary prevention of cerebrovascular disease, and in expanding their use in cerebrovascular disease without an evidence-based experience is probably not appropriate. IS is quite different from coronary heart disease in terms of physiopathology and both statins and aspirin have not shown a similar strong protective effect in primary prevention. [316] At the moment, suggesting CRP levels as a guide of statin therapy in cerebrovascular disease prevention is probably reckless.

Even in the absence of an obvious intervention to lower high CRP levels, proponents of CRP screening may argue that relatively high CRP levels identify individuals in whom we need to pay even more attention to so called traditional cerebrovascular risk factors. Whether this is a cost-effective approach or not remains to be determined. It is important that these unresolved issues will be fully resolved in the ongoing prospective studies studies before hs-CRP screening becomes widespread. Until these questions are resolved, it is not yet time for hs-CRP testing to become an accepted practice. Otherwise, large numbers of people could be needlessly alarmed and a great deal of money unnecessarily spent on tests, office visits, and medications. While strategy involving CRP screening for the primary and secondary prevention of coronary heart disease among middle-aged subjects have apparently showed to be relatively cost-effective and, in some cases, cost saving, [317-319] consistent data in stroke and elderly patients are still not available and very scant. [320]

Evidence Supporting C-Reactive Protein Use in Secondary Prevention of Stroke

In secondary prevention, the role of CRP is rapidly evolving. Multiple studies demonstrate that CRP levels predict future CVD events in stroke patients and add to the predictive value of usually prognostic markers. [51,207-210,235,237-241,321] Further, knowledge of inflammatory status has been shown effective in distinguishing patient subgroups more or less likely to benefit from an aggressive versus conservative management approach. [39] However, appropriate clinical cut-points for CRP in the setting of acute IS remain uncertain, as does the timing of CRP evaluation in relation to the onset of qualifying event. Before an extensive use, we should respond clearly to several questions.

Which is the value of CRP as a prognostic marker in IS? Although no large study has prospectively assessed the value of CRP for prognostic short- and long-term stratification of patients with IS, many data suggest that CRP might be of great value in this group of patients. [51,207-210,237-241,321] The data are strong and consistent for the mild to long-term prognosis, for which the relative risk (RR) observed in different studies is similar (RR≈2.5). [207-210,237-240,321] However, the data are less consistent for the in-hospital prognostic stratification of these patients, although it is reasonable to presume that CRP levels may also constitute a good marker in this condition. When studying patients with an acute IS, no value should be discharged as too high, because following stimulation, CRP levels can increase a thousand fold and there is evidence that in some patients constitutional hyper-responsiveness might lead to very high CRP levels even in the first hours after stroke (Figure 7). [39] Of course, in the presence of overt inflammatory and infection disease the data should be interpreted cautiously, a possibly CRP titration repeated at least 2 times after the underlying disease has resolved in a long-term stratification standpoint. The most foreseable use of CRP in the emergency room setting is actually not well defined. Current data suggest that patients with lower CRP levels in the emergency room setting are unlikely a worse prognosis. [322] Furthermore, observational data suggest possible differential benefits for antiplatelet agents such as aspirin, [36,245] ticlopidine [36] or clopidogrel, [323] lipid lowering [321,324] and anti-hypertensive agents [325] on the basis of CRP levels after IS.

When to sample? The available data suggest the utility of a sample taken at admission, within 12 to 24 hours after stroke onset. However, when samples were also taken at discharge, [208] CRP levels are better predictors of the mid to long-term prognosis than those at admission (Figure 8). This is probably due to the fact that discharge level more closely reflect the baseline inflammatory status of the patients and thus their intrinsic risk due to inflammatory activity. It is reasonable to assess the CRP levels at entry and when possible at discharge; 1 to 3 months later may be useful, because it is likely that the highest risk of future events is confined to patients with persistently elevated levels of CRP. [241]

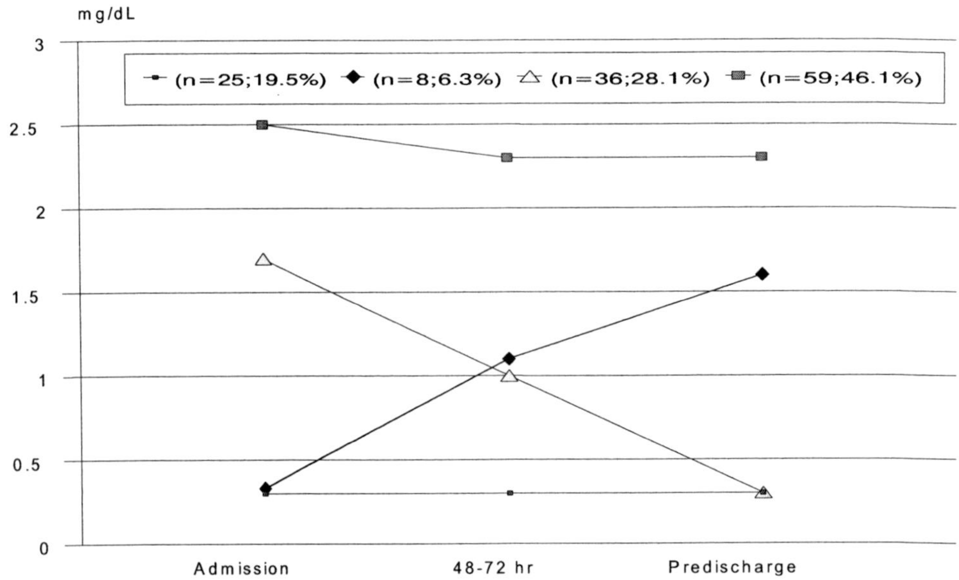

Figure 7. Changes in serum levels from admission through discharge. Different patterns are observed: persistently normal values, increasing values, decreasing values, and persistent elevation. Adapted from references 208 and 322.

What to do when CRP levels are elevated? The lack of a specific therapy which has been proved to reduce levels of CRP and risk makes this question quite questionable. However, the observation that statins [321] and angiotensin-converting enzyme inhibitors [325] are probably more effective in the presence of high CRP levels and that the efficacy of antiplatelet therapy [36] in secondary prevention appears to be directly related to level of inflammatory markers is already a first response. High CRP levels, associated with a higher risk, suggest a more aggressive medical therapy. The use of biochemical markers as a guide to the therapy will no longer be a controversial issue in the future and there is no doubt that CRP has all characteristics to be one of the ideal marker. However, additional well-designed epidemiological studies are needed to validate these findings.

Has the time come for including it in the risk profile? Despite the increasing number of studies on CRP in IS, it is still not clear which is the role of a marker of inflammation in the list of outcome predictors commonly used. To be of clinical utility CRP must be shown to add substantially to our ability to predict prognosis beyond that achievable by use of the traditional outcome predictors. CRP might be a good candidate. However, inflammation appears an important, common, but non necessary or a sufficient condition and hence the predictive accuracy of CRP measurement can only be limited, just like it is the case for isolated traditional prognostic factors. [326] Data are also lacking to show that interventions aimed at reducing CRP levels will lower the risk of subsequent CVD events. Without this information, use of hs-CRP assay either acutely or as a screening modality will be limited. In particular, routine inclusion of hs-CRP assay in risk factor profiling could result in a disproportionate number of patients with false-positive CRP elevations that are unrelated to prediction of future cerebrovascular events.

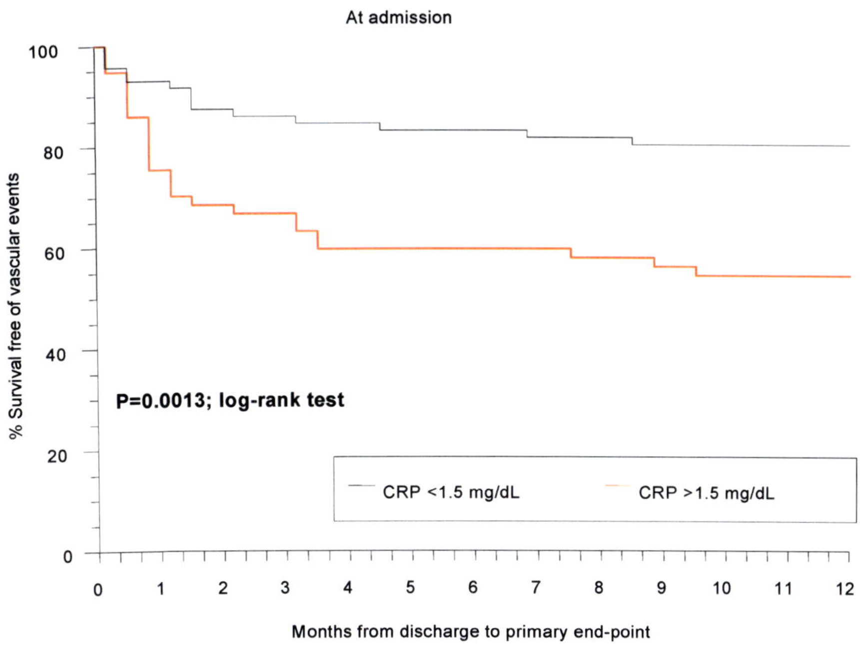

Figure 8. CRP provides prognostic information at different intervals after stroke onset. Cardiovascular event free survival among ischemic stroke patients according to CRP levels at hospital admission and at discharge. Data are cumulative freedom from risk of death or any new vascular event within 1-year in patients with CRP levels at admission and at discharge above or below an established validated cutoff point (1.5 mg/dL) between normal and elevated CRP. Adapted from reference 208.

Current Strategies to Reduce the Acute Inflammatory Response After Stroke. Antiplatelets Agents, Statins, Angiotensin Converting Enzime-Inhibitors

As documented above, CRP is a promising independent predictor of future cerebrovascular events that adds prognostic information to usual risk factor screening. At the moment, in the clinical practice settings of cerebrovascular disease, the extensive use of CRP testing should be discouraged in both primary and secondary prevention until more robust data will be available. For individuals for whom the AHA guidelines already call for therapeutic intervention, [327] a hs-CRP assay could be probably performed and high CRP level aggressively encourage physicians and patients to institute pharmacological therapy in those instances where none is currently being used or where compliance is poor. Risk factor assessment with attention to optimizing primary and secondary preventive measures for cerebrovascular disease should remain the essential objective of primary care clinicians. In most cases, assessment of standard risk factors should suffice to determine most patients who are at greatest risk. Interventions aimed at enacting healthy lifestyle changes should benefit all patients. These changes include smoking cessation, moderation of alcohol intake, achieving and maintaining appropriate body weight through proper dietary selection, and regular exercise. CRP levels will generally decrease as a natural consequence of implementing and enhancing beneficial lifestyle changes. Our newfound understanding of the role of inflammation helps us to comprehend the mechanisms by which a variety of interventions can reduce clinical events. Dietary modifications such as increased consumption of unsaturated fatty acids may act as an anti-inflammatory therapy by altering the pattern of prostanoids produced and/or by activating binding the nuclear receptor peroxisomal proliferation activating receptor-α (PPAR-α). [328,329] Dietary interventions may also limit postprandial hyperlipemia associated with triglyceride-rich lipoprotein particles, a recently recognized activator of inflammatory functions of endothelial cells. Exercise reduces CVD risk. By increasing NO production, elevating HDL, and augmenting insulin sensitivity, exercise may act in part by reducing inflammation. CVD risk might be further reduced by interventions aimed at correcting additional risk factors (ie, enhancing control of diabetes, lipid abnormalities, and blood pressure). Potential preventive measures, such as aspirin and clopidogrel, statins, angiotensin-converting enzyme inhibitors (ACE-I), β-blockers, and folate-vitamin B_{12} supplementation, should be actively considered and encouraged when appropriate. Hormone replacement should no longer be viewed as a protective measure for postmenopausal women. Beyond the lifestyle measures of exercise and diet, pharmacotherapy with statins, antiplatelet agents, and ACE-I may owe their clinical benefits in part to an anti-inflammatory action. Despite these advances in our understanding and intervention in regard to cerebrovascular risk, much remains to be done. Further in roads into reduction of cerebrovascular risk may well emerge as we begin to apply our recently acquired knowledge of the role that inflammation plays in atherosclerosis. In all likelihood, future basic research, including the application of functional genomics, will teach us new lessons about atherothrombosis and its complications and show the path to further ways to limit this disease. In coming years, we will see delineation of polymorphisms in the human genome, some of which will doubtless predict an individual's cerebrovascular risk. We believe that in the future we will target our preventive therapies by a combination of a panel of few serum tests, including traditional and a few nontraditional markers. These markers will provide an integrated assessment of the interaction between genotype and the environment, including individual behaviors (eg, smoking and diet). Genotyping, probably accomplished by high-throughput screening early in life, will identify genetic markers (eg, single nucleotide polymorphisms and haplotypes) that should predict individual responses to risk factors. The combination of the serum markers and hereditary predisposition revealed by genetic analysis should sharpen our ability to make a prescription for management of risks in individuals in a rational manner.

Multicenter, carefully controlled studies in stroke patients both ischemic and hemorrhagic are needed to determine whether CRP evaluation has utility in secondary prevention before recommending its use in common clinical practice. Appropriate clinical cut-points for CRP in the setting of acute stroke remain uncertain, as does the timing of CRP evaluation in relation to the onset of ischemia. An elevated CRP in this setting is associated with increased mild to long-term risks, [207-210,237-240,321] and thus additional evaluation modalities may be warranted. By contrast, current data suggest that patients with lower CRP levels in the emergency room setting are likely to have a benign prognosis in both IS [322] or ICH (Godoy D, 2004; unpublished results), but data are not conclusive.

Increasing evidence suggests that CRP may be directly involved in atherothrombogenesis that extends beyond its previously accepted role as an inflammatory marker. [330] CRP is present in the vessel wall, where it induces expression of the adhesion molecules E-selectin, VCAM-1 and ICAM-1 by endothelial cells, and serves as a chemo-attractant for monocytes as mediated by induction of MCP-1. [330] CRP opsonizes LDL and facilitates native LDL entry into macrophages. CRP binds to plasma membranes of damaged cells and activates complement via the classical pathway; [331] CRP is associated with endothelial cell dysfunction and progression of atherosclerosis, possibly by decreasing NO synthesis. [45] In line with these observations is the finding that CRP has the ability to sensitize endothelial cells to destruction by cytotoxic CD4+ T cells, [332] to facilitate thrombogenesis through stimulation of tissue factor biosynthesis by macrophages suggesting that high CRP plasma concentrations and the extent of its deposition in the atherosclerotic plaque are associated with plaque vulnerability and the occurrence of acute thrombotic events. [218,332]

Taken together, these recent findings on the pathophysiological role of CRP in atherogenesis may have several implications for future research, including the implementation of therapeutic strategies in CVD: (*i*) CRP plasma levels may become a target for intervention, e.g. by inhibiting hepatic biosynthesis; (*ii*) it is intriguing to speculate that direct interference with CRP-mediated effects either on the receptor level or on the level of CRP-mediated complement activation may influence progression of atherosclerosis and reduce tissue damage, leading to less severe disease. However, the primary cause for the accumulation and activation of inflammatory cells in the arterial subintimal space and the subsequent expression of pro-inflammatory cytokines and other mediators which play an important role in plaque progression and finally contribute to plaque destabilization and rupture, still remains largely unclear; (iii) the correlation of circulating CRP concentrations with stroke severity, [208-210] extent of ischemic lesion, [208-210] and the prognostic significance of these associations, [208-210] are consistent with CRP not just being a marker of disease but also contributing to pathogenesis of IS. A definitive way to test this concept will be the use of novel drugs that specifically block CRP binding and its proinflammatory effects in vivo. [218,332] If these compounds are effective, they may find very broad applicability. Such drugs would be a powerful tool for determining whether increased CRP production merely reflects atherosclerosis or does indeed participate in its pathogenesis and complications, and they could also have neuroprotective effects in acute IS. Knowledge of the structure and function of CRP — including its three dimensional structure alone and complexed with ligands [331] — establishes an excellent platform for future drug design.

References

[1] Stanimirovic D, Satoh K. Inflammatory mediators of cerebral endothelium: a role in ischemic brain inflammation. *Brain Pathol.* 2000; 10(1):113-126.

[2] del Zoppo G, Ginis I, Hallenbeck JM, Iadecola C, Wang X, Feuerstein GZ. Inflammation and stroke: putative role for cytokines, adhesion molecules and iNOS in brain response to ischemia. *Brain Pathol.* 2000; 10(1):95-112.

[3] del Zoppo GJ, Becker KJ, Hallenbeck JM. Inflammation after stroke: is it harmful? *Arch Neurol.* 2001; 58(4):669-672.

[4] American Heart Association. Stroke. Heart Disease and Stroke Statistics - 2003 Update. American Heart Association, 2003.

[5] Fassbender K, Bertsch T, Mielke O, Muhlhauser F, Hennerici M. Adhesion molecules in cerebrovascular diseases: evidence for an inflammatory endothelial activation in cerebral large- and small-vessel disease. *Stroke.* 1999; 30(8):1647-1650.

[6] Stary HC, Chandler AB, Glagov S, Guyton JR, Insull WJr, Rosenfeld ME et al. A definition of initial, fatty streak, and intermediate lesions of atherosclerosis: a report from the Committee on Vascular Lesions of the Council on Arteriosclerosis, American Heart Association. *Circulation.* 1994; 89(5):2462-2478.

[7] Napoli C, D'Armiento FP, Mancini FP, Postiglione A, Witztum JL, Palumbo G et al. Fatty streak formation occurs in human fetal aortas and is greatly enhanced by maternal hypercholesterolemia: intimal accumulation of low density lipoprotein and its oxidation precede monocyte recruitment into early atherosclerotic lesions. *J Clin Invest.* 1997; 100(11):2680-2690.

[8] Cesari M, Penninx BW, Newman AB, Kritchevsky SB, Nicklas BJ, Sutton-Tyrrell K et al. Inflammatory Markers and Onset of Cardiovascular Events. Results From the Health ABC Study. *Circulation.* 2003; 108(19):2317-2322.

[9] Blake GJ, Ridker PM. Inflammatory bio-markers and cardiovascular risk prediction. *J Intern Med.* 2002; 252(4):283-294.

[10] Lindsberg PJ, Grau AJ. Inflammation and infections as risk factors for ischemic stroke. *Stroke.* 2003; 34(10):2518-2532.

[11] Blann AD, Ridker PM, Lip GY. Inflammation, cell adhesion molecules, and stroke: tools in pathophysiology and epidemiology? *Stroke.* 2002; 33(9):2141-2143.

[12] del Zoppo G, Ginis I, Hallenbeck JM, Iadecola C, Wang X, Feuerstein GZ. Inflammation and stroke: putative role for cytokines, adhesion molecules and iNOS in brain response to ischemia. *Brain Pathol.* 2000; 10(1):95-112.

[13] Lowe GD. The relationship between infection, inflammation, and cardiovascular disease: an overview. *Ann Periodontol.* 2001; 6(1):1-8.

[14] Carr S, Farb A, Pearce WH, Virmani R, Yao JS. Atherosclerotic plaque rupture in symptomatic carotid artery stenosis. *J Vasc Surg.* 1996; 23(5):755-765.

[15] Guo Y, Jiang X, Zhou Z, Chen S, Zhao H, Li F. Relationship between levels of serum C-reactive protein, leucocyte count and carotid plaque in patients with ischemic stroke. *J Huazhong Univ Sci Technolog Med Sci.* 2003; 23(3):263-265.

[16] Iuliano L, Mauriello A, Sbarigia E, Spagnoli LG, Violi F. Radiolabeled native low-density lipoprotein injected into patients with carotid stenosis accumulates in macrophages of atherosclerotic plaque: effect of vitamin E supplementation. *Circulation.* 2000; 101(11):1249-1254.

[17] Tartiere JM, Henry OF, Safar H, Bureau JM, Girerd X, Safar ME et al. Carotid intima-media thickness and carotid and/or iliofemoral plaques: comparison of two markers of cardiovascular risk in hypertensive patients. *J Hypertens.* 2003; 21(4):739-746.

[18] Biasucci LM, Liuzzo G, Ciervo A, Petrucca A, Piro M, Angiolillo DJ et al. Antibody response to chlamydial heat shock protein 60 is strongly associated with acute coronary syndromes. *Circulation.* 2003; 107(24):3015-3017.

[19] Huittinen T, Leinonen M, Tenkanen L, Manttari M, Virkkunen H, Pitkanen T et al. Autoimmunity to human heat shock protein 60, Chlamydia pneumoniae infection, and inflammation in predicting coronary risk. *Arterioscler Thromb Vasc Biol.* 2002; 22(3):431-437.

[20] Kinjo K, Sato H, Sato H, Ohnishi Y, Hishida E, Nakatani D et al. Joint effects of Chlamydia pneumoniae infection and classic coronary risk factors on risk of acute myocardial infarction. *Am Heart J.* 2003; 146(2):324-330.

[21] Roivainen M, Viik-Kajander M, Palosuo T, Toivanen P, Leinonen M, Saikku P et al. Infections, inflammation, and the risk of coronary heart disease. *Circulation.* 2000; 101(3):252-257.

[22] Johnston SC, Messina LM, Browner WS, Lawton MT, Morris C, Dean D. C-reactive protein levels and viable Chlamydia pneumoniae in carotid artery atherosclerosis. *Stroke.* 2001; 32(12):2748-2752.

[23] Valtonen VV. Infection as a risk factor for infarction and atherosclerosis. *Ann Med.* 1991; 23(5):539-543.

[24] Tanne D, Haim M, Boyko V, Goldbourt U, Reshef T, Adler Y et al. Prospective study of Chlamydia pneumoniae IgG and IgA seropositivity and risk of incident ischemic stroke. *Cerebrovasc Dis.* 2003; 16(2):166-170.

[25] Tarnacka B, Gromadzka G, Czlonkowska A. Increased circulating immune complexes in acute stroke: the triggering role of Chlamydia pneumoniae and cytomegalovirus. *Stroke.* 2002; 33(4):936-940.

[26] Danesh J, Whincup P, Walker M, Lennon L, Thomson A, Appleby P et al. Low grade inflammation and coronary heart disease: prospective study and updated meta-analyses. *BMJ.* 2000; 321(7255):199-204.

[27] Blankenberg S, Rupprecht HJ, Poirier O, Bickel C, Smieja M, Hafner G et al. Plasma concentrations and genetic variation of matrix metalloproteinase 9 and prognosis of patients with cardiovascular disease. *Circulation.* 2003; 107(12):1579-1585.

[28] Montaner J, Alvarez-Sabin J, Barbera G, Angles A, Molina C, Abilleira S et al. [Correlation between the expression of proinflammatory cytokines and matrix metalloproteinases in the acute phase of an ischemic stroke]. *Rev Neurol.* 2001; 33(2):115-118.

[29] Zheng Z, Lee JE, Yenari MA. Stroke: molecular mechanisms and potential targets for treatment. *Curr Mol Med.* 2003; 3(4):361-372.

[30] Hsu HC, Mountz JD, Zhou T. Regulation of Fas-mediated apoptosis in CD2-fas transgenic mice. *Int Rev Immunol.* 1999; 18(4):309-327.

[31] Selmaj K, Raine C, Farooq M, Norton W, Brosan C. Apoptosis induced by lymphotoxin. *J Immun.* 1990; 147:1522-1529.

[32] Wojcik C. Regulation of apoptosis by the ubiquitin and proteasome pathway. *J Cell Mol Med.* 2002; 6(1):25-48.

[33] Bauvois B. Transmembrane proteases in cell growth and invasion: new contributors to angiogenesis? *Oncogene.* 2004; 23(2):317-329.

[34] de Jonge E, Dekkers PE, Creasey AA, Hack CE, Paulson SK, Karim A et al. Tissue factor pathway inhibitor does not influence inflammatory pathways during human endotoxemia. *J Infect Dis.* 2001; 183(12):1815-1818.

[35] Cushman M, Lemaitre RN, Kuller LH, Psaty BM, Macy EM, Sharrett AR et al. Fibrinolytic activation markers predict myocardial infarction in the elderly. The Cardiovascular Health Study. *Arterioscler Thromb Vasc Biol.* 1999; 19(3):493-498.

[36] Di Napoli M, Papa F. Inflammation, hemostatic markers, and antithrombotic agents in relation to long-term risk of new cardiovascular events in first-ever ischemic stroke patients. *Stroke.* 2002; 33(7):1763-1771.

[37] Gorelick PB. Stroke prevention therapy beyond antithrombotics: unifying mechanisms in ischemic stroke pathogenesis and implications for therapy: an invited review. *Stroke.* 2002; 33(3):862-875.

[38] Tohgi H, Konno S, Takahashi S, Koizumi D, Kondo R, Takahashi H. Activated coagulation/fibrinolysis system and platelet function in acute thrombotic stroke patients with increased C-reactive protein levels. *Thromb Res.* 2000; 100(5):373-379.

[39] Di Napoli M. Early inflammatory response in ischemic stroke. *Thromb Res.* 2001; 103(3):261-264.

[40] Tohgi H, Takahashi H, Tamura K, Konno S, Kawamorita A, Nozaki Y. Ischemic stroke among inpatients with preceding inflammatory response. *Thromb Res.* 2001; 104(5):375-377.

[41] Haapaniemi E, Tatlisumak T, Soinne L, Syrjala M, Kaste M. Plasminogen activator inhibitor-1 in patients with ischemic stroke. *Acta Neurochir.* 2000; 76(Suppl):277-278.

[42] Olah L, Misz M, Kappelmayer J, Ajzner E, Csepany T, Fekete I et al. Natural coagulation inhibitor proteins in young patients with cerebral ischemia. *Cerebrovasc Dis.* 2001; 12(4):291-297.

[43] Theuma P, Fonseca VA. Inflammation and emerging risk factors in diabetes mellitus and atherosclerosis. *Curr Diab Rep.* 2003; 3(3):248-254.

[44] Gram J, Bladbjerg EM, Moller L, Sjol A, Jespersen J. Tissue-type plasminogen activator and C-reactive protein in acute coronary heart disease. A nested case-control study. *J Intern Med.* 2000; 247(2):205-212.

[45] Libby P, Aikawa M. Effects of statins in reducing thrombotic risk and modulating plaque vulnerability. *Clin Cardiol.* 2003; 26(Suppl 1):I11-I14.

[46] Macfelda K, Weiss TW, Kaun C, Breuss JM, Zorn G, Oberndorfer U et al. Plasminogen activator inhibitor 1 expression is regulated by the inflammatory mediators interleukin-1alpha, tumor necrosis factor-alpha, transforming growth factor-beta and oncostatin M in human cardiac myocytes. *J Mol Cell Cardiol.* 2002; 34(12):1681-1691.

[47] McDermott MM, Green D, Greenland P, Liu K, Criqui MH, Chan C et al. Relation of levels of hemostatic factors and inflammatory markers to the ankle brachial index. *Am J Cardiol.* 2003; 92(2):194-199.

[48] Baidoshvili A, Nijmeijer R, Lagrand WK, Hack CE, Niessen HW. Localisation of C reactive protein in infarcted tissue sites of multiple organs during sepsis. *J Clin Pathol.* 2002; 55(2):152-153.

[49] Lagrand WK, Visser CA, Hermens WT, Niessen HW, Verheugt FW, Wolbink GJ et al. C-reactive protein as a cardiovascular risk factor: more than an epiphenomenon? *Circulation.* 1999; 100(1):96-102.

[50] Sellmayer A, Limmert T, Hoffmann U. High sensitivity C-reactive protein in cardiovascular risk assessment. CRP mania or useful screening? *Int Angiol.* 2003; 22(1):15-23.

[51] Guo Y, Jiang X, Chen S, Zhao HW, Gu KY. [C-reactive protein as an important prognostic marker for ischemic stroke]. *Zhonghua Yu Fang Yi Xue Za Zhi.* 2003; 37(2):102-104.

[52] Kang SM, Chung N, Kim JY, Koo BK, Choi D, Jang Y et al. Relation of vasodilator response of the brachial artery to inflammatory markers in patients with coronary artery disease. *Echocardiography.* 2002; 19(8):661-667.

[53] Kimoto-Kinoshita S, Nishida S, Tomura TT. Decrease of endothelial nitric oxide synthase in stroke-prone spontaneously hypertensive rat cerebral cortex. *Neurosci Lett.* 2000; 288(2):103-106.

[54] Kawashima S, Yamashita T, Miwa Y, Ozaki M, Namiki M, Hirase T et al. HMG-CoA reductase inhibitor has protective effects against stroke events in stroke-prone spontaneously hypertensive rats. *Stroke.* 2003; 34(1):157-163.

[55] Christman JW, Blackwell TS, Juurlink BH. Redox regulation of nuclear factor kappa B: therapeutic potential for attenuating inflammatory responses. *Brain Pathol.* 2000; 10(1):153-162.

[56] Di Napoli M, Papa F. The proteasome system and proteasome inhibitors in stroke: controlling the inflammatory response. *Curr Opin Invest Drug.* 2003; 4(11):1333-1342.

[57] Clemens JA. Cerebral ischemia: gene activation, neuronal injury, and the protective role of antioxidants. *Free Radic Biol Med.* 2000; 28(10):1526-1531.

[58] Kato H, Kogure K. Biochemical and molecular characteristics of the brain with developing cerebral infarction. *Cell Mol Neurobiol.* 1999; 19(1):93-108.

[59] Barber PA, Auer RN, Buchan AM, Sutherland GR. Understanding and managing ischemic stroke. *Can J Physiol Pharmacol.* 2001; 79(3):283-296.

[60] Graham SH, Chen J. Programmed cell death in cerebral ischemia. *J Cereb Blood Flow Metab.* 2001; 21(2):99-109.

[61] Mattson MP, Duan W, Pedersen WA, Culmsee C. Neurodegenerative disorders and ischemic brain diseases. *Apoptosis.* 2001; 6(1-2):69-81.

[62] Bartko D, Lesicky O, Buc M. [Cerebral infarct and the immune response]. *Bratisl Lek Listy.* 1997; 98(6):321-329.

[63] Becker KJ. Targeting the central nervous system inflammatory response in ischemic stroke. *Curr Opin Neurol.* 2001; 14(3):349-353.

[64] Stoll G, Jander S, Schroeter M. Inflammation and glial responses in ischemic brain injury. *Prog Neurobiol.* 1998; 56:149-171.

[65] Ginsberg MD. Adventures in the pathophysiology of brain ischemia: penumbra, gene expression, neuroprotection: the 2002 Thomas Willis Lecture. *Stroke*. 2003; 34(1):214-223.

[66] Bednar MM, Dooley RH, Zamani M, Howard DB, Gross CE. Neutrophil and platelet activity and quantification following delayed tPA therapy in a rabbit model of thromboembolic stroke. *J ThrombThrombolysis*. 1995; 1(2):179-185.

[67] Kogure K, Yamasaki Y, Matsuo Y, Kato H, Onodera H. Inflammation of the brain after ischemia. *Acta Neurochir (Wien)*. 1996; 66(Suppl):40-43.

[68] Lehrmann E, Christensen T, Zimmer J, Diemer NH, Finsen B. Microglial and macrophage reactions mark progressive changes and define the penumbra in the rat neocortex and striatum after transient middle cerebral artery occlusion. *J Comp Neurol*. 1997; 386(3):461-467.

[69] Schurer L, Grogaard B, Gerdin B, Kempski O, Arfors KE. Leucocyte depletion does not affect post-ischaemic nerve cell damage in the rat. *Acta Neurochir (Wien)*. 1991; 111(1-2):54-60.

[70] Lopez O, Lanthorn T. Anti-neutrophil antiserum reduces infarct volume after mouse permanent middle cerebral artery occlusion without producing neutropenia. *Neurosci Res Commun*. 1993; 13(1):45-53.

[71] Shimakura A, Kamanaka Y, Ikeda Y, Kondo K, Suzuki Y, Umemura K. Neutrophil elastase inhibition reduces cerebral ischemic damage in the middle cerebral artery occlusion. *Brain Res*. 2000; 858(1):55-60.

[72] Zhang RL, Chopp M, Jiang N, Tang WX, Prostak J, Manning AM et al. Anti-intercellular adhesion molecule-1 antibody reduces ischemic cell damage after transient but not permanent middle cerebral artery occlusion in the Wistar rat. *Stroke*. 1995; 26(8):1438-1442.

[73] Zhang RL, Chopp M, Zaloga C, Zhang ZG, Jiang N, Gautam SC et al. The temporal profiles of ICAM-1 protein and mRNA expression after transient MCA occlusion in the rat. *Brain Res*. 1995; 682(1-2):182-188.

[74] Chopp M, Zhang ZG. Anti-adhesion molecule and nitric oxide protection strategies in ischemic stroke. *Curr Opin Neurol*. 1996; 9(1):68-72.

[75] Yanaka K, Camarata PJ, Spellman SR, Skubitz AP, Furcht LT, Low WC. Laminin peptide ameliorates brain injury by inhibiting leukocyte accumulation in a rat model of transient focal cerebral ischemia. *J Cereb Blood Flow Metab*. 1997; 17(6):605-611.

[76] Phillips JB, Williams AJ, Adams J, Elliott PJ, Tortella FC. Proteasome inhibitor PS519 reduces infarction and attenuates leukocyte infiltration in a rat model of focal cerebral ischemia. *Stroke*. 2000; 31(7):1686-1693.

[77] Connolly ES, Jr., Winfree CJ, Springer TA, Naka Y, Liao H, Yan SD et al. Cerebral protection in homozygous null ICAM-1 mice after middle cerebral artery occlusion. Role of neutrophil adhesion in the pathogenesis of stroke. *J Clin Invest*. 1996; 97(1):209-216.

[78] Kitagawa K, Matsumoto M, Mabuchi T, Yagita Y, Ohtsuki T, Hori M et al. Deficiency of intercellular adhesion molecule 1 attenuates microcirculatory disturbance and infarction size in focal cerebral ischemia. *J Cereb Blood Flow Metab*. 1998; 18(12):1336-1345.

[79] Soriano SG, Lipton SA, Wang YF, Xiao M, Springer TA, Gutierrez-Ramos JC et al. Intercellular adhesion molecule-1-deficient mice are less susceptible to cerebral ischemia-reperfusion injury. *Ann Neurol.* 1996; 39(5):618-624.

[80] Kochanek PM, Hallenbeck JM. Polymorphonuclear leukocytes and monocytes/macrophages in the pathogenesis of cerebral ischemia and stroke. *Stroke.* 1992; 23(9):1367-1379.

[81] Garcia JH, Liu KF, Yoshida Y, Lian J, Chen S, del Zoppo GJ. Influx of leukocytes and platelets in an evolving brain infarct (Wistar rat). *Am J Pathol.* 1994; 144(1):188-199.

[82] Clark RK, Lee EV, Fish CJ, White RF, Price WJ, Jonak ZL et al. Development of tissue damage, inflammation and resolution following stroke: an immunohistochemical and quantitative planimetric study. *Brain Res Bull.* 1993; 31(5):565-572.

[83] Schroeter M, Jander S, Witte OW, Stoll G. Local immune responses in the rat cerebral cortex after middle cerebral artery occlusion. *J Neuroimmunol.* 1994; 55(2):195-203.

[84] Clark RK, Lee EV, White RF, Jonak ZL, Feuerstein GZ, Barone FC. Reperfusion following focal stroke hastens inflammation and resolution of ischemic injured tissue. *Brain Res Bull.* 1994; 35(4):387-392.

[85] Zhang RL, Chopp M, Chen H, Garcia JH. Temporal profile of ischemic tissue damage, neutrophil response, and vascular plugging following permanent and transient (2H) middle cerebral artery occlusion in the rat. *J Neurol Sci.* 1994; 125(1):3-10.

[86] Kato H, Kogure K, Liu XH, Araki T, Itoyama Y. Progressive expression of immunomolecules on activated microglia and invading leukocytes following focal cerebral ischemia in the rat. *Brain Res.* 1996; 734(1-2):203-212.

[87] del Zoppo GJ, Schmid-Schonbein GW, Mori E, Copeland BR, Chang CM. Polymorphonuclear leukocytes occlude capillaries following middle cerebral artery occlusion and reperfusion in baboons. *Stroke.* 1991; 22(10):1276-1283.

[88] Matsuo Y, Onodera H, Shiga Y, Shozuhara H, Ninomiya M, Kihara T et al. Role of cell adhesion molecules in brain injury after transient middle cerebral artery occlusion in the rat. *Brain Res.* 1994; 656(2):344-352.

[89] Morikawa E, Zhang SM, Seko Y, Toyoda T, Kirino T. Treatment of focal cerebral ischemia with synthetic oligopeptide corresponding to lectin domain of selectin. *Stroke.* 1996; 27(5):951-955.

[90] Hartl R, Schurer L, Schmid-Schonbein GW, del Zoppo GJ. Experimental antileukocyte interventions in cerebral ischemia. *J Cereb Blood Flow Metab.* 1996; 16(6):1108-1119.

[91] Okada Y, Copeland BR, Mori E, Tung MM, Thomas WS, del Zoppo GJ. P-selectin and intercellular adhesion molecule-1 expression after focal brain ischemia and reperfusion. *Stroke.* 1994; 25(1):202-211.

[92] Haring HP, Berg EL, Tsurushita N, Tagaya M, del Zoppo GJ. E-selectin appears in nonischemic tissue during experimental focal cerebral ischemia. *Stroke.* 1996; 27(8):1386-1391.

[93] Liu T, Young PR, McDonnell PC, White RF, Barone FC, Feuerstein GZ. Cytokine-induced neutrophil chemoattractant mRNA expressed in cerebral ischemia. *Neurosci Lett.* 1993; 164(1-2):125-128.

[94] Watanabe K, Konishi K, Fujioka M, Kinoshita S, Nakagawa H. The neutrophil chemoattractant produced by the rat kidney epithelioid cell line NRK-52E is a protein related to the KC/gro protein. *J Biol Chem.* 1989; 264(33):19559-19563.

[95] Yamagami S, Tamura M, Hayashi M, Endo N, Tanabe H, Katsuura Y et al. Differential production of MCP-1 and cytokine-induced neutrophil chemoattractant in the ischemic brain after transient focal ischemia in rats. *J Leukoc Biol.* 1999; 65(6):744-749.

[96] Wang X, Yue TL, Barone FC, Feuerstein GZ. Monocyte chemoattractant protein-1 messenger RNA expression in rat ischemic cortex. *Stroke.* 1995; 26(4):661-665.

[97] Kim JS, Gautam SC, Chopp M, Zaloga C, Jones ML, Ward PA et al. Expression of monocyte chemoattractant protein-1 and macrophage inflammatory protein-1 after focal cerebral ischemia in the rat. *J Neuroimmunol.* 1995; 56(2):127-134.

[98] Kreutzberg GW. Microglia: A sensor for pathological events in the CNS. *Trends Neurosci.* 1996; 19(8):312-318.

[99] Emsley HC, Tyrrell PJ. Inflammation and infection in clinical stroke. *J Cereb Blood Flow Metab.* 2002; 22(12):1399-1419.

[100] Sairanen TR, Lindsberg PJ, Brenner M, Siren AL. Global forebrain ischemia results in differential cellular expression of interleukin-1beta (IL-1beta) and its receptor at mRNA and protein level. *J Cereb Blood Flow Metab.* 1997; 17(10):1107-1120.

[101] Thomas A, Gasque P, Vaudry D, Gonzalez B, Fontaine M. Expression of a complete and functional complement system by human neuronal cells in vitro. *Int Immunol.* 2000; 12(7):1015-1023.

[102] Zhang Z, Chopp M, Goussev A, Powers C. Cerebral vessels express interleukin 1beta after focal cerebral ischemia. *Brain Res.* 1998; 784(1-2):210-217.

[103] Asea A, Kraeft SK, Kurt-Jones EA, Stevenson MA, Chen LB, Finberg RW et al. Hsp70 stimulates cytokine production through a CD14-dependant pathway, demonstrating its dual role as a chaperone and cytokine. *Nat Med.* 2000; 6(4):435-442.

[104] Kol A, Lichtman AH, Finberg RW, Libby P, Kurt-Jones EA. Cutting edge: Heat shock protein (Hsp) 60 activates the innate immune response: CD14 is an essential receptor for Hsp60 activation of mononuclear cells. *J Immunol.* 2000; 164(1):13-17.

[105] Fassbender K, Rossol S, Kammer T, Daffertshofer M, Wirth S, Dollman M et al. Proinflammatory cytokines in serum of patients with acute cerebral ischemia: kinetics of secretion and relation to the extent of brain damage and outcome of disease. *J Neurol Sci.* 1994; 122(2):135-139.

[106] Chrousos GP. The hypothalamic-pituitary-adrenal axis and immune-mediated inflammation. *N Engl J Med.* 1995; 332(20):1351-1362.

[107] Perini F, Morra M, Alecci M, Galloni E, Marchi M, Toso V. Temporal profile of serum anti-inflammatory and pro-inflammatory interleukins in acute ischemic stroke patients. *Neurol Sci.* 2001; 22(4):289-296.

[108] Vila N, Castillo J, Davalos A, Chamorro A. Proinflammatory cytokines and early neurological worsening in ischemic stroke. *Stroke.* 2000; 31(10):2325-2329.

[109] Castellanos M, Castillo J, Garcia MM, Leira R, Serena J, Chamorro A et al. Inflammation-mediated damage in progressing lacunar infarctions: a potential therapeutic target. *Stroke.* 2002; 33(4):982-987.

[110] Boutin H, LeFeuvre RA, Horai R, Asano M, Iwakura Y, Rothwell NJ. Role of IL-1alpha and IL-1beta in ischemic brain damage. *J Neurosci.* . 2001; 21(15):5528-5534.

[111] Liu T, McDonnell PC, Young PR, White RF, Siren AL, Hallenbeck JM et al. Interleukin-1 beta mRNA expression in ischemic rat cortex. *Stroke.* 1993; 24(11):1746-1750.

[112] Relton JK, Rothwell NJ. Interleukin-1 receptor antagonist inhibits ischaemic and excitotoxic neuronal damage in the rat. *Brain Res Bull.*1992; 29(2):243-246.

[113] Garcia J, Liu K, Relton J. Interleukin-1 receptor antagonist decreases the number of necrotic neurons in rats with middle cerebral artery occlusion. *Am J Pathol.* 1995; 147(5):1477-1486.

[114] Yang GY, Zhao YJ, Davidson BL, Betz AL. Overexpression of interleukin-1 receptor antagonist in the mouse brain reduces ischemic brain injury. *Brain Res.* 1997; 751(2):181-188.

[115] Huang Q, Tatro JB. Alpha-melanocyte stimulating hormone suppresses intracerebral tumor necrosis factor-alpha and interleukin-1beta gene expression following transient cerebral ischemia in mice. *Neurosci Lett.* 2002; 334(3):186-190.

[116] Barone FC, Arvin B, White RF, Miller A, Webb CL, Willette RN et al. Tumor necrosis factor-alpha. A mediator of focal ischemic brain injury. *Stroke.* 1997; 28(6):1233-1244.

[117] Arvin B, Neville LF, Barone FC, Feuerstein GZ. The role of inflammation and cytokines in brain injury. *Neurosci Biobehav Rev.* 1996; 20(3):445-452.

[118] Feuerstein GZ, Wang X, Barone FC. The role of cytokines in the neuropathology of stroke and neurotrauma. *Neuroimmunomodulation.* 1998; 5(3-4):143-159.

[119] Lavine SD, Hofman FM, Zlokovic BV. Circulating antibody against tumor necrosis factor-alpha protects rat brain from reperfusion injury. *J Cereb Blood Flow Metab.* 1998; 18(1):52-58.

[120] Wang X, Yue TL, Barone FC, White RF, Gagnon RC, Feuerstein GZ. Concomitant cortical expression of TNF-alpha and IL-1 beta mRNAs follows early response gene expression in transient focal ischemia. *Mol Chem Neuropathol.* 1994; 23(2-3):103-114.

[121] Cheng B, Christakos S, Mattson MP. Tumor necrosis factors protect neurons against metabolic-excitotoxic insults and promote maintenance of calcium homeostasis. *Neuron.* 1994; 12(1):139-153.

[122] Wang X, Yue TL, Young PR, Barone FC, Feuerstein GZ. Expression of interleukin-6, c-fos, and zif268 mRNAs in rat ischemic cortex. *J Cereb Blood Flow Metab.* 1995; 15(1):166-171.

[123] Baumann H, Gauldie J. The acute phase response. *Immunol Today.* 1994; 15(2):74-80.

[124] Dziedzic T, Bartus S, Klimkowicz A, Motyl M, Slowik A, Szczudlik A. Intracerebral hemorrhage triggers interleukin-6 and interleukin-10 release in blood. *Stroke.* 2002; 33(9):2334-2335.

[125] Acalovschi D, Wiest T, Hartmann M, Farahmi M, Mansmann U, Auffarth GU et al. Multiple levels of regulation of the interleukin-6 system in stroke. *Stroke.* 2003; 34(8):1864-1869.

[126] Mackiewicz A, Schooltink H, Heinrich PC, Rose-John S. Complex of soluble human IL-6-receptor/IL-6 up-regulates expression of acute-phase proteins. *J Immunol.* 1992; 149(6): 2021-2027.

[127] Iadecola C. Bright and dark sides of nitric oxide in ischemic brain injury. *Trends Neurosci.* 1997; 20(3):132-139.

[128] Fehsel K, Kolb-Bachofen V, Kolb H. Analysis of TNF alpha-induced DNA strand breaks at the single cell level. *Am J Pathol.* 1991; 139(2):251-254.

[129] Zheng L, Fisher G, Miller RE, Peschon J, Lynch DH, Lenardo MJ. Induction of apoptosis in mature T cells by tumour necrosis factor. *Nature.* 1995; 377(6547):348-351.

[130] Pelidou SH, Kostulas N, Matusevicius D, Kivisakk P, Kostulas V, Link H. High levels of IL-10 secreting cells are present in blood in cerebrovascular diseases. *Eur J Neurol.*1999; 6(4):437-442.

[131] van Exel E, Gussekloo J, de Craen AJ, Bootsma-van der Wiel A, Frolich M, Westendorp RG. Inflammation and stroke: the Leiden 85-Plus Study. *Stroke.* 2002; 33(4):1135-1138.

[132] Vila N, Castillo J, Davalos A, Esteve A, Planas AM, Chamorro A. Levels of anti-inflammatory cytokines and neurological worsening in acute ischemic stroke. *Stroke.* 2003; 34(3):671-675.

[133] Pantoni L, Sarti C, Inzitari D. Cytokines and cell adhesion molecules in cerebral ischemia: experimental bases and therapeutic perspectives. *Arterioscler Thromb Vasc Biol.* 1998; 18(4):503-513.

[134] Beech JS, Reckless J, Mosedale DE, Grainger DJ, Williams SC, Menon DK. Neuroprotection in ischemia-reperfusion injury: an antiinflammatory approach using a novel broad-spectrum chemokine inhibitor. *J Cereb Blood Flow Metab.* 2001; 21(6):683-689.

[135] Kostulas N, Kivisakk P, Huang Y, Matusevicius D, Kostulas V, Link H. Ischemic stroke is associated with a systemic increase of blood mononuclear cells expressing interleukin-8 mRNA. *Stroke.* 1998; 29(2):462-466.

[136] Yamagami S, Tamura M, Hayashi M, Endo N, Tanabe H, Katsuura Y et al. Differential production of MCP-1 and cytokine-induced neutrophil chemoattractant in the ischemic brain after transient focal ischemia in rats. *J Leukoc Biol.* 1999; 65(6):744-749.

[137] Dawson J, Miltz W, Mir AK, Wiessner C. Targeting monocyte chemoattractant protein-1 signalling in disease. *Expert Opin Ther Targets.* 2003; 7(1):35-48.

[138] Bates S, Read SJ, Harrison DC, Topp S, Morrow R, Gale D et al. Characterisation of gene expression changes following permanent MCAO in the rat using subtractive hybridisation. *Brain Res Mol Brain Res.* 2001; 93(1):70-80.

[139] Losy J, Zaremba J. Monocyte chemoattractant protein-1 is increased in the cerebrospinal fluid of patients with ischemic stroke. *Stroke.* 2001; 32(11):2695-2696.

[140] Sakamoto M, Fujisawa Y, Nishioka K. Physiologic role of the complement system in host defense, disease, and malnutrition. *Nutrition.* 1998; 14(4):391-398.

[141] Laufer J, Katz Y, Passwell JH. Extrahepatic synthesis of complement proteins in inflammation. *Mol Immunol.* 2001; 38(2-3):221-229.

[142] Vasthare US, Barone FC, Sarau HM, Rosenwasser RH, DiMartino M, Young WF et al. Complement depletion improves neurological function in cerebral ischemia. *Brain Res Bull.* 1998; 45(4):413-419.

[143] Huang J, Kim LJ, Mealey R, Marsh HC, Jr., Zhang Y, Tenner AJ et al. Neuronal protection in stroke by an sLex-glycosylated complement inhibitory protein. *Science.* 1999; 285(5427):595-599.

[144] De Simoni MG, Storini C, Barba M, Catapano L, Arabia AM, Rossi E et al. Neuroprotection by complement (C1) inhibitor in mouse transient brain ischemia. *J Cereb Blood Flow Metab.* 2003; 23(2):232-239.

[145] Akita N, Nakase H, Kaido T, Kanemoto Y, Sakaki T. Protective effect of C1 esterase inhibitor on reperfusion injury in the rat middle cerebral artery occlusion model. *Neurosurgery.* 2003; 52(2):395-400.

[146] Lindsberg PJ, Ohman J, Lehto T, Karjalainen-Lindsberg ML, Paetau A, Wuorimaa T et al. Complement activation in the central nervous system following blood-brain barrier damage in man. *Ann Neurol.*1996; 40(4):587-596.

[147] Hirschl RB. Oxygen delivery in the pediatric surgical patient. *Curr Opin Pediatr.* 1994; 6(3):341-347.

[148] Furie MB, Randolph GJ. Chemokines and tissue injury. *Am J Pathol.* 1995; 146(6):1287-1301.

[149] Frijns CJ, Kappelle LJ. Inflammatory cell adhesion molecules in ischemic cerebrovascular disease. *Stroke.* 2002; 33(8):2115-2122.

[150] Beray-Berthat V, Palmier B, Plotkine M, Margaill I. Neutrophils do not contribute to infarction, oxidative stress, and NO synthase activity in severe brain ischemia. *Exp Neurol.* 2003; 182(2):446-454.

[151] Iadecola C, Alexander M. Cerebral ischemia and inflammation. *Curr Opin Neurol.* 2001; 14(1):89-94.

[152] Lerouet D, Beray-Berthat V, Palmier B, Plotkine M, Margaill I. Changes in oxidative stress, iNOS activity and neutrophil infiltration in severe transient focal cerebral ischemia in rats. *Brain Res.* 2002; 958(1):166-175.

[153] Zhang R, Wang L, Zhang L, Chen J, Zhu Z, Zhang Z et al. Nitric oxide enhances angiogenesis via the synthesis of vascular endothelial growth factor and cGMP after stroke in the rat. *Circ Res.* 2003; 92(3):308-313.

[154] Barthwal MK, Srivastava N, Nag D, Seth PK, Srimal RC, Dikshit M. Antioxidant levels in the rat brain after nitric oxide synthase inhibition: a preliminary report. *Redox Rep.* 2000; 5(2-3):75-80.

[155] Ducrocq S, Benjelloun N, Plotkine M, Ben Ari Y, Charriaut-Marlangue C. Poly(ADP-ribose) synthase inhibition reduces ischemic injury and inflammation in neonatal rat brain. *J Neurochem.* 2000; 74(6):2504-2511.

[156] Batot g, Martel C, Capdeville N, Wientjes F, Morel F. Characterization of neutrophil NADPH oxidase activity reconstituted in a cell-free assay using specific monoclonal antibodies raised against cytochrome b558. *Eur J Biochem.* 1995; 234(1):208-215.

[157] Babior BM, Lambeth JD, Nauseef W. The neutrophil NADPH oxidase. *Arch Biochem Biophys.* 2002; 397(2):342-344.

[158] Walder CE, Green SP, Darbonne WC, Mathias J, Rae J, Dinauer MC. Ischemic stroke injury is reduced in mice lacking a functional NADPH oxidase. *Stroke.* 1997; 28(11):2252-2258.

[159] Planas AM, Soriano MA, Berruezo M, Justicia C, Estrada A, Pitarch S et al. Induction of Stat3, a signal transducer and transcription factor, in reactive microglia following transient focal cerebral ischaemia. *Eur J Neurosci.* 1996; 8(12):2612-2618.

[160] Ruscher K, Isaev N, Trendelenburg G, Weih M, Iurato L, Meisel A et al. Induction of hypoxia inducible factor 1 by oxygen glucose deprivation is attenuated by hypoxic preconditioning in rat cultured neurons. *Neurosci Lett.* 1998; 254(2):117-120.

[161] O'Neill LA, Kaltschmidt C. NF-kappa B: a crucial transcription factor for glial and neuronal cell function. *Trends Neurosci.* 1997; 20(6):252-258.

[162] Kimura C, Oike M, Ito Y. Hypoxia-induced alterations in Ca(2+) mobilization in brain microvascular endothelial cells. *Am J Physiol Heart Circ Physiol.* 2000; 279(5):H2310-H2318.

[163] Barone FC, White RF, Spera PA, Ellison J, Currie RW, Wang X et al. Ischemic preconditioning and brain tolerance: temporal histological and functional outcomes, protein synthesis requirement, and interleukin-1 receptor antagonist and early gene expression. *Stroke.* 1998; 29(9):1937-1950.

[164] Villringer A, Dirnagl U. [Pathophysiology of cerebral ischemia]. *Z Arztl Fortbild Qualitatssich.* 1999; 93(3):164-168.

[165] Dirnagl U, Iadecola C, Moskowitz MA. Pathobiology of ischaemic stroke: an integrated view. *Trends Neurosci.* 1999; 22(9):391-397.

[166] Tang Y, Lu A, Aronow BJ, Wagner KR, Sharp FR. Genomic responses of the brain to ischemic stroke, intracerebral haemorrhage, kainate seizures, hypoglycemia, and hypoxia. *Eur J Neurosci.* 2002; 15(12):1937-1952.

[167] Iadecola C, Salkowski CA, Zhang F, Aber T, Nagayama M, Vogel SN et al. The transcription factor interferon regulatory factor 1 is expressed after cerebral ischemia and contributes to ischemic brain injury. *J Exp Med.* 1999; 189(4):719-727.

[168] Buchan AM, Li H, Blackburn B. Neuroprotection achieved with a novel proteasome inhibitor which blocks NF-kappaB activation. *Neuroreport.* 2000; 11(2):427-430.

[169] Di Napoli M, Papa F. MLN-519. Millennium/PAION. *Curr Opin Investig Drugs.* 2003; 4(3):333-341.

[170] Stephenson D, Yin T, Smalstig EB, Hsu MA, Panetta J, Little S et al. Transcription factor nuclear factor-kappa B is activated in neurons after focal cerebral ischemia. *J Cereb Blood Flow Metab.* 2000; 20(3):592-603.

[171] Priller J, Dirnagl U. Inflammation in stroke — a potential target for neuroprotection? *Ernst Schering Res Found Workshop.* 2002;(39):133-157.

[172] Amir RE, Iwai K, Ciechanover A. The NEDD8 pathway is essential for SCF(beta - TrCP)-mediated ubiquitination and processing of the NF-kappa B precursor p105. *J Biol Chem.* 2002; 277(26):23253-23259.

[173] Chen Z, Hagler J, Palombella VJ, Melandri F, Scherer D, Ballard D et al. Signal-induced site-specific phosphorylation targets I kappa B alpha to the ubiquitin-proteasome pathway. *Genes Dev.* 1995; 9(13):1586-1597.

[174] Perkins ND. The Rel/NF-kappa B family: friend and foe. *Trends Biochem Sci.* 2000; 25(9):434-440.

[175] Schmedtje JF, Ji YS, Liu WL, Dubois RN, Runge MS. Hypoxia induces cyclooxygenase-2 via the NF-kappa-B p65 transcription factor in human vascular endothelial cells. *J Biol Chem.* 1997; 272(1):601-608.

[176] Kyriakis JM, Avruch J. Mammalian mitogen-activated protein kinase signal transduction pathways activated by stress and inflammation. *Physiol Rev.* 2001; 81(2):807-869.

[177] Legos JJ, Erhardt JA, White RF, Lenhard SC, Chandra S, Parsons AA et al. SB 239063, a novel p38 inhibitor, attenuates early neuronal injury following ischemia. *Brain Res.* 2001; 892(1):70-77.

[178] American College of Chest Physicians, Society of Critical Care Medicine Consensus Conference. Definitions for Sepsis and organ failure and guidelines for the use of innovative therapies in sepsis. *Crit Care Med.* 1992; 20(6):864-874.

[179] Bone RC. Systemic Inflammatory response syndrome : a unifying concept of systemic inflammation. In: Fein A, (Ed). Sepsis and multiorgan failure. Baltimore: Williams and Wilkins, 1997: 3-10.

[180] Coimbra C, Drake M, Boris-Moller F, Wieloch T. Long-lasting neuroprotective effect of postischemic hypothermia and treatment with an anti-inflammatory/antipyretic drug. Evidence for chronic encephalopathic processes following ischemia. *Stroke.* 1996; 27(9):1578-1585.

[181] Emsley HC, Smith CJ, Gavin CM, Georgiou RF, Vail A, Barberan EM et al. An early and sustained peripheral inflammatory response in acute ischaemic stroke: relationships with infection and atherosclerosis. *J Neuroimmunol.* 2003; 139(1-2):93-101.

[182] Slowik A, Turaj W, Pankiewicz J, Dziedzic T, Szermer P, Szczudlik A. Hypercortisolemia in acute stroke is related to the inflammatory response. *J Neurol Sci.* 2002; 196(1-2):27-32.

[183] Yoshimoto Y, Tanaka Y, Hoya K. Acute Systemic Inflammatory Response Syndrome in Subarachnoid Hemorrhage. *Stroke.* 2001; 32(9):1989-1993.

[184] Godoy D, Boccio A, Nafissi H. [Systemic Inflammatory Response Syndrome and Spontaneous Intracerebral hemorrhage]. *Rev Neurol.* 2002; 35(12):1101-1105.

[185] Castillo J, Davalos A, Alvarez-Sabin J, Pumar JM, Leira R, Silva Y et al. Molecular signatures of brain injury after intracerebral hemorrhage. *Neurology.* 2002; 58(4):624-629.

[186] Pozzilli C, Lenzi GL, Argentino C, Bozzao L, Rasura M, Giubilei F et al. Peripheral white blood cell count in cerebral ischemic infarction. *Acta Neurol Scand.* 1985; 71(5):396-400.

[187] Kazmierski R, Guzik P, Ambrosius W, Kozubski W. [Leukocytosis in the first day of acute ischemic stroke as a prognostic factor of disease progression]. *Wiad Lek.* 2001; 54(3-4):143-151.

[188] Kostulas N, Pelidou SH, Kivisakk P, Kostulas V, Link H. Increased IL-1beta, IL-8, and IL-17 mRNA expression in blood mononuclear cells observed in a prospective ischemic stroke study. *Stroke.* 1999; 30(10):2174-2179.

[189] Grau AJ, Reis A, Buggle F, Al Khalaf A, Werle E, Valois N et al. Monocyte function and plasma levels of interleukin-8 in acute ischemic stroke. *J Neurol Sci.* 2001; 192(1-2):41-47.

[190] Arakelian A, Boiadzhian A, Pogosian A, Bakunts G, Sil'vanian G, Egiian L. [Circulating immune complexes in ischemic and hemorrhagic strokes]. *Zh Nevrol Psikhiatr Im S S Korsakova*. 2003; Suppl 8:44-47.
[191] Voice JK, Lachmann PJ. Neutrophil Fc gamma and complement receptors involved in binding soluble IgG immune complexes and in specific granule release induced by soluble IgG immune complexes. *Eur J Immunol*. 1997; 27(10):2514-2523.
[192] Nezlin R. A quantitative approach to the determination of antigen in immune complexes. *J Immunol Methods*. 2000; 237(1-2):1-17.
[193] Hatashita S, Hoff JT. Brain edema and cerebrovascular permeability during cerebral ischemia in rats. *Stroke*. 1990; 21(4):582-588.
[194] Buttner T, Weyers S, Postert T, Sprengelmeyer R, Kuhn W. S-100 protein: serum marker of focal brain damage after ischemic territorial MCA infarction. *Stroke*. 1997; 28(10):1961-1965.
[195] Zhang ZG, Zhang L, Jiang Q, Zhang R, Davies K, Powers C et al. VEGF enhances angiogenesis and promotes blood-brain barrier leakage in the ischemic brain. *J Clin Invest*. 2000; 106(7):829-838.
[196] Huber JD, Witt KA, Hom S, Egleton RD, Mark KS, Davis TP. Inflammatory pain alters blood-brain barrier permeability and tight junctional protein expression. *Am J Physiol Heart Circ Physiol*. 2001; 280(3):H1241-H1248.
[197] Brillault J, Berezowski V, Cecchelli R, Dehouck MP. Intercommunications between brain capillary endothelial cells and glial cells increase the transcellular permeability of the blood-brain barrier during ischaemia. *J Neurochem*. 2002; 83(4):807-817.
[198] Rothwell NJ, Hopkins SJ. Cytokines and the nervous system II: Actions and mechanisms of action. *Trends Neurosci*. 1995; 18(3):130-136.
[199] Grau AJ, Buggle F, Becher H, Zimmermann E, Spiel M, Fent T et al. Recent bacterial and viral infection is a risk factor for cerebrovascular ischemia: clinical and biochemical studies. *Neurology*. 1998; 50(1):196-203.
[200] Ramadori G, Christ B. Cytokines and the hepatic acute-phase response. *Semin Liver Dis*. 1999; 19(2):141-155.
[201] Luheshi G, Rothwell N. Cytokines and fever. *Int Arch Allergy Immunol*. 1996; 109(4):301-307.
[202] Elneihoum AM, Falke P, Axelsson L, Lundberg E, Lindgarde F, Ohlsson K. Leukocyte activation detected by increased plasma levels of inflammatory mediators in patients with ischemic cerebrovascular diseases. *Stroke*. 1996; 27(10):1734-1738.
[203] Murros K, Fogelholm R, Kettunen S, Vuorela AL. Serum cortisol and outcome of ischemic brain infarction. *J Neurol Sci*. 1993; 116(1):12-17.
[204] Chamorro A, Vila N, Ascaso C, Saiz A, Montalvo J, Alonso P et al. Early prediction of stroke severity. Role of the erythrocyte sedimentation rate. *Stroke*. 1995; 26(4):573-576.
[205] Czlonkowska A, Ryglewicz D, Lechowicz W. Basic analytical parameters as the predictive factors for 30-day case fatality rate in stroke. *Acta Neurol Scand*. 1997; 95(2):121-124.
[206] Hajat C, Hajat S, Sharma P. Effects of poststroke pyrexia on stroke outcome : a meta-analysis of studies in patients. *Stroke*. 2000; 31(2):410-414.

[207] Muir KW, Weir CJ, Alwan W, Squire IB, Lees KR. C-reactive protein and outcome after ischemic stroke. *Stroke.* 1999; 30(5):981-985.

[208] Di Napoli M, Papa F, Bocola V. C-reactive protein in ischemic stroke: an independent prognostic factor. *Stroke.* 2001; 32(4):917-924.

[209] Winbeck K, Poppert H, Etgen T, Conrad B, Sander D. Prognostic relevance of early serial C-reactive protein measurements after first ischemic stroke. *Stroke.* 2002; 33(10):2459-2464.

[210] Di Napoli M, Papa F, Bocola V. Prognostic influence of increased C-reactive protein and fibrinogen levels in ischemic stroke. *Stroke.* 2001; 32(1):133-138.

[211] Marz P, Cheng JG, Gadient RA, Patterson PH, Stoyan T, Otten U et al. Sympathetic neurons can produce and respond to interleukin 6. *Proc Natl Acad Sci U S A.* 1998; 95(6):3251-3256.

[212] Tarkowski E, Rosengren L, Blomstrand C, Wikkelso C, Jensen C, Ekholm S et al. Early intrathecal production of interleukin-6 predicts the size of brain lesion in stroke. *Stroke.* 1995; 26(8):1393-1398.

[213] Ferrarese C, Mascarucci P, Zoia C, Cavarretta R, Frigo M, Begni B et al. Increased cytokine release from peripheral blood cells after acute stroke. *J Cereb Blood Flow Metab.* 1999; 19(9):1004-1009.

[214] Smith CJ, Emsley HC, Gavin CM, Georgiou RF, Vail A, Barberan EM et al. Peak plasma interleukin-6 and other peripheral markers of inflammation in the first week of ischaemic stroke correlate with brain infarct volume, stroke severity and long-term outcome. *BMC Neurol.* 2004; 4(1):2.

[215] Shainkin-Kestenbaum R, Zimlichman S, Lis M, Lidor C, Pomerantz M, Knyszynski A et al. Effect of serum amyloid A, HDL-apolipoprotein, on endothelial cell proliferation. Implication of an enigmatic protein to atherosclerosis. *Biomed Pept Proteins Nucleic Acids.* 1996; 2(3):79-84.

[216] Ilzecka J, Stelmasiak Z. Prognostic importance of monitoring Serum Amyloid A protein (SAA) in patients with cerebral infarction. *Acta clin Croat.* 2000; 39(3):139-146.

[217] Pepys MB, Berger A. The renaissance of C reactive protein. *BMJ.* 2001; 322(7277):4-5.

[218] Pepys MB, Hirschfield GM. C-reactive protein: a critical update. *J Clin Invest.* 2003; 111(12):1805-1812.

[219] Kuta AE, Baum LL. C-reactive protein is produced by a small number of normal human peripheral blood lymphocytes. *J Exp Med.* 1986; 164(1):321-326.

[220] Robey FA, Jones KD, Tanata T, Liu T-H. Binding of C-reactive protein to chromatin and nucleosome core particles: a possible physiological role of C-reactive protein. *J Biol Chem.* 1984; 259(11):7311-7316.

[221] Rost NS, Wolf PA, Kase CS, Kelly-Hayes M, Silbershatz H, Massaro JM et al. Plasma concentration of C-reactive protein and risk of ischemic stroke and transient ischemic attack: the Framingham study. *Stroke.* 2001; 32(11):2575-2579.

[222] Di Napoli M. Systemic complement activation in ischemic stroke. *Stroke.* 2001; 32(6):1443-1448.

[223] Takagi K, Tsuchiya Y, Ohwaki K, Okinaga K, Nagashima Y, Ishii T et al. [Body temperature in the super-acute phase of the cerebrovascular disorders: mainly focused on the subarachnoid hemorrhage]. *No To Shinkei*. 2002; 54(2):139-145.

[224] Gong C, Hoff JT, Keep RF. Acute inflammatory reaction following experimental intracerebral hemorrhage in rat. *Brain Res*. 2000; 871(1):57-65.

[225] Xue M, Del Bigio MR. Intracortical hemorrhage injury in rats : relationship between blood fractions and brain cell death. *Stroke*. 2000; 31(7):1721-1727.

[226] Xue M, Del Bigio MR. Intracerebral injection of autologous whole blood in rats: time course of inflammation and cell death. *Neurosci Lett*. 2000; 283(3):230-232.

[227] Del Bigio MR, Yan HJ, Campbell TM, Peeling J. Effect of fucoidan treatment on collagenase-induced intracerebral hemorrhage in rats. *Neurol Res*. 1999; 21(4):415-419.

[228] Power C, Henry S, Del Bigio MR, Larsen PH, Corbett D, Imai Y et al. Intracerebral hemorrhage induces macrophage activation and matrix metalloproteinases. *Ann Neurol*. 2003; 53(6):731-742.

[229] Zimmerman M. Endothelin and subarachnoid hemorrhage: an overview. *Neurosurgery*. 2003; 43(4):863-875.

[230] Ridker PM, Buring JE, Shih J, Matias M, Hennekens CH. Prospective study of C-reactive protein and the risk of future cardiovascular events among apparently healthy women. *Circulation*. 1998; 98(8):731-733.

[231] Ridker PM. C-reactive protein and risks of future myocardial infarction and thrombotic stroke. *Eur Heart J*. 1998; 19(1):1-3.

[232] Ford ES, Giles WH. Serum C-reactive protein and self-reported stroke: findings from the Third National Health and Nutrition Examination Survey. *Arterioscler Thromb Vasc Biol*. 2000; 20(4):1052-1056.

[233] Curb JD, Abbott RD, Rodriguez BL, Sakkinen P, Popper JS, Yano K et al. C-reactive protein and the future risk of thromboembolic stroke in healthy men. *Circulation*. 2003; 107(15):2016-2020.

[234] Ridker PM, Hennekens CH, Buring JE, Rifai N. C-reactive protein and other markers of inflammation in the prediction of cardiovascular disease in women. *N Engl J Med*. 2000; 342(12):836-843.

[235] Canova CR, Courtin C, Reinhart WH. C-reactive protein (CRP) in cerebro-vascular events. *Atherosclerosis*. 1999; 147(1):49-53.

[236] Di Napoli M, Di Gianfilippo G, Bocola V. C-Reactive protein, serum amyloid A protein, and coronary events. *Circulation*. 1999; 100(15):e66.

[237] Di Napoli M, Di Gianfilippo G, Sollecito A, Bocola V. C-reactive protein and outcome after first-ever ischemic stroke. *Stroke*. 2000; 31(1):238-239.

[238] Anuk T, Assayag EB, Rotstein R, Fusman R, Zeltser D, Berliner S et al. Prognostic implications of admission inflammatory profile in acute ischemic neurological events. *Acta Neurol Scand*. 2002; 106(4):196-199.

[239] Ceccarelli E, Donati C, Forconi S, Cappelli R, Masotti L. C-reactive protein, physical disability, and prognosis in very old patients with ischemic stroke. *J Gerontol A Biol Sci Med Sci*. 2002; 57(8):M520-M522.

[240] Iyigun I, Bakirci Y. Plasma concentrations of C-reactive protein and fibrinogen in ischaemic stroke. *J Int Med Res*. 2002; 30(6):591-596.

[241] Arenillas JF, Alvarez-Sabin J, Molina CA, Chacon P, Montaner J, Rovira A et al. C-reactive protein predicts further ischemic events in first-ever transient ischemic attack or stroke patients with intracranial large-artery occlusive disease. *Stroke*. 2003; 34(10):2463-2468.

[242] Guo Y, Jiang X, Zhou Z, Chen S, Zhao H, Li F. Relationship between levels of serum C-reactive protein, leucocyte count and carotid plaque in patients with ischemic stroke. *J Huazhong Univ Sci Technolog Med Sci*. 2003; 23(3):263-265.

[243] Cao JJ, Thach C, Manolio TA, Psaty BM, Kuller LH, Chaves PH et al. C-reactive protein, carotid intima-media thickness, and incidence of ischemic stroke in the elderly: the Cardiovascular Health Study. *Circulation*. 2003; 108(2):166-170.

[244] Libby P, Ridker PM. Novel inflammatory markers of coronary risk: theory versus practice. *Circulation*. 1999; 100(11):1148-1150.

[245] Ridker PM, Cushman M, Stampfer MJ, Tracy RP, Hennekens CH. Inflammation, aspirin, and the risk of cardiovascular disease in apparently healthy men. *N Engl J Med*. 1997; 336(14):973-979.

[246] Gussekloo J, Schaap MC, Frolich M, Blauw GJ, Westendorp RG. C-reactive protein is a strong but nonspecific risk factor of fatal stroke in elderly persons. *Arterioscler Thromb Vasc Biol*. 2000; 20(4):1047-1051.

[247] Strandberg TE, Tilvis RS. C-reactive protein, cardiovascular risk factors, and mortality in a prospective study in the elderly. *Arterioscler Thromb Vasc Biol*. 2000; 20(4):1057-1060.

[248] Ridker PM, Rifai N, Rose L, Buring JE, Cook NR. Comparison of C-reactive protein and low-density lipoprotein cholesterol levels in the prediction of first cardiovascular events. *N Engl J Med*. 2002; 347(20):1557-1565.

[249] Ridker PM. High-sensitivity C-reactive protein: potential adjunct for global risk assessment in the primary prevention of cardiovascular disease. *Circulation*. 2001; 103(13):1813-1818.

[250] Horowitz GL, Beckwith BA. C-reactive protein in the prediction of cardiovascular disease. *N Engl J Med*. 2000; 343(7):512-513.

[251] Chung MK, Martin DO, Sprecher D, Wazni O, Kanderian A, Carnes CA et al. C-reactive protein elevation in patients with atrial arrhythmias: inflammatory mechanisms and persistence of atrial fibrillation. *Circulation*. 2001; 104(24):2886-2891.

[252] Takahashi T, Anzai T, Yoshikawa T, Maekawa Y, Asakura Y, Satoh T et al. Serum C-reactive protein elevation in left ventricular remodeling after acute myocardial infarction--role of neurohormones and cytokines. *Int J Cardiol*. 2003; 88(2-3):257-265.

[253] Shlipak MG, Fried LF, Crump C, Bleyer AJ, Manolio TA, Tracy RP et al. Elevations of inflammatory and procoagulant biomarkers in elderly persons with renal insufficiency. *Circulation*. 2003; 107(1):87-92.

[254] Zebrack JS, Anderson JL, Beddhu S, Horne BD, Bair TL, Cheung A et al. Do associations with C-reactive protein and extent of coronary artery disease account for the increased cardiovascular risk of renal insufficiency? *J Am Coll Cardiol*. 2003; 42(1):57-63.

[255] Colhoun HM, Schalkwijk C, Rubens MB, Stehouwer CD. C-reactive protein in type 1 diabetes and its relationship to coronary artery calcification. *Diabetes Care*. 2002; 25(10):1813-1817.

[256] Connelly PW, Hanley AJ, Harris SB, Hegele RA, Zinman B. Relation of waist circumference and glycemic status to C-reactive protein in the Sandy Lake Oji-Cree. *Int J Obes Relat Metab Disord*. 2003; 27(3):347-354.

[257] Freeman DJ, Norrie J, Caslake MJ, Gaw A, Ford I, Lowe GD et al. C-reactive protein is an independent predictor of risk for the development of diabetes in the West of Scotland Coronary Prevention Study. *Diabetes*. 2002; 51(5):1596-1600.

[258] Jager A, van Hinsbergh VW, Kostense PJ, Emeis JJ, Yudkin JS, Nijpels G et al. von Willebrand factor, C-reactive protein, and 5-year mortality in diabetic and nondiabetic subjects: the Hoorn Study. *Arterioscler Thromb Vasc Biol*. 1999; 19(12):3071-3078.

[259] Matsumoto K, Sera Y, Abe Y, Ueki Y, Tominaga T, Miyake S. Inflammation and insulin resistance are independently related to all-cause of death and cardiovascular events in Japanese patients with type 2 diabetes mellitus. *Atherosclerosis*. 2003; 169(2):317-321.

[260] Thorand B, Lowel H, Schneider A, Kolb H, Meisinger C, Frohlich M et al. C-reactive protein as a predictor for incident diabetes mellitus among middle-aged men: results from the MONICA Augsburg cohort study, 1984-1998. *Arch Intern Med*. 2003; 163(1):93-99.

[261] Wolf M, Sandler L, Hsu K, Vossen-Smirnakis K, Ecker JL, Thadhani R. First-trimester C-reactive protein and subsequent gestational diabetes. *Diabetes Care*. 2003; 26(3):819-824.

[262] Shamsuzzaman AS, Winnicki M, Lanfranchi P, Wolk R, Kara T, Accurso V et al. Elevated C-reactive protein in patients with obstructive sleep apnea. *Circulation*. 2002; 105(21):2462-2464.

[263] Teramoto S, Yamamoto H, Ouchi Y. Increased C-reactive protein and increased plasma interleukin-6 may synergistically affect the progression of coronary atherosclerosis in obstructive sleep apnea syndrome. *Circulation*. 2003; 107(5):E40.

[264] Bellomo G, Lippi G, Saronio P, Reboldi G, Verdura C, Timio F et al. Inflammation, infection and cardiovascular events in chronic hemodialysis patients: a prospective study. *J Nephrol*. 2003; 16(2):245-251.

[265] Chul SK, Suh JY, Kim BS, Kang JH, Kim H, Lee MH et al. High sensitivity c-reactive protein as an independent risk factor for essential hypertension. *Am J Hypertens*. 2003; 16(6):429-433.

[266] Di Napoli M, Papa F. Association Between Blood Pressure and C-Reactive Protein Levels in Acute Ischemic Stroke. *Hypertension*. 2003; 42(6):1117-1123.

[267] Chambers JC, Eda S, Bassett P, Karim Y, Thompson SG, Gallimore JR et al. C-reactive protein, insulin resistance, central obesity, and coronary heart disease risk in Indian Asians from the United Kingdom compared with European whites. *Circulation*. 2001; 104(2):145-150.

[268] Cook DG, Mendall MA, Whincup PH, Carey IM, Ballam L, Morris JE et al. C-reactive protein concentration in children: relationship to adiposity and other cardiovascular risk factors. *Atherosclerosis*. 2000; 149(1):139-150.

[269] De Maat MP, Kluft C. Determinants of C-reactive protein concentration in blood. *Ital Heart J.* 2001; 2(3):189-195.

[270] Gillum RF. Association of serum C-reactive protein and indices of body fat distribution and overweight in Mexican American children. *J Natl Med Assoc.* 2003; 95(7):545-552.

[271] Pieroni L, Bastard JP, Piton A, Khalil L, Hainque B, Jardel C. Interpretation of circulating C-reactive protein levels in adults: body mass index and gender are a must. *Diabetes Metab.* 2003; 29(2 Pt 1):133-138.

[272] Han TS, Sattar N, Williams K, Gonzalez-Villalpando C, Lean ME, Haffner SM. Prospective study of C-reactive protein in relation to the development of diabetes and metabolic syndrome in the Mexico City Diabetes Study. *Diabetes Care.* 2002; 25(11):2016-2021.

[273] Ridker PM, Buring JE, Cook NR, Rifai N. C-reactive protein, the metabolic syndrome, and risk of incident cardiovascular events: an 8-year follow-up of 14 719 initially healthy American women. *Circulation.* 2003; 107(3):391-397.

[274] Sattar N, Gaw A, Scherbakova O, Ford I, O'Reilly DS, Haffner SM et al. Metabolic syndrome with and without C-reactive protein as a predictor of coronary heart disease and diabetes in the West of Scotland Coronary Prevention Study. *Circulation.* 2003; 108(4):414-419.

[275] Tracy RP. Inflammation, the metabolic syndrome and cardiovascular risk. *Int J Clin Pract Suppl.* 2003; (134):10-17.

[276] Wakatsuki A, Okatani Y, Fukaya T. Effect of transdermal estradiol and oral conjugated equine estrogen on C-reactive protein in retinoid-placebo trial in healthy women. *Circulation.* 2003; 107(18):e127-e128.

[277] Decensi A, Omodei U, Robertson C, Bonanni B, Guerrieri-Gonzaga A, Ramazzotto F et al. Effect of transdermal estradiol and oral conjugated estrogen on C-reactive protein in retinoid-placebo trial in healthy women. *Circulation.* 2002; 106(10):1224-1228.

[278] Silvestri A, Gebara O, Vitale C, Wajngarten M, Leonardo F, Ramires JA et al. Increased levels of C-reactive protein after oral hormone replacement therapy may not be related to an increased inflammatory response. *Circulation.* 2003; 107(25):3165-3169.

[279] Abramson JL, Vaccarino V. Relationship between physical activity and inflammation among apparently healthy middle-aged and older US adults. *Arch Intern Med.* 2002; 162(11):1286-1292.

[280] Ford ES. Does exercise reduce inflammation? Physical activity and C-reactive protein among U.S. adults. *Epidemiology.* 2002; 13(5):561-568.

[281] Isasi CR, Deckelbaum RJ, Tracy RP, Starc TJ, Berglund L, Shea S. Physical fitness and C-reactive protein level in children and young adults: the Columbia University BioMarkers Study. *Pediatrics.* 2003; 111(2):332-338.

[282] Rothenbacher D, Hoffmeister A, Brenner H, Koenig W. Physical activity, coronary heart disease, and inflammatory response. *Arch Intern Med.* 2003; 163(10):1200-1205.

[283] Albert MA, Glynn RJ, Ridker PM. Alcohol consumption and plasma concentration of C-reactive protein. *Circulation.* 2003; 107(3):443-447.

[284] Bermudez EA, Rifai N, Buring J, Manson JE, Ridker PM. Interrelationships among circulating interleukin-6, C-reactive protein, and traditional cardiovascular risk factors in women. *Arterioscler Thromb Vasc Biol.* 2002; 22(10):1668-1673.

[285] Brenner H, Rothenbacher D, Bode G, Marz W, Hoffmeister A, Koenig W. Coronary heart disease risk reduction in a predominantly beer-drinking population. *Epidemiology.* 2001; 12(4):390-395.

[286] Miller GE, Stetler CA, Carney RM, Freedland KE, Banks WA. Clinical depression and inflammatory risk markers for coronary heart disease. *Am J Cardiol.* 2002; 90(12):1279-1283.

[287] Steptoe A, Kunz-Ebrecht SR, Owen N. Lack of association between depressive symptoms and markers of immune and vascular inflammation in middle-aged men and women. *Psychol Med.* 2003; 33(4):667-674.

[288] Tiemeier H, Hofman A, van Tuijl HR, Kiliaan AJ, Meijer J, Breteler MM. Inflammatory proteins and depression in the elderly. *Epidemiology.* 2003; 14(1):103-107.

[289] Slade GD, Offenbacher S, Beck JD, Heiss G, Pankow JS. Acute-phase inflammatory response to periodontal disease in the US population. *J Dent Res.* 2000; 79(1):49-57.

[290] Slade GD, Ghezzi EM, Heiss G, Beck JD, Riche E, Offenbacher S. Relationship between periodontal disease and C-reactive protein among adults in the Atherosclerosis Risk in Communities study. *Arch Intern Med.* 2003; 163(10):1172-1179.

[291] Wehrmacher WH. Periodontal disease predicts and possibly contributes to acute myocardial infarction. *Dent Today.* 2001; 20(4):80-81.

[292] De Maat MP, Kluft C. The association between inflammation markers, coronary artery disease and smoking. *Vascul Pharmacol.* 2002; 39(3):137-139.

[293] Brull DJ, Serrano N, Zito F, Jones L, Montgomery HE, Rumley A et al. Human CRP Gene Polymorphism Influences CRP Levels. Implications for the Prediction and Pathogenesis of Coronary Heart Disease. *Arterioscler Thromb Vasc Biol.* 2003; 23(11):2063-2069.

[294] Chatha K, Anderson NR, Gama R. Ethnic variation in C-reactive protein: UK resident Indo-Asians compared with Caucasians. *J Cardiovasc Risk.* 2002; 9(3):139-141.

[295] Hubacek JA, Stavek P, Pit'ha J, Skodova Z, Poledne R. [CD14 (C-159-->T) polymorphism and levels of C-reactive protein]. *Cas Lek Cesk.* 2003; 142(3):174-176.

[296] Retterstol L, Eikvar L, Berg K. A twin study of C-Reactive Protein compared to other risk factors for coronary heart disease. *Atherosclerosis.* 2003; 169(2):279-282.

[297] Herbeth B, Siest G, Henny J. High sensitivity C-reactive protein (CRP) reference intervals in the elderly. *Clin Chem Lab Med.* 2001; 39(11):1169-1170.

[298] Schmidt R, Schmidt H, Curb JD, Masaki K, White LR, Launer LJ. Early inflammation and dementia: a 25-year follow-up of the Honolulu-Asia Aging Study. *Ann Neurol.* 2002; 52(2):168-174.

[299] Yaffe K, Lindquist K, Penninx BW, Simonsick EM, Pahor M, Kritchevsky S et al. Inflammatory markers and cognition in well-functioning African-American and white elders. *Neurology.* 2003; 61(1):76-80.

[300] Yu H, Rifai N. High-sensitivity C-reactive protein and atherosclerosis: from theory to therapy. *Clin Biochem.* 2000; 33(8):601-610.

[301] Danesh J, Pepys MB. C-reactive protein in healthy and in sick populations. *Eur Heart J*. 2000; 21(19):1564-1565.

[302] Ford ES, Giles WH, Myers GL, Mannino DM. Population distribution of high-sensitivity C-reactive protein among US men: findings from National Health and Nutrition Examination Survey 1999-2000. *Clin Chem*. 2003; 49(4):686-690.

[303] Hutchinson WL, Koenig W, Frohlich M, Sund M, Lowe GD, Pepys MB. Immunoradiometric assay of circulating C-reactive protein: age-related values in the adult general population. *Clin Chem*. 2000; 46(7):934-938.

[304] Imhof A, Frohlich M, Loewel H, Helbecque N, Woodward M, Amouyel P et al. Distributions of C-reactive protein measured by high-sensitivity assays in apparently healthy men and women from different populations in Europe. *Clin Chem*. 2003; 49(4):669-672.

[305] Kayaba K, Ishikawa S, Gotoh T, Nago N, Kajii E, Nakamura Y et al. Five-year intra-individual variability in C-reactive protein levels in a Japanese population-based study: the Jichi Medical School Cohort Study at Yamato, 1993-1998. *Jpn Circ J*. 2000; 64(4):303-308.

[306] Primatesta P, Falaschetti E, Poulter NR. Influence of hormone replacement therapy on C-reactive protein: population-based data. *J Cardiovasc Risk*. 2003; 10(1):57-60.

[307] Rifai N, Ridker PM. Population distributions of C-reactive protein in apparently healthy men and women in the United States: implication for clinical interpretation. *Clin Chem*. 2003; 49(4):666-669.

[308] Chenillot O, Henny J, Steinmetz J, Herbeth B, Wagner C, Siest G. High sensitivity C-reactive protein: biological variations and reference limits. *Clin Chem Lab Med*. 2000; 38(10):1003-1011.

[309] Kluft C, De Maat MP. Determination of the habitual low blood level of C-reactive protein in individuals. *Ital Heart J*. 2001; 2(3):172-180.

[310] Ledue TB, Rifai N. Preanalytic and analytic sources of variations in C-reactive protein measurement: implications for cardiovascular disease risk assessment. *Clin Chem*. 2003; 49(8):1258-1271.

[311] Ockene IS, Matthews CE, Rifai N, Ridker PM, Reed G, Stanek E. Variability and classification accuracy of serial high-sensitivity C-reactive protein measurements in healthy adults. *Clin Chem*. 2001; 47(3):444-450.

[312] Middleton J. Effect of analytical error on the assessment of cardiac risk by the high-sensitivity C-reactive protein and lipid screening model. *Clin Chem*. 2002; 48(11):1955-1962.

[313] Manson JE, Hsia J, Johnson KC, Rossouw JE, Assaf AR, Lasser NL et al. Estrogen plus progestin and the risk of coronary heart disease. *N Engl J Med*. 2003; 349(6):523-534.

[314] Pradhan AD, Manson JE, Rossouw JE, Siscovick DS, Mouton CP, Rifai N et al. Inflammatory biomarkers, hormone replacement therapy, and incident coronary heart disease: prospective analysis from the Women's Health Initiative observational study. *JAMA*. 2002; 288(8):980-987.

[315] Gotto AM, Jr. Statins and C-reactive protein: considering a novel marker of cardiovascular risk. *Prev Cardiol*. 2002; 5(4):200-203.

[316] Di Napoli M. Benefits of statins in cerebrovascular disease. *Curr Opin Investig Drugs*. 2004; 5(3):295-305.

[317] Blake GJ, Ridker PM, Kuntz KM. Potential cost-effectiveness of C-reactive protein screening followed by targeted statin therapy for the primary prevention of cardiovascular disease among patients without overt hyperlipidemia. *Am J Med.* 2003; 114(6):485-494.

[318] Ess SM, Szucs TD. Medical-economical aspects of high sensitivity C-reactive protein assay for the prediction of coronary heart disease. An analysis in Germany and Italy. *Ital Heart J.* 2001; 2(3):181-188.

[319] Ridker PM. Clinical application of C-reactive protein for cardiovascular disease detection and prevention. *Circulation.* 2003; 107(3):363-369.

[320] Di Napoli M, Papa F. Clinical use of C-reactive protein for prognostic stratification in ischemic stroke: has the time come for including it in the patient risk profile? *Stroke.* 2003; 34(2):375-376.

[321] Di Napoli M, Papa F. Inflammation, statins, and outcome after ischemic stroke. *Stroke.* 2001; 32(10):2446-2447.

[322] Di Napoli M, Papa F, Bocola V. Periodontal disease, C-reactive protein, and ischemic stroke. *Arch Intern Med.* 2001; 161(9):1234-1235.

[323] Cha JK, Jeong MH, Lee KM, Bae HR, Lim YJ, Park KW et al. Changes in platelet p-selectin and in plasma C-reactive protein in acute atherosclerotic ischemic stroke treated with a loading dose of clopidogrel. *J Thromb Thrombolysis.* 2002; 14(2):145-150.

[324] Lalouschek W, Lang W, Greisenegger S, Mullner M. Determination of lipid profiles and use of statins in patients with ischemic stroke or transient ischemic attack. *Stroke.* 2003; 34(1):105-110.

[325] Di Napoli M, Papa F. Angiotensin-Converting Enzyme Inhibitor Use Is Associated With Reduced Plasma Concentration of C-Reactive Protein in Patients With First-Ever Ischemic Stroke. *Stroke.* 2003; 34(12):2922-2924.

[326] Di Napoli M. Editorial comment--C-reactive protein and vascular risk in stroke patients: potential use for the future. *Stroke.* 2003; 34(10):2468-2470.

[327] Gorelick PB, Sachar R, Smith DB, Alberts M, Mustone-Alexander L, Rader D et al. Prevention of a first stroke: a review of guidelines and a multidisciplinary consensus statement from the National Stroke Association. *JAMA.* 1999; 281(12):1112-1120.

[328] Deplanque D, Gele P, Petrault O, Six I, Furman C, Bouly M et al. Peroxisome proliferator-activated receptor-alpha activation as a mechanism of preventive neuroprotection induced by chronic fenofibrate treatment. *J Neurosci.* 2003; 23(15):6264-6271.

[329] Frohlich KU, Fries HW, Rudiger M, Erdmann R, Botstein D, Mecke D. Yeast cell cycle protein CDC48p shows full-length homology to the mammalian protein VCP and is a member of a protein family involved in secretion, peroxisome formation, and gene expression. *J Cell Biol.* 1991; 114(3):443-453.

[330] Koenig W. Update on C-reactive protein as a risk marker in cardiovascular disease. *Kidney Int Suppl.* 2003;(84):S58-S61.

[331] Szalai AJ. The biological functions of C-reactive protein. *Vascul Pharmacol.* 2002; 39(3):105-107.

[332] Pepys MB, Hirschfield GM. C-reactive protein and atherothrombosis. *Ital Heart J.* 2001; 2(3):196-199.

In: Progress in Inflammation Research
Editor: James A. Pitzer, pp. 147-163

ISBN 1-59454-277-5

Chapter IV

Nitric Oxide Metabolism in Muscle Mitochondria in Endotoxic and Septic Shock

Silvia Alvarez* and Alberto Boveris
Laboratory of Free Radical Research, School of Pharmacy and Biochemistry, University of Buenos Aires, Buenos Aires, Argentina

Abstract

Endotoxemia and septic shock occur with an exacerbated inflammatory response that damages tissue mitochondria. Skeletal muscle appears as one of the main target organs in septic shock, showing an increased nitric oxide (NO) production and an early oxidative stress. Heart and diaphragm mitochondria produced, in normal conditions, 67 and 24% of maximal total cellular NO production, and endotoxemic rats showed 30-90% increased mtNOS activity. Heart and diaphragm mitochondrial $O_2^{\bullet -}$ and H_2O_2 production were 2-3 increased during endotoxemia and Mn-SOD activity showed a 2 fold increase in treated animals. One of the current hypothesis for the molecular mechanisms underlying the complex condition of septic shock is that the enhanced NO production by mtNOS and cytosolic iNOS leads to excessive peroxynitrite production and protein nitration in the mitochondrial matrix, causing mitochondrial dysfunction and contractile failure. The available data suggest that impairment of mitochondrial function based on the pathological alteration of NO metabolism and on the production of toxic oxidative and nitrosative species, constitutes the basis of the molecular mechanism of organ dysfunction in endotoxic and septic shock. The high NO production by mtNOS and mitochondrial dysfunction, which are characteristics of the septic shock syndrome, open new avenues for experimentation and for the analisis of clinical data.

* Corresponding author:Silvia Alvarez, Physical-Chemistry Division, School of Pharmacy and Biochemistry, University of Buenos Aires, Junin 956, C1113AAD, Buenos Aires, Argentina, salvarez@ffyb.uba.ar

Keywords: endotoxemia, LPS, mitochondria, mitochondrial nitric oxide synthase, heart, diaphragm

Septic Shock

Septic shock constitutes a major cause of death following trauma and a persistent problem in surgical patients. Three related syndromes, with the common background of sepsis, are recognized in increasing order of severity: systemic inflammatory response syndrome (SIRS), septic shock, and multiple organ failure (MOF). The onset of sepsis is characterized by fever, usually accompanied by shrivering or hypothermia, tachycardia and tachypnea. These symptoms characterize SIRS, and evolve to septic shock when hypotension and loss of concience appears, and to MOF when organ dysfunction develops. The mortality of sepsis increases dramatically when the situation is assiciated to MOF. The prevalent hypothesis regarding the mechanism of the three related syndromes is that they are caused by an excessive defensive and inflammatory response. Recently, inflammation has been defined as a state with increased concentrations of NO and of inflammatory cytokines, mainly interleukin 1-β (IL-1) and tumor necrosis factor-α (TNF-α), in this way leading to a new operational concept (Dianzani, 1996), that replaced the old one describing inflammation with the macroscopic characteristics of redness, heat, pain and swelling. Nitric oxide influences many aspects of the inflammatory cascade ranging from its own increased production by sensitive and immunocompetent cells, to the recruitment of leukocytes and macrophages. Septic shock constitutes a paradigm of acute whole body inflammation, with massive increases of NO and inflammatory cytokines in the biological fluids, with systemic damage to vascular endothelium, and with impaired tissue and whole body respiration despite adequate oxygen supply (Goris, 1985; Pinsky, 2001; De Angelo, 1999).

Septic shock is initiated by components of the cell wall of gram-positive or gram-negative bacteria. Gram-negative bacteria contain an endotoxin (lipopolisaccharide or LPS), which is the cell wall component responsible for the early events leading to a massive inflammatory response and septic shock. The cell wall of gram-positive bacteria contains lipoteichoic acid (LTA) and peptidoglycan (PepG). The LPS from *Escherichia coli* is extensively used in experimental septic shock and consists of a polysaccharide, an oligosaccharide core and a highly conserved lipid A portion. The lipid A moiety is understood as responsible for the toxic proinflammatory properties of LPS (Raetz, 1990; Darveau, 1998). LPS induces a receptor-mediated signaling cascade in the sensitive and immunocompetent cells, that leads to NF-κB activation, the transcription and subsequent release of cytokines and other proinflammatory mediators by monocytes and macrophages. This situation induces the expression or mRNA of a variety of pro-inflammatory mediators including TNF-α, ILs, adhesion molecules and enzymes, such as cyclooxygenase-2 (COX-2) and iNOS, which are implicated in the pathogenesis of septic shock (Christman, 1998; Cadenas, 2002). The intracellular factors that regulate the degree of activation of NF-κB following LPS activation are complex and seem to be controlled by the cellular redox status (Flohé, 1997). An incresing number of reports indicate that antioxidants, as vitamin E-derivatives, α-lipoic acid, DMSO or glutathione, abolish NF-κB activation in response to

LPS strongly supporting involvement of reactive oxygen species in NF-κB activation. Moreover, patients with sepsis present increased concentrations of markers of oxidative damage (as ascorbyl radical content, TBARS, conjugated dienes or xanthine oxidase activity) and low concentrations of plasma antioxidants (vitamin E, selenium and glutathione peroxidase) (Ogilvie, 1991; Galley, 1996). During the last decade, significant advances have been made in clarifying the LPS signalling pathway that leads to NF-κB activation and proinflammatory gene transcription. The NF-κB pathway represents an attractive therapeutic target in strategies for controlling acute and excessive inflammation (Goode, 1995; Borrelli, 1996; Spapen, 1998).

Treatment of septic shock usually includes respiratory support to optimize tissue oxygenation, intravenous fluid administration, broad-spectrum antimicrobial therapy and anti-inflammatory agents (glucocorticoids and nonsteroidal anti-inflammatory drugs), and vasoppressor support; all of wich are limited in their effectiveness. Competitive inhibitors of NOS activity were considered as potentially useful in the treatment of the severe hypotension of septic shock (Gray, 1990; Kilbourn 1990; Wei, 1995, Hobbs, 1999). However, clinical trials using L-NMMA (targinine) failed to show a beneficial effect in septic shock patients (Ruetten, 2000). The new inhibitors of CXCL-8 receptors, that reduce neutrophil recruitment and activation (Cutrin, 2004), seem at the moment the best pharmacological approach for septic shock.

Cellular and Mitochondrial Production of Superoxide Radical, Hydrogen Peroxide and Nitric Oxide

Superoxide anion radical ($O_2^{\bullet-}$) and hydrogen peroxide (H_2O_2) are products of the partial reduction of oxygen normally produced as by-products of mitochondrial respiration and as products of cytosolic and peroxisomal enzyme activities. The main quantitative intracellular sources of H_2O_2 are: mitochondria, endoplasmic reticulum and peroxisomes in hepatocytes; mitochondria and peroxisomes in kidney cortex, mitochondria and endoplasmic reticulum in lung and mitochondria in all other cell types. Of course, phagocytes are effective sources of intracellular H_2O_2. In mitochondria, $O_2^{\bullet-}$ is the stoichiometric precursor of H_2O_2, by a reaction catalyzed by the matrix enzyme manganese-superoxide dismutase (Mn-SOD). In the endoplasmic reticulum both $O_2^{\bullet-}$ and H_2O_2 are primarily generated and in similar amounts. Peroxisomal oxidases produce H_2O_2 as final product and $O_2^{\bullet-}$ as a intraperoxisomal metabolite, is negligible. The concentration of $O_2^{\bullet-}$ in mitochondria and in bacteria (10^{-10} M) (Boveris, 1997) are similar and about ten-times higher than in the cytosol, where it is about 10^{-11} M. The production of $O_2^{\bullet-}$ in mitochondria is a normal consequence of aerobic metabolism due to the autoxidation of electron transfer intermediates, such as ubisemiquinone and the semiquinone of the flavin moiety of NADH-dehydrogenase whose occurrence is inherent to mitochondrial function. In fact, diversion of electrons to reduce oxygen by direct one-electron transfer is a thermodynamically favored and kinetically unfavoured process for the reduced states of all the components of the mitochondrial respiratory chain. Some intermediates such as the mentioned ubisemiquinone and the flavin semiquinone of NADH-dehydrogenase are kinetically able to undergo collisional and noncatalyzed reactions with one-electron transfer to the O_2 molecule (Boveris, 1982). These autoxidation rates, with turnover numbers of 0.5 and 2 min^{-1} for the quinone and the flavin, respectively, are 200-400 times slower than the rates of electron transfer between the components of the respiratory chain that exhibit turover numbers of 100 and 800 min^{-1} for the quinone and the flavin, respectively. The majority of mitochondrial $O_2^{\bullet-}$ (70-80%) is vectorially released to the mitochondrial matrix, but recently it was found that a 20-30% is released to the mitochondrial intermembrane space (Han, 2001). The process of mitochondrial production of H_2O_2 is strongly modulated by the mitochondrial metabolic state and by the intramitochondrial concentration of NO (Boveris, 2000). The mitochondrial rates of H_2O_2 production are 6-10 times higher in the resting mitochondrial state 4 than in the active mitochondrial state 3. The exposure of mitochondria or submitochondrial particles to NO initiates or markedly increases the mitochondrial production of both $O_2^{\bullet-}$ and H_2O_2 (Poderoso, 1996, Packer, 1996); the molecular mechanism is afforded by the NO-inhibition of electron transfer at ubiquinol-cytochrome c reductase.

The discovery of NO by Ignarro (1987) opened a broad perspective in vascular regulation and pharmacology, but also allowed to explore the NO effects in inflammation and cellular metabolism. Nitric oxide is now recognized as a ubiquitous signaling molecule, acting both as an intecellular messenger and as intracellular regulator. Three different genomic nitric oxide synthases (NOS) have been identified: the neuronal NOS (nNOS or NOS-I), the inducible or macrophague NOS (iNOS or NOS-II) and the endothelial NOS (eNOS or NOS-III) (Ignarro, 2000). A fourth type, mitochondrial NOS (mtNOS), differentiated by its subcellular localization in the mitochondrial inner membrane, was simultaneously reported in rat liver mitochondria by Ghafourifar and Richter (1997) and Giulivi (1998a). NO production was reported in rat brain (Lores-Arnaiz, 1999; Lacza, 2001), kidney (Boveris, 2002), heart (French, 2001; Kanai, 2001) and diaphragm (Boczkowski, 1999; Boveris, 2002) mitochondria. Mitochondria and submitochondrial preparations yield rates of 0.5-1.0 nmol NO/min. mg prot. The finding that mitochondria contain their own isoform of NOS (mtNOS), is consistent with the view of the regulation of mitochondrial energy production by NO. The protein identity of mtNOS deserves a special comment. During the last five years, variants of NOS located in mitochondria (mtNOS) have been immunologically described. Results have not been consistent: a protein with iNOS reactivity was reported in the liver mitochondria from rat, mouse and pig (Tatoyan, 1998; Lacza, 2001), an eNOS reacting enzime was observed in mouse heart mitochondria (Kanai, 2001) and rat liver (Elfering, 2002). Cross reactions due to homology are the best explanation, otherwise mtNOS should encompass a broad spectrum of stucturally and immunologically different proteins resulting from transcriptional or translational variants targeted to mitochondria.

The optimum pH for mtNOS activity is 6.5 and 7.0 for diaphragm and heart mitochondria. In normal animals, the activity in the mitochondrial fraction (mtNOS) accounted for 67% (heart) and 24% (diaphragm) of the maximal total cellular NOS activity. Total cellular NOS activity was calculated as the sum of the mitochondrial activity and the activity of the post mitochondrial isolation supernatantat (cytosol) at each corresponding physiological pH (7.8 for the mitochondrial matrix and 7.0 for the cytosol). Kinetic studies and double-reciprocal plots yielded K_M values for O_2 of 4.6 μM (diaphragm) and 3.3 μM (heart), and K_M values for L-arg of 37 μM (diaphragm) and 36 μM (heart).

The subcellular distribution of NOS activities and their complementation for physiological function is just starting to be understood. In liver and thymus, an mtNOS and an endoplasmic reticulum NOS with different properties and immunoreactivity have been described (Bustamante, 2002). In brain an mtNOS coexists with a cytosolic-synaptosomal NOS, both with different properties and similar immunoreactivity (Riobó, 2002; Lores-Arnaiz, 2004).

The Effects of NO and Peroxynitrite in Mitochondrial Electron Transfer

The property of NO of inhibiting mitochondrial electron transfer was first recognized in 1994 by two British research groups (Cleeter, 1994; Brown and Cooper, 1994) that reported the inhibition of brain and muscle cytochrome oxidase (complex IV) activity by low NO concentrations in a reversible and O_2-competitive manner. The observation was rapidly confirmed by other groups using NO donors and pure NO and liver, heart and brown fat mitochondria (Poderoso 1996; Takehara 1995; Koivisto 1997; Nizoli, 2003). Nitric oxide levels of 0.1-0.2 μM decreased mitochondrial respiration to one half, at O_2/NO ratios of about 150 (Boveris, 2000).

A second point in the mitochondrial respiratory chain that is sensitive to NO, is complex III, ubiquinol-cytochrome c reductase, where a reversible inhibition of electron transfer occurs between cytochromes b and c, and initiates or enhances mitochondrial $O_2^{\bullet-}$ and H_2O_2 production (Poderoso, 1996). Complex III is less sensitive to NO inhibition (IC_{50} = 0.25 μM) than complex IV (IC_{50} = 0.15 μM). An irreversible inhibition of complex III activity by peroxynitrite has been reported by Cassina and Radi (1996).

The third sensitive point is mitochondrial complex I; in this case the involved nitrogen reactive species is peroxynitrite. A selective inhibition of NADH-dehydrogenase (complex I) activity in submitochondrial particles by $ONOO^-$ has been reported (Riobó, 2001). Peroxynitrite is produced in the mitochondrial matrix by the termination reaction of two free radicals, $O_2^{\bullet-}$ and NO (Beckman, 1996) in the fastest reaction known in biological systems ($k = 1.9 \times 10^{10}\ M^{-1}s^{-1}$), except for the neutralization reaction of H^+ and HO^- ($k = 14 \times 10^{10}\ M^{-1}s^{-1}$). Peroxynitrite is a powerful oxidant, that when produced in excess leads to tyrosine nitration of the intramitochondrial proteins. Intramitochondrial levels of 3-5 nM $ONOO^-$ have been estimated for physiological conditions, and levels above 20-30 nM are considered cytotoxic.

The effects of NO and peroxynitrite on the electron transfer activities of the mitochondrial respiratory chain are illustrated in Fig. 1. The actions of NO on complexes III and IV are likely to occur under physiological conditions and to constitute regulatory devices of the energy supply and cell signaling biochemical devices for mitochondrial function. At variance, the effects of peroxynitrite in complexes I and III are likely to constitute toxic actions that would be determinant of mitochondrial and cell dysfunction in inflammation and septic shock and, through cumulative effects, of mitochondrial and cell aging.

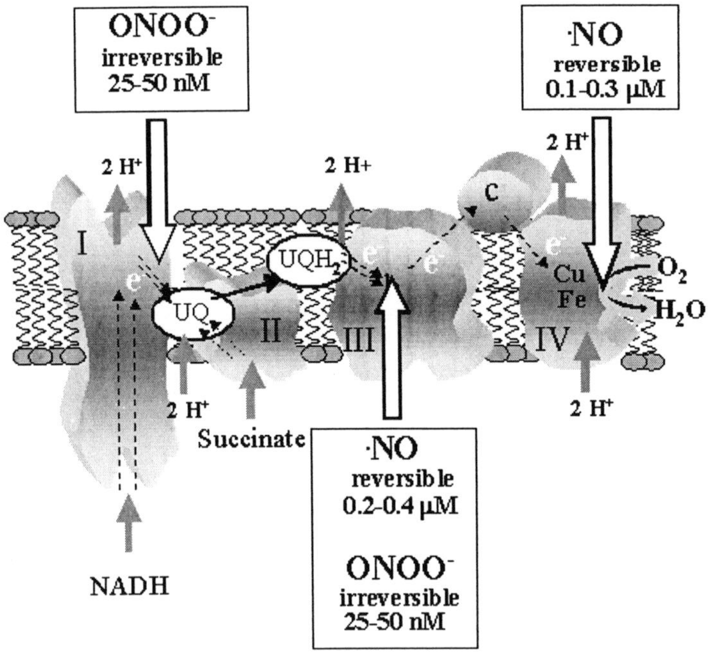

Figure 1. Sites of action of nitric oxide and peroxynitrite in the mitochondrial respiratory chain. Reversible and irreversible indicate the type of inhibition and are understood as regulatory or toxic processes, respectively. The indicated steady-state concentrations were determined or estimated to reduce enzymatic activity to one half, at a concentration of 100-150 □M.

The effects of NO on complexes III and IV can be reproduced by activation of mtNOS in isolated mitochondria. When the organelles are supplemtend with the NOS substrate arginine show a significant decrease in their respiratory rates (Giulivi, 1998b; Boveris, 2003; Lores Arnaiz, 2004). Moreover, mitochondria added with NOS inhibitors, such as L-NMMA or nitro-arginine, exhibit a significant increase in their respiration (Giulivi, 1998b; Boveris, 2003; Lores Arnaiz, 2004).). These two effects are explained by the continous production of NO by mtNOS and by the reversible, oxygen-competitive inhibition and high affinity of cytochrome oxidase by NO (Brown, 1994; Cleeter, 1994; Poderoso, 1996; Koivisto, 1997; Brunori, 1999). The contemporary concept is that mitochondrial and cellular oxygen uptake are regulated by adenosine diphosphate (ADP), O_2, and NO (Brunori, 1999; Boveris, 2001). The biological effect of a given NO concentration due to the O_2-competitive inhibition of cytochrome oxidase will depend on the simultaneous O_2 concentration; lowering the pO_2 increases and extends the effects of NO (Takehara, 1995). Isolated mitochondria supplemented with arginine show increased production of $O_2^{\bullet-}$, H_2O_2 and peroxinitrite. The increase in $O_2^{\bullet-}$ and H_2O_2 production is due to the inhibition of complex III by the mtNOS-produced NO, and the enhanced peroxinitrite formation a consequence of the enhanced intramitochondrial levels of $O_2^{\bullet-}$ and NO. Nitrosylation/nitration of mitochondrial components has been observed in these conditions. Alteration of mitochondrial proteins, complex I for instance, resticts energy output, further increases $O_2^{\bullet-}$ and H_2O_2 generation, and changes cell signalling for proliferation and apoptosis through the redox effects on the specific pathways. These mechanisms are prototypically operating in generalized diseases like sepsis with multiple organ failure, or area-limited neurodegenerative disorders like Parkinsons´disease (Carreras, 2004).

The steady-state concentration of NO in the mitochondrial matrix, is mainly determined by its reactions with $O_2^{\bullet-}$ and ubiquinol. The mitochondrial pathways of $O_2^{\bullet-}$ and NO metabolism are shown in Fig. 2, that also gives the steady-state concentrations of both metabolites and related species in mammalian mitochondria.

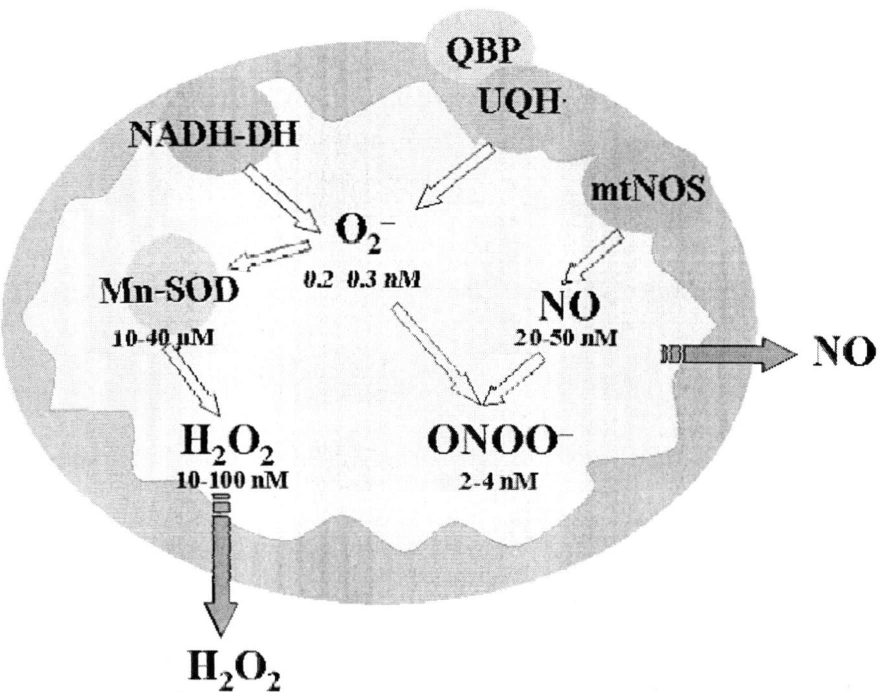

Figure 2. Metabolism of superoxide radical and nitric oxide in the mitochondrial matrix. The number below the symbols indicate the approximate steady-state concentrations for mammalian organs under physiological conditions. The arrows reaching outside the mitochondrion indicate diffusion of H2O2 and NO to the cytosol. QBP: ubiquinone binding protein; NADH-DH: NADH-dehydrogenase.

Nitric Oxide and Superoxide Radical Production in Sepsis

A series of findings led to the concept that NO plays a central role in the molecular mechanism of the cardiovascular alterations of septic shock. These findings are: an elevated circulating nitrite/nitrate, the stable byproducts of NO, in septic patients; a reduction in vascular tone after endotoxin or proinflammatory cytokine administration; and the absolute identification of endothelium-derived relaxing factor (EDRF) as NO. The pathogenic role of

NO in sepsis and septic shock can, in fact, encompass both vascular alterations and the direct cellular toxic effects of NO, peroxynitrite and other NO-derived products.

The free radical view describes the process and consequences of inflammation as a network, involving three radicals: NO, $O_2^{\bullet-}$ and ROO (as produced by cyclo-oxygenases). The role of NO in the pathophysiology of septic shock was advanced by Thiemermann and Vane, who observed that administration of the NOS inhibitor L-NMMA to rats decreased the severe hypotension produced by administration of LPS (Thiemermann, 2000; Ruetten, 2000).

Several studies in experimental animals have shown that NO synthesized by the inducible isoform of the NOS (iNOS) is an important mediator of the decreased force of respiratory and locomotor muscles in sepsis (Boczkowski, 1996; El Dwairi, 1998; Gath, 1996). This seems related to muscular oxidative stress, secondary to the local generation of peroxynitrite (Boczkowski, 1999). In vivo nitration of the iNOS of skeletal muscle from patients with sepsis was shown to occur on four tyrosine residues; a fingerprint of increased $ONOO^-$ formation (Lanone, 2002). Therefore, iNOS-derived peroxynitrite was considered as the main mediators of the deletereous effects of septic shock in muscles (Boczkowski, 2000), although other mediators, as intracellular Ca^{2+}, are not ruled out.

Muscle is one of the target organs in septic shock due to its large contribution to the vascular space and to the extensive vasodilation and hypotension, which are characteristic of septic shock. Increased spontaneous muscle chemiluminescence is an early indicator, simultaneous with hypotermia, of the multiple dysfunction of septic shock in rats (Llesuy, 1994). Moreover, skeletal muscle failure, with impaired respiration and movements, is frequently associated with sepsic shock and MOF. It was early recognized that endotoxic and septic shock produce dramatic metabolic changes in skeletal muscle metabolism (Clowes, 1983; Raymond, 1982). The most entertained contemporary view concerning the molecular mechanism of septic shock pathogenesis is that a markedly increased NO production affords the primary event, that leads to increased peroxynitrite formation, nitration, nitrosylation and to a series of secondary metabolic and functional alterations, according to the observations in rat diaphragm (Boczkowski, 1999; Lanone, 2000), human muscle (Lanone, 2000), and dog heart (Preiser, 2001). Significant increases in iNOS mRNA, protein and enzyme activity have been reported in rat diaphragm and human skeletal muscle (Boczkowski, 1999; Lanone, 2000), in the latter case the expression of iNOS protein correlated with sepsis severity.

Mitochondrial Dysfunction and Septic Shock

The concept of a bioenergetic failure due to muscle mitochondrial dysfunction as part of the pathogenic mechanism of septic shock was introduced about 35 years ago (Shumer, 1970; Mela, 1971). This phenomenon is now considered as derived from increased NO and peroxynitrite levels in both the vascular smooth muscle and in skeletal and heart muscle. The whole syndome of mitochondrial dysfunction is characterized by decreased rates of state 3 respiration and ATP synthesis, decreased respiratory controls and membrane potential, increased rates of state 4 respiration, and increased mitochondrial size and fragility.

An association between NO overproduction, antioxidant depletion, mitochondrial dysfunction, and decreased ATP concentrations was recently related to organ failure and eventual outcome (Brealey, 2002). These indicators that correlate with the severity of disease and outcome, support the notion that the mitochondrial dysfunction resulting in bioenergetic failure is the critical factor in the pathophysiology of septic shock and MOF (Brealey, 2003).

Mitochondria isolated from skeletal muscle in endotoxic and septic shocks exhibit impaired respiration. These dysfunctional mitochondria show a decreased active state 3 oxygen uptake, more marked with NAD-linked substrates where the inhibition is in the 30-60% range, than with succinate where the respiration is decreased by 10-40%. Table I summarizes data from a few studies that show that the mitochondrial respiratory rates supported by NAD-linked substrates are significantly decreased in rat and human skeletal muscle during sepsis and in rat heart and diaphragm after LPS administration (Boczkowski, 1999; Llesuy, 1994; Poderoso, 1978; Fukumoto, 2003). The respiratory impairment is due to an inhibition of electron transfer, as it can be inferred from the decreased state 3 respiratory rate, simultaneous with an unchanged state 4 respiration; meaning abscence of uncoupling and normal ADP:O ratios (Callahan, 2001).

Table I. Mitochondrial Respiration Supported by NAD-Linked Substrates in Septic and Endotoxic Shock

	Oxygen Uptake (natom O/ min/mg prot)		
Mitochondria/Condition	state 3	state 4	respiratory control
Rat muscle/septic shock[a]			
Control	149 ± 5	23 ± 2	6.5 ± 0.2
Sepsis, 6 h	120 ± 8	24 ± 3	5.0 ± 0.2
Sepsis, 12 h	97 ± 6	24 ± 8	4.0 ± 0.1
Rat diaphragm/endotoxin[b]			
Control	200 ± 10	32 ± 2	6.2 ± 0.7
Endotoxin, 12 h	183 ± 7	33 ± 3	5.5 ± 0.6
Endotoxin, 24 h	120 ± 10	28 ± 2	4.3 ± 0.2
Rat heart/endotoxin[c]			
Control	117 ± 5	33 ± 4	3.5 ± 0.5
Endotoxin, 2 h	112 ± 7	38 ± 3	2.9 ± 0.3
Endotoxin, 6 h	91 ± 3	39 ± 4	2.3 ± 0.2
Human muscle/septic shock[d]			
Normal patients	171 ± 21	57 ± 10	3.5 ± 0.4
Severe sepsis	81 ± 12	42 ± 8	1.9 ± 0.2
Septic shock	65 ± 16	37 ± 9	1.7 ± 0.2
Cardiogenic shock	119 ± 12	43 ± 7	2.9 ± 0.3

[a]Taken from Llesuy et al, 1994; 6 mM malate and 6 mM glutamate as substrates.

[b]Taken and modified from Boczkowski et al, 1999; 2.5 mM malate and 10 mM pyruvate as substrates.

[c]Taken from Fukumoto et al, 2002 and recalculated according to Lores Arnaiz et al, 2004; 1 mM malate and 10 mM glutamate as substrates.

[d]Taken from Poderoso et al, 1979 and unpublished results; 6 mM malate and 6 mM glutamate as substrates.

The inhibition of electron transfer is now considered as derived by an excessive production of NO by mtNOS and cytosolic iNOS, which leads to: a) inhibition of cytochrome oxidase (complex IV); the excessive production of NO leads to excessive peroxynitrite generation, that in turn leads to b) the inhibition of ubiquinol-cytochrome c reductase (complex III) and, c) inhibition of NADH-ubiquinone reductase (complex I).

This concept of dysfunctional mitochondria is also adessed in other situations or diseases such as ischemia/reperfusion (Gonzalez-Flecha, 1993), aging (Beckman, 1998), Parkinson´s disease and other neurodegenerative disorders (Navarro, 2002).

The decreased mitochondrial respiratory rate agrees with the decreased whole animal oxygen uptake (about 30%) and body temperature, which are associated to septic shock (Llesuy, 1994; Poderoso, 1994). The inhibition of in vitro mitochondrial oxygen uptake was found partly reversible by the addition of serum albumin, meaning that the impairment is also partly due to increased free fatty acid levels. Mitochondrial dysfunction in vivo in human sepsis is reversible as observed in sucessive muscle samples taken from recovering patients (Poderoso, 1978).

Muscle mitochondria isolated from rats with septic shock show a 2.5-2.8 times increased rate of H_2O_2 formation (table II), which appears to reflect the effects of both NO and $ONOO^-$ in ubiquinol-cytochrome c reductase (complex III) (Poderoso, 1996; Cassina, 1996).

Nitric Oxide and Superoxide Radical Production by Heart and Diaphragm Mitochondria During Septic Shock

During the last five years significant and novel findings have been described for NO metabolism in muscle mitochondria during sepsis. The main findings for this syndrome are: a) a marked increase in mtNOS activity and NO production in heart and diaphragm (Boveris 2002; Boczkowski, 1999); b) the mitochondrial productions of $O_2^{\bullet-}$, H_2O_2 and $ONOO^-$ are enhanced (Boczkowski, 1999); c) the increases of the stready-state concentrations of $O_2^{\bullet-}$,H_2O_2 and $ONOO^-$ secondary to a given increase in NO steady state levels, have been described (Alvarez, 2003); d) mtNOS and Mn-SOD show a parallel increase in activity in sepsis (Alvarez, 2003); e) contactile failure follows mitochondrial impairment (Boczkowski, 1999; Escames, 2002); f) a mechanism of translocation of iNOS (determined as a Ca^{2+}-independent activity) to mitochondria was described (Lisdero, 2004).

Experimental endotoxic shock produces a marked increase in the activity of rat diaphragm and heart mtNOS. The production of NO by submitochondrial membranes increased by 122% (diaphragm) and 32% (heart) after 6 h of LPS (10 mg/kg) administration (Table II). The mechanism of mtNOS induction in muscle by endotoxin is not fully understood; however, there is an standing hypothesis that this process involves a protein tyrosyne kinase, NF-κB and nuclear NOS gene activation, mRNA transcription, novel protein biosynthesis, and exportation to mitochondria (Boveris, 2002).

Significant increases in iNOS mRNA, protein and enzyme activity, have been reported in rat diaphragm and human skeletal muscle (Boczkowski, 1999; Lanone, 2000). On the other hand, experimental endotoxic shock was observed to produce a marked increase in the activity of rat diaphragm mtNOS (Boveris, 2002).

The mitochondrial $O_2^{\bullet-}$ and H_2O_2 productions were found increased in endotoxic shock in rats. Preincubation with 1nitroso-glutathione determined an about 80% inhibition of cytochrome *b*-cytochrome *c* electron transfer in complex III with a measurable rate of $O_2^{\bullet-}$ production that was 3 times increased by endotoxic shock in heart mitochondria and 1.8 times in diaphragm mitochondria (Table II). The mitochondrial production of H_2O_2 in mitochondrial state 4 (resting mitochondria with maximal physiological H_2O_2 rates), was also markedly increased in endotoxic shock; 2.6 times in heart mitochondria and 1.8 in diaphragm mitochondria (Table II). High mitochondrial $O_2^{\bullet-}$ and H_2O_2 production during endotoxemia seem due to the irreversible inhibition of the respiratory chain by peroxinitrite (Boveris, 2002; Escames, 2003) Added NO inhibits cytochrome oxidase (complex IV) (Brown, 1995; Brown, 1994) and complex III (Cleeter, 1994) in vitro and increases $O_2^{\bullet-}$ and H_2O_2 production in submitochondrial particles and mitochondria, but these effects that occur in vivo, are lost during mitochondrial isolation.

Diaphragm mitochondria isolated from LPS-treated rats were reported uncoupled with a 7 and 33 % decrease in respiratory control, 3 h and 6 h after LPS inoculation (Boczkowski, 1999). Western blot analysis of diaphragm mitochondrial exhibit a pattern of protein nitration with several bands, similar to the one observed after 30 min of exposure of mitochondria to 1 mM SIN-1 (Lanone, 2002). Nitration of mitochondrial proteins and maximal impairment of mitochondrial function are associated with a significant decrease in diaphragmatic force generation.

Table II. Effect of Endotoxic Shock on NO, $O_2^{\bullet-}$ and H_2O_2 Production in Heart and Diaphragm Mitochondria♦

ORGAN	NO PRODUCTION (nmol /min mg prot.) mitochondria	$O_2^{\bullet-}$ PRODUCTION (nmol /min mg prot.) cytosol	H_2O_2 PRODUCTION (nmol /min mg prot.) mitochondria	mitochondria
		Heart		
Control	0.69 ± 0.04	0.64 ± 0.05	0.86 ± 0.09	0.40 ± 0.07
LPS	0.91 ± 0.08*	0.67 ± 0.05	2.55 ± 0.18*	1.03 ± 0.12*
		Diaphragm		
Control	0.76 ± 0.08	1.13 ± 0.05	1.88 ± 0.12	1.02 ± 0.10
LPS	1.70 ± 0.12*	1.77 ± 0.15*	3.40 ± 0.25*	1.57 ± 0.14*

* ($p<0.01$)

♦ NO production was measured in submitochondrial membranes (SMM) and in cytosol; H_2O_2 production was measured in intact mitochondria; O_2^- production, was measured in SMM. The assay of O_2^- production was carried out after 3 min preincubation with GSNO 100 μM with effective 2 μM NO.

The observed increase in H_2O_2 production (Table II) is in a way in agreement with the observation of higher Mn-SOD activity in endotoxic shock. An increased $O_2^{\bullet-}$ dismutation rate to H_2O_2 catalized by Mn-SOD, is expected to better compete with the $O_2^{\bullet-}$ and NO reaction to yield peroxynitrite. The LPS endotoxin and TNF-α were reported to increase the Mn-SOD content in endothelial cells (Shiki, 1987; Shaffer, 1990).

A correlation of mtNOS and Mn-SOD activity was observed for heart and diaphragm mitochondria during the development of endotoxic shock. A similar pattern was observed during rat brain development (Riobó, 2002). These reports support the idea of a shared genomic expression mechanism for mtNOS and Mn-SOD.

Concluding Remarks

Mitochondria play a central role in the intracellular events associated with inflammation and septic shock, as active sources and sensitive targets of NO. Muscle mitochondria show with a fast time course, a marked increase in mtNOS activity and a reduced respiration (characterized by inhibition of electron transfer) that seem to define the pathological state of the dysfunctional mitochondria, observed in inflammation.

Although the concept of a bipolar distribution of NOS in diaphragm and heart muscle cells has been addressed here, the relative contributions of mtNOS and of NOS cytosolic isoforms to the pathogenesis of inflammation and septic shock constitutes an open and challenging question. Our analysis of the relative contribution of mitochondria to the total cellular capacity of NO synthesis in mammalian organs indicate that the mitochondrial contribution is far from being negligible, with the 60-70% range in heart and in the 20-30% range in diaphragm.

The observations presented here, suggest that the impairment of mitochondrial function based on an increased NO production and on an altered NO metabolism, as well as on the production of oxidative and nitrosative species, constitutes the basis of the molecular mechanism of organ dysfunction in endotoxic and septic shock. Moreover, the observations of high NO production by mtNOS and of mitochondrial dysfunction, which are among the main characteristics of septic shock, open new avenues for experimentation and interpretation of the clinical data.

Acknowledgements

Supported by research grants of University of Buenos Aires (B075), ANPCYT (PICT 00-8710) and CONICET (PIP 02271-00)

References

Alvarez, S., Boveris, A. Muscle mitochondria dysfunction in endotoxemia: NO metabolism. *Free. Rad. Biol. Med.* 35: S51, 2003.

Beckman, K. B.; Ames, B. N. Mitochondrial aging: open questions.*Ann. NY Acad. Sci.* 854: 118-127, 1998.

Beckman, K. B., Koppenol, W. H. Nitric oxide, superoxide, and peroxynitrite: the good, the bad, and the ugly. *Am. J. Physiol.* 271: 1424-1437, 1996.

Boczkowski, J., Lanone, S., Ungureanu-Longrois, D., Danialou, G., Fournier, T., Aubier, M. Induction of diaphragmatic nitric oxide synthase after endotoxin administration in rats. *J. Clin. Invest.* 98: 1550-1559.

Boczkowski, J.; Lisdero, C. L.; Lanone, S.; Samb, A.; Carreras, M. C.; Boveris, A.; Aubier, M.; Poderoso, J. J., Endogenous peroxynitrite mediates mitochondrial dysfunction in rat diaphragm during endotoxemia. *FASEB J.* **13:** 1637-1646;1999.Borrelli, E., Roux-Lombard, P., Grau, G. E., Girardin, E., Ricou, B., Dayer, J., Suter, PM. Plasma concentrations of cytokines, their soluble receptors, and the antioxidant vitamins can predict the development of multiple organ failure in patients at risk. *Crit. Care Med.* 24: 392-397, 1996.

Boveris, A., Cadenas, E. Cellular sources and steady-state levels of reactive oxygen species. In: Biadasz-clerch, L., Massaro, D. (eds.) Oxygen, Gene Expression and Cellular Function, Marcel Dekker, New York, pp. 1-25, 1997.

Boveris, A., Poderoso, J. J. Regulation of oxygen metabolism by nitric oxide. In: Ignarro, L. J. (ed.) *Nitric Oxide: Biology and Pathology*, Academic Press, New York, pp. 355-368, 2000.

Boveris, A., Cadenas, E. Production of superoxide radicals and hydrogen peroxide in mitochondria. In: Oberley, L. W. (ed.) *Superoxide Dismutase*, CRC Press, Boca Ratón, Florida. Pp 15-30, 1982.

Boveris, A., Costa, L. E., Poderoso, J. J., Carreras, M. C., Cadenas, E. Regulation of mitochondrial respiration by oxygen and nitric oxide. *Ann. New York Acad. Sci.* 899: 121-135; 2001.

Boveris, A.; Alvarez, S.; Navarro, A. The role of mitochondrial nitric oxide synthase in inflammation and septic shock. *Free Rad. Biol. Med.* 33: 1186-1193, 2002.

Boveris, A., Valdez, L. B., Alvarez, S., Zaobornyj, T., Boveris, A. D., Navarro, A. Kidney mitochondrial nitric oxide synthase. *Antioxid. Redox. Signal.* 5: 265-271, 2003a.

Brealey, D. Association between mitochondrial dysfunction and severity and outcome of septic shock. *The Lancet* 360: 219-223, 2002.

Brealey, D., Singer, M. Mitochondrial dysfunction in sepsis. *Curr. Infect. Dis. Resp.* 5: 365-371, 2003.

Brown, G. C., Cooper, C. E. Nanomolar concentrations of nitric oxide reversibly inhibits synaptosomal respiration by competing with oxygen at cytochrome oxidase. *FEBS Lett.* 356: 50-54; 1994.

Brown, G.C. Nitric oxide regulates mitochondrial respiration and cell functions by inhibiting cytochrome oxidase. *FEBS Lett.* 369: 136-139, 1995.

Brunori, M., Giuffre, A., Sarti, P., Stubauer, G., Wilson, M. T. Nitric oxide and cellular respiration. *Cell Mol. Life Sci.* 56: 549-557;1999.

Bustamante, J., Bersier, G., Aron Badin, R., Cymering, C., Parodi, A., Boveris, A. Sequential NO production by mitochondria and endoplasmic reticulum during induced apoptosis. *Nitric Oxide* 6: 333-341, 2002.

Cadenas, S., Cadenas, A. M. Fighting the stranger-antioxidant protection against endotoxin toxicity. *Toxicol.* 180:45-63, 2002.

Callahan, L. A., Stofan, D. A., Szweda, L. I., Nethery, D. E., Supinski, G. S. Free radicals alter maximal diaphragmatic mitochondrial oxygen consumption in endotoxin-induced sepsis. *Free Rad. Biol. Med.* 30: 129-138; 2001.

Carreras, M. C.; Franco, M. C.; Peralta, J. C.; Poderoso, J. J. Nitric oxide, complex I, and the modulation of mitochondrial reactive species in biology and disease. *Mol. Aspects Med.* 2004, in press.

Cassina, A., Radi, R. Differential inhibitory action of nitric oxide and peroxynitrite on mitochondrial electron transport. *Arch Biochem Biophys.* 328: 309-316; 1996.

Christman, J. W., Lancaster, L. H., Blackwell, T. S. Nuclear factor-kB: a pivotal role in the systemic inflammation response syndrome and new target for therapy. *Intens. Care Med.* 24: 1131-1138, 1998.

Cleeter, M. W. J., Cooper, V. M., Darley-Usmar, V. M., Moncada, S., Schapira, A. H. V. Reversible inhibition of cytochrome c oxidase, the terminal enzyme of the mitochondrial respiratory chain, by nitric oxide: implications for neurodegenerative diseases. *FEBS Lett.* 356: 295-298; 1994.

Clowes, G. H., George, B. C., Vellee, C. A., Savaris, C. A. Muscle proteolisis induced by a circulating peptide in patients with sepsis of trauma. *N. Engl. J. Med.* 308: 545-552; 1983.

Cutrín, J. C. Repertaxin, a novel non-competitive allosteric inhibitor of the CXCL-8 receptors, reduces the neutrophil recruitment in the rat liver submitted to ischemia/reperfusion injury. *Free Rad. Biol. Med.*, in press, 2004.

Darveau, R. P. Lipid A diversity and the innate host response to bacterial infection. *Curr. Opin. Microbiol.* 1: 36-42, 1998.

De Angelo, J. Nitric oxide scavengers in the treatment of shock associated with systemic inflammatory response syndrome. *Expert. Opin. Pharmacother.* 1: 19-29; 1999.

Dianzani, M. U.; *Trattato di Patologia generale.* Torino: Unione Tipografico-Editrice Torinese; 1996, 1230-1348.

El Dwairi, Q., Comtois, A., Guo, Y., Hussain, S. N. Endotoxin-induced skeletal muscle contractile dysfunction: contribution of nitric oxide synthases. *Am. J. Physiol.* 274: 770-779, 1998.

Elfering, S. L.; Sarkela, T. M.; Giulivi, C. Biochemistry of mitochondrial nitric oxide synthase. *J. Biol. Med.* 277: 38079-38086; 2002.

Escames, G.; León, J.; Macías, L.; Khaldy, H.; Acuña-Castroviejo, D. Melatonin counteracts lipoplosaccharide-induced expresion and activity of mitochondrial nitric oxide synthase in rats. *FASEB J.* 17: 932-934; 2003.

Flohe, L., Brigelius-Flohe, R., Saliou, C., Traber, M., Packer, L. Redox regulation of NF-kappaB activation. *Free Rad. Biol. Med.* 22, 1115-1126, 1997.

French, S., Giulivi, C., Balaban, R. S. Nitric oxide synthase in porcine heart mitochondria: evidence for low physiological activity. *Am. J. Heart Circ. Physiol.* 280: 2863-2867; 2001.

Fukumoto, K., Pierro, A. Spitz, L., Eaton, S. Neonatal endotoxemia affects heart but not kidney bioenergetics. *J. Pediat. Surg.* 38: 690-693, 2003.

Galley, H. F., Davies, M. J., Webster, N. R. Ascorbyl radical formation in patients with sepsis: effect of ascorbate loading. *Free Rad. Biol. Med.* 20: 139-143, 1996.

Ghafourifar, P.; Richter, C. Nitric oxide synthase activity in mitochondria. *FEBS Lett.* 418: 291-296;1997.

Gath, I., Cloos, E. I., Godtel-Armbrust, U., Schmitt, S., Nakane, M., Wessler, I., Fostermann, U. Inducible NO synthase II and neuronal NO synthase I are constitutively expressed in different structures of guinea pig skeletal muscle: implications for contractile function. *FASEB J.* 10: 1614-1620, 1996.

Giulivi, C. Functional implications of nitric oxide produced by mitochondria in mitochondrial metabolism. *Biochem. J.* 332: 673-679; 1998.

Giulivi, C.; Poderoso, J. J.; Boveris, A., Production of nitric oxide by mitochondria. *J Biol Chem.* 273: 11038-11043; 1998.

Gonzalez-Flecha, B.; Cutrín, J. C.; Boveris, A. Time course and mechanism of oxidative stress and tissue damage in rat liver subjected to in vivo ischemia-reperfusion. *J. Clin. Invest.* 91: 456-464, 1993.

Goode, H. F., Cowley, H. C., Walker, B. E., Howde, P. D., Webster, N. R. Decreased antioxidant status and increased lipid peroxidation in patients with septic shock and secondary organ dysfunction. *Crit. Care. Med.* 23: 646-651, 1995.

Goris, R.J., Boekhorst, T.P., Nuytinck, J.K., Gimbere, J.S. Multiple-organ failure. Generalized autodestructive inflammation. *Arch. Surg.* 120: 1109-1115; 1985.

Gray, G. A., Julou-Schaeffer, G., Oury, K., Fleming, I., Parrat, J. R., Stoclet, J. C. An L-arginine-derived factor mediates endotoxin induced vascular hyposensitivity to calcium. *Eur. J. Pharmacol.* 191: 89-92, 1990.

Han, D., Williams, E., Cadenas, E. Mitochondrial respiratory chain-dependent generation of superoxide anion and its release to the intermembrane space. *Biochem. J.* 353: 411-416, 2001.

Hobbs, A. J., Higgs, A., Moncada, S. Inhibition of nitric oxide synthase as a potential therapeutic target. *Annu. Rev. Pharmacol. Toxicol.* 39: 191-220, 1999.

Ignarro, L., Buga, G. M., Wood, K. S., Byrns, R. E., Chaudhuri, G. Endothelium-derived relaxing factor produced and released from artery and vein is nitric oxide. *Proc. Natl. Acad. Sci. USA.* 84: 9265-9269, 1987.

Ignarro, L. J. Introduction and overview. In: Ignarro, L. J. (ed.) *Nitric Oxide: Biology and Pathology*, Academic Press, New York, pp. 3-22, 2000.

Kanai, A. J.; Pearce, L. L.; Clemens, P. R.; Birder, L. A.; Van Bibber, M.M.; Choi, S. I.; de Groat, W. C.; Peterson, J. Identification of a neuronal nitric oxide sinthase in isolated cardiac mitochondria using electrochemical detection. *Proc. Natl. Acad. Sci. USA* 98: 14126-14131; 2001.

Kilbourn, R. G., Jubran, A., Gross, S. S., Grifith, O. W., Levi, R., Adams. Reversal of endotoxin-mediated shock by Ng-methyl-L-arginine, an inhibitor of nitric oxide synthesis. *Biochem. Biophys. Res. Commun.* 172: 1132-1138, 1990.

Koivisto, A., Matthias, A., Bronnikov, G., Nedergard, J. Kinetics of the inhibition of mitochondrial respiration by NO. *FEBS Lett.* 417: 75-80; 1997.

Lacza, Z., Puskar, M., Figueroa, J. P., Zhang, J., Rajapakse, N., Busua, D. W. Mitochondrial nitric oxide synthase is constitutively active and is functionally upregulated in hypoxia. *Free Rad. Biol. Med.* 31: 1609-1615; 2001.

Lanone, S., Mebazaa, A., Heymes, C., Henin, D., Poderoso, J. J., Panis, Y., Zedda, C., Billiar, T., Payen, D., Aubier, M., Boczkowski, J. Muscular contractile failure in septic patients: role of the inducible nitric oxide synthase pathway. *Am. J. Respir. Crit. Care Med.* 162: 2308-2315;2000.

Lanone, S., Manivet, P., Callebert, J., Launay, J. M., Payen, D., Aubier, M., Mebazaa, A. Inducible nitric oxide synthase (NOS2) expressed in septic patients is nitrated on selected tyrosine residues: implications for enzyme activity. *Biochem. J.* 366: 399-404; 2002.

Llesuy, S.; Evelson, P.; Gonzalez-Flecha, B.; Peralta, J.; Carreras, M. C.; Poderoso, J. J.; Boveris, A. Oxidative stress in muscle and liver of rats with septic syndrome. *Free Radic Biol Med.* 16: 445-451;1994

Lores-Arnaiz, S.; Coronel, M. F.; Boveris, A., Nitric oxide, superoxide, and hydrogen peroxide production in brain mitochondria after haloperidol treatment. *Nitric Oxide* 3: 235-243;1999.

Lores-Arnaiz, S., D'Amico, G., Bustamante, J., Boveris, A. Brain mitochondrial nitric oxide synthase: in vitro and in vivo inhibition by chlorpromazine. *Arch. Biochem. Biophys.* In press, 2004.

Mela, L.; Bacalzo, L. V.; Miller, L. D. Defective oxidative metabolism of rat liver mitochondria in hemorrhagic and endotoxemic shock. *Am. J. Physiol.* 220: 571-577; 1971.

Navarro, A.; Sanchez del Pino, M. J.; Gómez, C.; Peralta, J. L.; Boveris, A. Behavioral dysfunction, brain oxidative stress, and impaired mitochondrial electron transfer in aging mice. *Am. J. Physiol. Regulatory Integrative Comp. Physiol.* 282: 985-992, 2002.

Nisoli, E., Clementi, E., Paolucci, C., Cozzi, V., Tonello, C., Sciorati, C., Bracale, R., Valerio, A., Francolini, M., Moncada, S., Carruba, M. Mitochondrial biogenesis in mammals: the role of endogenous nitric oxide. *Science* 299: 896-899, 2003.

Ogilvie, A. C., Groenveld, A. B., Straub, J. P., Thijs, L. G. Plasma lipid peroxides and antioxidants in human septic shock. *Intens. Care Med.* 17: 40-44, 1991.

Packer, M. A., Porteous, C. M., Murphy, M. P. Superoxide production by mitochondria in the presence of nitric oxide forms peroxynitrite. *Biochem. Mol. Biol. Int.* 40: 527-534, 1996.

Pinsky, M. R. Sepsis: a pro- and anti-inflammatory disequilibrium syndrome. *Contrib. Nephrol.* 132: 354-366; 2001.

Poderoso, J. J., Carreras, M. C. Lisdero, C., Riobo, N., Schopfer, F., Boveris, A. Nitric oxide inhibits electron transfer and increases superoxide radical production in rat heart mitochondria and submitochondrial particles. *Arch.Biochem.Biophys.* 328: 85-92; 1996.

Poderoso, J. J.; Boveris, A.; Jorge, M. A.; Gherardi, C. R.; Caprile, A. W.; Turrens, J.; Stoppani, A. O.M. Funcion mitocondrial en el shock septico. *Medicina (B Aires).* 38: 371-377;1978.

Poderoso, J. J.; Lisdero, C.; Schopfer, F.; Riobó, N.; Carreras, M. C.; Cadenas, E.; Boveris, A. The regulation of mitochondrial oxygen uptake by redox reactions involving nitric oxide and ubiquinol. *J. Biol. Chem.* 274: 37709-37716; 1999.

Poderoso, J.J., Fernandez, S., Carreras, M. C., Tchercanski, D., Acevedo, C., Rubio, M., Peralta, J., Boveris, A. Liver oxygen uptake dependence and mitochondrial function in septic rats. *Circ. Shock* 44: 175-182; 1994.

Preiser, J. C., Zhang, H., Vray, B., Hrabak, A., Vincent, J. L. Time course of inducible nitric oxide synthase activity following endotoxin administration in dogs. *Nitric Oxide,* 5: 208-211; 2001.

Raetz, C. R. Biochemistry of endotoxins. *Annu. Rev. Biochem.* 59: 129-170, 1990.

Raymond, R. M., Rosenfeld, G. A., Emerson T. E. Direct effect of insulin and endotoxin on glucose uptake by skeletal muscle during high cardiac index sepsis. *Surg. Gynecol. Obstet.* 88: 87-96; 1982.

Riobó, N. A.; Clementi, E.; Melani, M.; Boveris, A.; Cadenas, E.; Moncada, S.; Poderoso, J. J. Nitric oxide inhibits mitochondrial NADH:ubiquinone reductase activity through peroxinitrite formation. *Biochem. J.* 277: 42447-42455, 2001.

Riobó, N.; Melani, M.; Sanjuán, N.; Fiszman, M.; Gravielle, M. C.; Carreras, M. C.; Cadenas, E.; Poderoso, J. J. The modulation of mitochondrial nitrc oxyde synthase activity in rat brain development. *J. Biol. Chem.* 277: 42447-42455; 2002.

Ruetten, H., Thiemermann, C. Nitric oxide and septic shock. In: Ignarro, L., ed. *Nitric Oxide: Biology and Pathobiology*. San Diego: Academic Press; 2000: 747-758.

Schopfer, F.; Riobó, N. A.; Carreras, M. C.; Alvarez, B.; Radi, R.; Boveris, A.; Cadenas, E.; Poderoso, J. J. Oxidation of ubiquinol by peroxynitrite:implications for protection of mitochondria against nitrosative damage. *Biochem. J.* 349:35-42, 2000.

Shaffer, J. B., Treanor, C. P., Del Vecchio, P. J. Expression of bovine and mouse endothelial cell antioxidant enzymes following TNF-a exposure. *Free Rad. Biol. Med.* 8: 497-502, 1990.

Shiki, Y., Meyrick, B. O., Brigham, K. L., Burr, I. M. Endotoxin increases superoxide dismutase in cultured bovine pulmonary endothelial cells. *Am. J. Physiol.* 252: 436-440, 1987.

Shumer, W., Gupta, T. K., Moss, G. S., Nyhus, L. Effect of endotoxemia on liver cell mitochondria in man. *Ann. Surg.* 171: 875-882; 1970.

Spapen, H., Zhang, H., Demanet, C., Vleminckx, W., Vincent, J. L., Huyghens, L. Does N-acetyl-L-cysteine influence cytokine response during early human septic shock? *Chest* 113: 1616-1624, 1998.

Takehara, Y., Kanno, T., Yoshioka, T., Inoue, M., Utsumi, K. Oxygen-dependent regulation of mitochondrial energy metabolism by nitric oxide. *Arch. Biochem. Biophys.* 323: 27-32; 1995.

Tatoyan, A., Giulivi, C. Purification and characterization of a nitric oxide synthase from rat liver mitochondria. *J. Biol. Chem.* 273: 11044-11048, 1998.

Thiemermann, C., Vane, J. R. Inhibition of nitric oxide synthesis reduces the hypotension induced by bacterial lipopolysaccharide in the rat in vivo. *Eur. J. Pharmacol.* 182: 591-595; 1990.

Valdez, L. B.; Zaobornyj, T.; Boveris, A. Characterization of rat liver and kidney mitochondrial nitric oxide synthase. *Free Rad. Biol. Med.* 35: S97 abstr. (2003)

Wei, X. Q. Charles, I. G., Smith, A., Ure, J., Feng, G. J., Huang, F. P. Altered immune response in mice lacking inducible nitric oxide synthase. *6* 375:408-411, 1995

In: Progress in Inflammation Research
Editor: James A. Pitzer, pp. 165-182
ISBN 1-59454-277-5

Chapter V

A New Hypothesis for the Origin of Shock: Self-Digestion of the *Ischemic Intestine* by Pancreatic Enzymes

***Florian Fitzal*[*1,2,3], *Erik Kistler*[3], *Hiroshi Mitsuoka*[3], *Tony E. Hugli*[4] *and Geert W. Schmid-Schönbein*[3]**

[1]Department of Surgery, General Hospital University Vienna, Austria
[2]Ludwig Boltzmann Institute for Traumatology, Vienna, Austria
[3]Department of Bioengineering, Whitaker Institute of Biomedical Engineering University of California San Diego, La Jolla, CA, USA
[4] California Toxicology Research Institute, Carlsbad, CA, USA

Abstract

The gut has long been suspected of being involved in the pathology of shock. It seems to contribute in a significant way to the development of SIRS and sepsis. In the past, the proposed mechanisms of action were typically based on one of two hypotheses. The first hypothesis is that bacterial and endotoxin translocation in the intestine contribute to the morbidity and mortality seen in shock. The second hypothesis is that a major part of the pathophysiology seen in patients with sepsis is due to an production of secondarily induced inflammatory mediators. Our recent investigations have served to demonstrate that *pancreatic enzymes* appear to be directly involved in the production of the inflammatory mediators which have been observed in the blood of animals during experimental shock.

* Please address all correspondence to: Dr Florian Fitzal Department of Surgery, General Hospital, University Vienna Medical School, Waehringer Guertel 18-20, 1090 Vienna, Austria, Europe, Phone: 40400 5621, Fax: 40400 5641, florian.fitzal@akh-wien.ac.at None of the authors have a commercial conflict of interest with the reagents mentioned in this review.

The Origin of Inflammation in Shock

In critically ill patients, the systemic inflammatory response syndrome [SIRS] and sepsis are common complications with an incidence of up to 20% [1]and a mortality rate between 30 and 50% in ICU patients [2]. The key mechanisms leading to SIRS and sepsis in patients without an identifiable focus of infection are still unresolved.

The gut has long been suspected of being involved in the pathology of shock. It seems to contribute in a significant way to the development of SIRS and sepsis [3]. In the past, the proposed mechanisms of action were typically based on one of two hypotheses. The first hypothesis is that bacterial and endotoxin translocation in the intestine contribute to the morbidity and mortality seen in shock [4]. The second hypothesis is that a major part of the pathophysiology seen in patients with sepsis is due to an production of secondarily induced inflammatory mediators [5]. Although many interventions, such as anti-endotoxin and anti-cytokines have been protective in animals, clinical studies have proven no significant benefit in shock-induced mortality [6]. Data from several clinical experiments do not support a significant role for bacterial and endotoxin translocation either. Thus, there is a need to re-examine the original hypothesis for shock and our thinking about the development of multiple-organ-failure [7].

Past experience has shown that treatment directed against one specific mediator in shock does not lead to successful outcomes; instead it appears that a more efficacious target for a new therapy may be aimed at stopping the production of several endogenous released cell inflammatory mediators.

Increased cellular activation in SIRS, sepsis and shock is an early event which can be detected by leukocyte pseudopod formation, endothelial oxygen free radical production and expression of membrane adhesion molecules [8] and is directly correlated with survival [9]. Our results suggest that among these inflammatory mediators are candidates with molecular weight less than 3 kDa [10]. Moreover some of these factors are hydrophobic while others are hydrophilic [11]. These mediators, rather than solely endotoxin and cytokines may be involved in cell activation during shock [6].

Furthermore, our recent investigations have served to demonstrate that *pancreatic enzymes* appear to be directly involved in the production of the inflammatory mediators which have been observed in the blood of animals during experimental shock.

Pancreatic Enzymes and Splanchnic Pathology

The splanchnic organs including intestine and pancreas constitute a large blood volume of about 70ml/kg body weight equivalent to about 25% of the total blood volume. During shock blood flow falls and reaches low flow conditions in these organs. A low splanchnic perfusion can be observed particularly in patients with increased levels of catecholamines [12], characteristic for critically ill patients. Low flow states trigger the inflammatory cascade with an initial innocent elevation of permeability, enhanced leukocyte-endothelial interaction, to eventual cell apoptosis and organ failure. The pancreas and the intestine are highly susceptible to hypoxia during clinical and experimental shock. Ischemic damage of these particular organs has been observed in various shock studies.

Intestinal ischemia and reperfusion has been hypothesized to play an important role in the development of SIRS after trauma and hemorrhage. Intestinal damage itself correlates with cytokine production and increased mortality during shock [13]. In an interesting study by Evans et al., the exclusion of the small intestine from the bowel followed by an anastomosis between the duodenum and the colon served to decrease intestinal damage and appeared to protect animals from septic shock [14]. The mechanism for this protective effect has not been elucidated. These results, however, already suggest that pancreatic enzymes entering the small intestine from the duodenum may contribute to mortality in shock.

In a series of experiments Bounous et al. demonstrated that pancreatic enzymes are capable of aggravating intestinal damage by proteolytic cleavage [15]. Pancreatic duct ligation or pancreatectomy at least 5 days prior to shock induction seemed to be protective in animal experiments [1618]. A fibrotic pancreas, accomplished by duct ligation 2.5 months prior to shock induction, significantly increased the blood flow to several splanchnic organs during shock [17]. Oral administration of Trasylol, a selective blocker of pancreatic proteases, provided limited protection of the intestinal mucosa from necrosis [19]. Animals with duct ligation several days before hemorrhage had reduced intestinal mucosa necrosis as well [18, 20]. Improvement of morphological damage in the mucosa correlated with survival in this experiment [20].

Pancreatic Enzymes and Inflammatory Mediators

The mechanism by which oral protease inhibition increased survival in Bounous` study is unresolved. In related experiments, Lefer and colleagues demonstrated that pancreatic enzymes play a special role in the development of an unknown myocardial depressant factor [MDF] within the blood [2123]. They proposed the release of MDF in form of a peptide from the ischemic pancreas during shock. This peptide was estimated to have a molecular weight in the range of 500 to 1000 Da [24]. Splanchnic blood flow has been found to be inversely related to MDF levels [23]. Conversely, increasing splanchnic blood flow during endotoxic shock reduced MDF levels in blood [23]. Pancreatectomy prior to shock nearly abolishes the MDF activity [22]. Perhaps the strongest evidence supporting the pancreatic origin of MDF is its production by incubating homogenates of splanchnic tissue. Pancreatic homogenates produce MDF, whereas intestinal, hepatic and splenic homogenates fail to generate significant quantities [25]. The MDF may be transported in the intestinal lymph [26]. Mitsuoka et al. found decreased levels of inflammatory mediators in portal effluent as well as more systemically following intestinal protease inhibition in a splanchnic artery occlusion shock model. These results suggest that the pancreas may be involved in the production of endogenous inflammatory factors followed by SIRS during shock [Fig.1].

Kistler and Schmid-Schönbein were the first to demonstrate that pancreatic enzymes posses the ability to activate human leukocytes, as well as other cell subtypes, such as endothelium and interstitial cells [27]. They mixed pancreatic homogenates with naive human leukocytes and determined formation of pseudopods and free radicals as measures for cell activation. Pancreatic homogenate but neither physiological levels of trypsin alone nor other organ homogenates [intestine, lung, liver, heart, brain, spleen, thymus, aorta, kidney, skeletal muscle] without pancreatic enzymes were able to significantly activate human leukocytes [28]. Interestingly, all organs including intestine, liver and lung digested by pancreatic enzymes, however, activated human leukocytes. Thus, Kistler and Schmid-Schönbein hypothesized that activated pancreatic enzymes may cross the mucosal barrier during intestinal ischemic and low flow states [including shock] and produce inflammatory mediators by tissue cleavage [10]. Their results suggested that there may be a close relationship between pancreatic enzymes, intestinal damage, cell activation, and shock-induced SIRS.

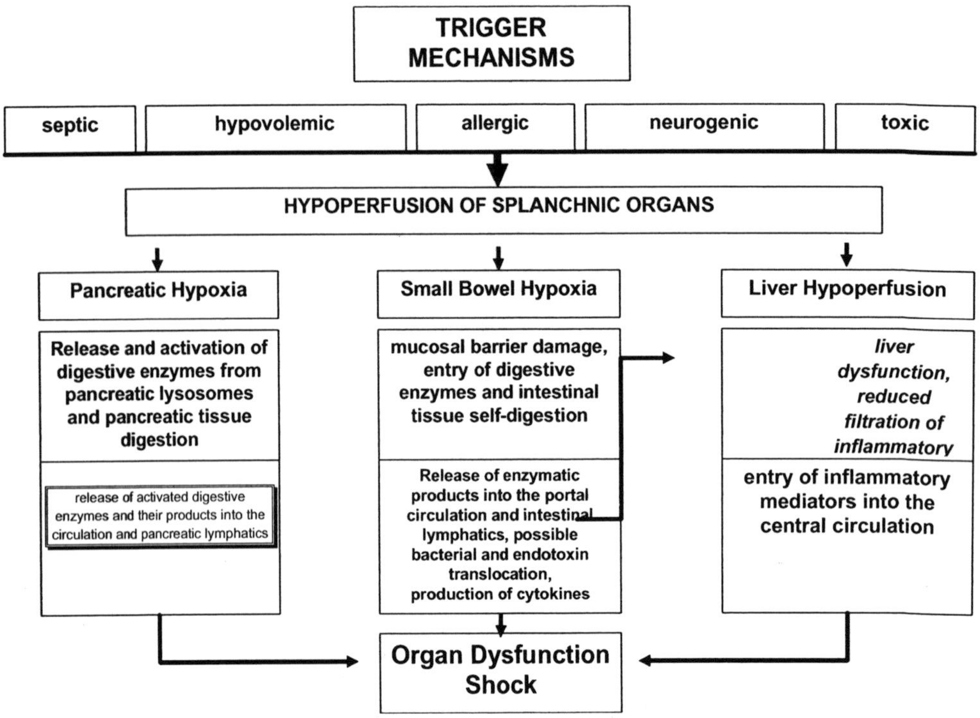

Figure 1. Hypothesis of the impact of the pancreas and the gut during shock for the development of a systemic inflammation.

Intestinal Protease Inhibition [IPI] as Protection Against Shock

Schmid-Schönbein et al. investigated the role of the serine protease and lipase inhibitor 6-amidino-2-naphtyl p-guanidinobenzoate dimethanesulfate [ANGD, Futhan®] as a therapeutic option in intestinal ischemia-induced shock. Although the authors were able to increase blood pressure during these experiments and significantly decrease leukocyte activation, systemic inflammation and symptoms of shock were still present [29]. It appears that inhibition of leukocyte activating factors in the blood after their production in the intestine may not be sufficient to block the inflammatory cascade started by proteolytic cleavage of the intestine by pancreatic digestive enzymes. In light of the fact that digestive enzymes are fully activated in the lumen of the intestine as part of normal digestion, an alternative approach is required to block the production of the inflammatory mediators.

Schmid-Schönbein and colleagues developed a method for *intra-intestinal* digestive enzyme inhibition [IPI] by lavage with ANGD [Futhan®] during intestinal ischemia and reperfusion-induced shock. Using intra-intestinal lavage with ANGD they were able to significantly reduce pancreatic digestive enzyme activity within the gut [30]. This protection was not achieved by intestinal lavage with saline alone, but required the presence of the pancreatic enzyme inhibitor ANGD during lavage. Mitsuoka and Schmid-Schönbein also demonstrated that the protective effects of IPI during shock could be reproduced with another broad-spectrum pancreatic enzyme inhibitor, gabexate mesilate [FOY®] [31]. In both sets of experiments, IPI significantly attenuated typical symptoms of shock, such as central hemodynamic dysfunction, the production of systemic leukocyte activating factors in portal and central venous blood, or infiltration of inflammatory cells into the intestinal, hepatic or pulmonary circulation [30-32]. The experiments also showed that IPI reduces lung damage and thus is useful to attenuate multiple organ failure.

Intravenous administration of enzyme inhibitors provided only a modest improvement in blood pressure in response to hypotension in shock. This observation supports the hypothesis that intra-intestinal blockade of digestive enzymes in the lumen of the intestine is required to improve survival and decrease production of inflammatory mediators in shock produced by intestinal ischemia. Intravenous enzyme inhibition is less effective since it only indirectly targets digestive enzymes instead of blocking them at their site of action, i.e. in the lumen of the intestine.

Digestive enzymes are fully activated in the lumen of the intestine as part of normal digestion. A breakdown of the mucosal epithelial brush-border barrier, for example by intestinal ischemia, leads to entry of digestive enzymes into the wall of the intestine [33]. The entry of pancreatic digestive enzymes may lead to self-digestion of extracellular and cellular elements of the intestinal wall, a process that may lead to production of inflammatory mediators, which in turn enter the portal venous circulation and intestinal lymphatics.

IPI Reduces Production of Inflammatory Mediators in the Gut

The hypothesis remained to be tested that intestinal proteases digest the intestinal wall during shock followed by cleavage of intestinal tissue and the production of factors that may in fact be responsible for a systemic inflammatory response. Thus, we examined the role of IPI in blocking mucosal damage and generation of leukocyte activating factors within the intestinal wall. We also characterized leukocyte activation and microcirculatory dysfunction in a peripheral organ as an indicator of systemic inflammation during intestinal ischemia and reperfusion [34].

These experiments demonstrated that IPI prior to intestinal ischemia and reperfusion significantly improved central blood pressure [Fig.2], decreased intestinal damage [Fig.3], reduced the production of leukocyte activating factors within the gut, as well as increasing the release of inflammatory factors in the circulation [Fig.4]. The results suggest that intestinal enzymes are important cofactors in producing cell-inflammatory mediators within the gut during shock. We further demonstrated that TNF alpha levels within the intestine are not reduced by IPI, suggesting that the factors produced by entry of digestive enzymes into the wall of the intestine may be different from cytokines [35]. The hypothesis is supported by the observation that the enzyme-induced leukocyte activating factors are hydrophobic in nature, many of which with a molecular weight below 3kDa [11].

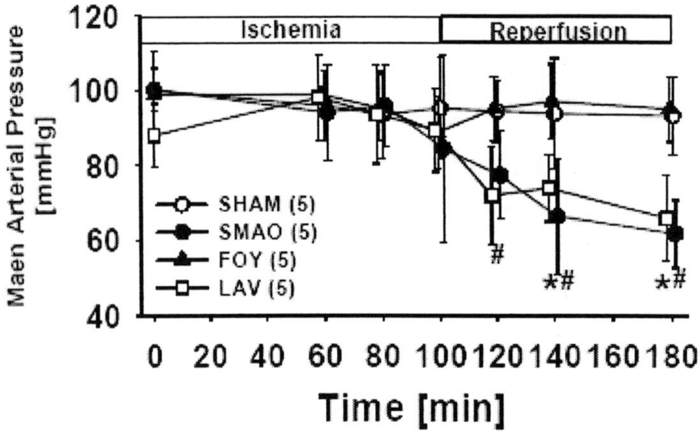

Figure 2. Mean arterial blood pressure during ischemia [from time zero until 100 min] and reperfusion [100 min until 180 min]. After reperfusion the blood pressure fell significantly in animals subjected to superior mesenteric artery occlusion [SMAO] and in animals with intestinal lavage before ischemia [LAV]. Intestinal lavage with the protease inhibitor FOY before ischemia and reperfusion significantly attenuated the blood pressure reduction. #P<0.05 compared with baseline. *P<0.05 compared with the SHAM or FOY group. Reproduced by permission from Karger Publishers from the article: Intestinal pancreatic protease inhibition attenuates intestinal-ischemia-induced shock by reducing cell activation and gut injury J Vasc Res Vol.39 2002 [34].

Intraluminal washout provides protection and minimizes morphological damage to the intestine after ischemia and reperfusion [36]. In light of the evidence that ischemia-induced gut damage and the formation of activating factors within the intestinal wall are reduced by IPI, it is possible that pancreatic protease-induced disruption of intestinal cells [6] or extracellular matrix proteins [37] may be involved in the patho-physiological generation of inflammatory mediators. Intravenous application of the pancreatic protease inhibitor only modestly improved intestinal ischemia-induced hypotension and the formation of leukocyte activating factors [29]. In contrast, IPI almost completely abolished intestinal ischemia-induced shock, suggesting again that intra-luminal rather than intravascular enzyme inhibition reduces the formation of inflammatory mediators.

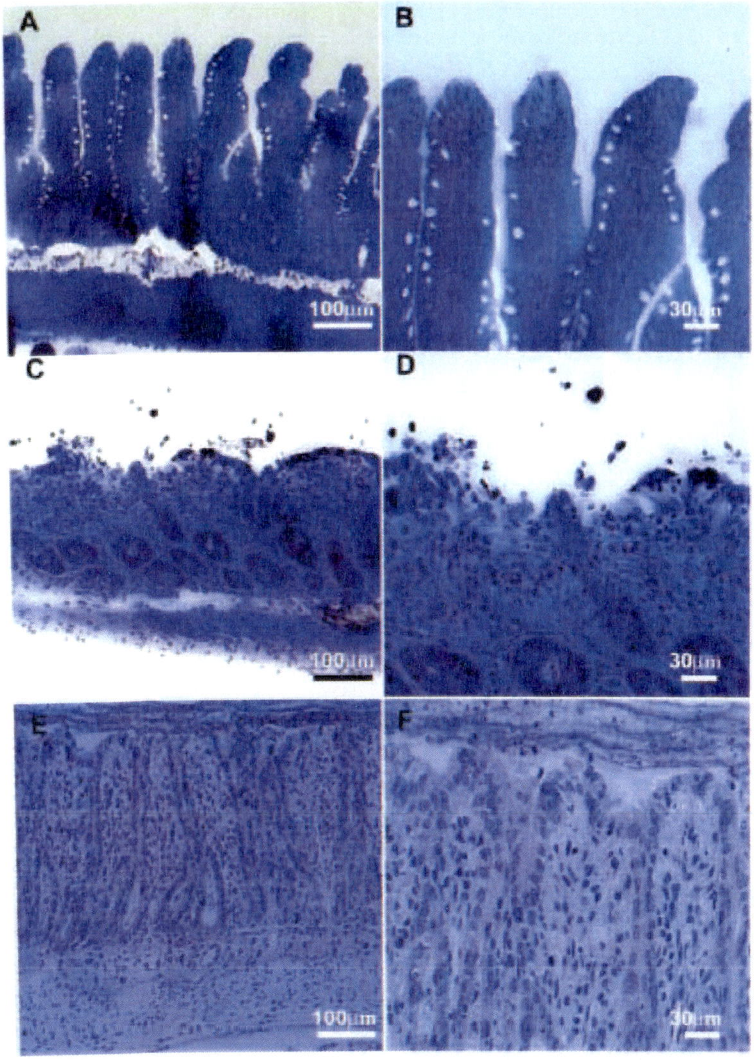

Figure 3. Histological sections of the small intestine from SHAM [panels A and B] and from rats undergoing intestinal buffer lavage [panels C and D] or lavage with protease inhibitor gabexate mesilate [FOY] [panels E and F]. Sections are from tissue collected at the end of 80 min of reperfusion after 100 min of superior mesenteric artery occlusion. SHAM animals show typical villi structure with low leukocyte infiltration [A] and a regular brush border [panel B]. LAV animals demonstrate ulcerations and loss of villi architecture with a high amount of leukocyte infiltrating the whole intestine [panels C and D]. Intra-intestinal pancreas protease inhibition further reduced gut damage as indicated by intact villi and partially intact brush border but with infiltrating leukocytes [panels E and F]. Reproduced by permission from Karger Publishers from the article: Intestinal pancreatic protease inhibition attenuates intestinal-ischemia-induced shock by reducing cell activation and gut injury J Vasc Res Vol.39 2002 [34].

Other mechanisms that may provide the beneficial effect of IPI must also be considered. It may be possible that IPI reduces endotoxin translocation. In our studies IPI did not reduce endotoxin activity in intestinal fluid. Inflammatory mediators other than endotoxin, are abundant in post-hemorrhagic plasma [29] and mesenteric lymph [38, 39]. These mediators increase lung permeability and endothelial cell damage during hemorrhage and after resuscitation. In our studies no significant correlation between endotoxin activity or TNF alpha levels and leukocyte activation could be identified, in line with earlier observations [40]. While IPI did not change intestinal endotoxin activity, the intervention significantly decreased endotoxin translocation. The mechanism by which IPI serves to prevent leukocyte activation may be less dependent on endotoxin or TNF alpha in plasma because these parameters did not correlate with one another.

IPI serves to rinse the intestinal content and thereby may reduce the level of inflammatory mediators within the intestinal [intraluminal] fluid. However, the ability of inflammatory mediators to activate human leukocytes in-vitro is not attenuated by the addition of an enzyme inhibitor [27]. Thus, it is less likely that the enzyme inhibitors themselves block leukocyte activation in-vivo. Since we observed an initial drop in mean arterial blood pressure and no reduction in functional capillary density in the intestinal microcirculation during and after intestinal lavage, with or without a pancreatic enzyme inhibitor [unpublished results from pilot studies with sham-shocked animals], we concluded that intestinal washout itself has no direct effect in improving cardiovascular hemodynamics. Some studies have suggested that FOY®, given intravenously, reduces reperfusion damage by inhibiting leukocyte activation and TNF production [41]. In our experiments, FOY® has been given intra-intestinally, thus our results are primarily based on intestinal enzyme inhibition by FOY®. The rapid application of the inhibitor [0.37mM = 8mg/50ml buffer over 1 min] limits intestinal uptake, which requires about 15 min [42]. Only about 10 ml of the buffer solution [1.6 mg FOY®] remained in the intestine after lavage. Even if the remaining FOY® has been absorbed from the intestine and reached the circulation, this dosage is much lower than that used for intravenous treatment. Moreover we demonstrated that intravenous application of a pancreatic enzyme inhibitor during intestinal ischemia/reperfusion had only modest effects on blood pressure and systemic cell activation [29]. Thus the evidence suggests that the mechanism by which FOY® reduces reperfusion-induced intestinal injury, shock and leukocyte cell activation may be based on intestinal enzyme inhibition.

FOY® has been found to reduce production of oxygen radicals [43] and nitric oxide synthesis [NOS] [44]. However, Mitsuoka et al. showed that intra-intestinal application of allopurinol to Futhan did not significantly improve intestinal injury, blood pressure and systemic circulation above the protection provided by ANGD itself, suggesting that oxygen radicals may not play a major role in this respect [32]. Regarding NOS inhibition, we measured the intestinal microcirculation during lavage with and without FOY® in sham animals with an intravital microscope. FOY® did not reduce capillary or postcapillary perfusion, suggesting that FOY®, in our protocol, did not influence intestinal iNOS [data not shown]. iNOS plays a minor role in our studies because its synthesis requires several hours and our experiments were based on shorter time courses.

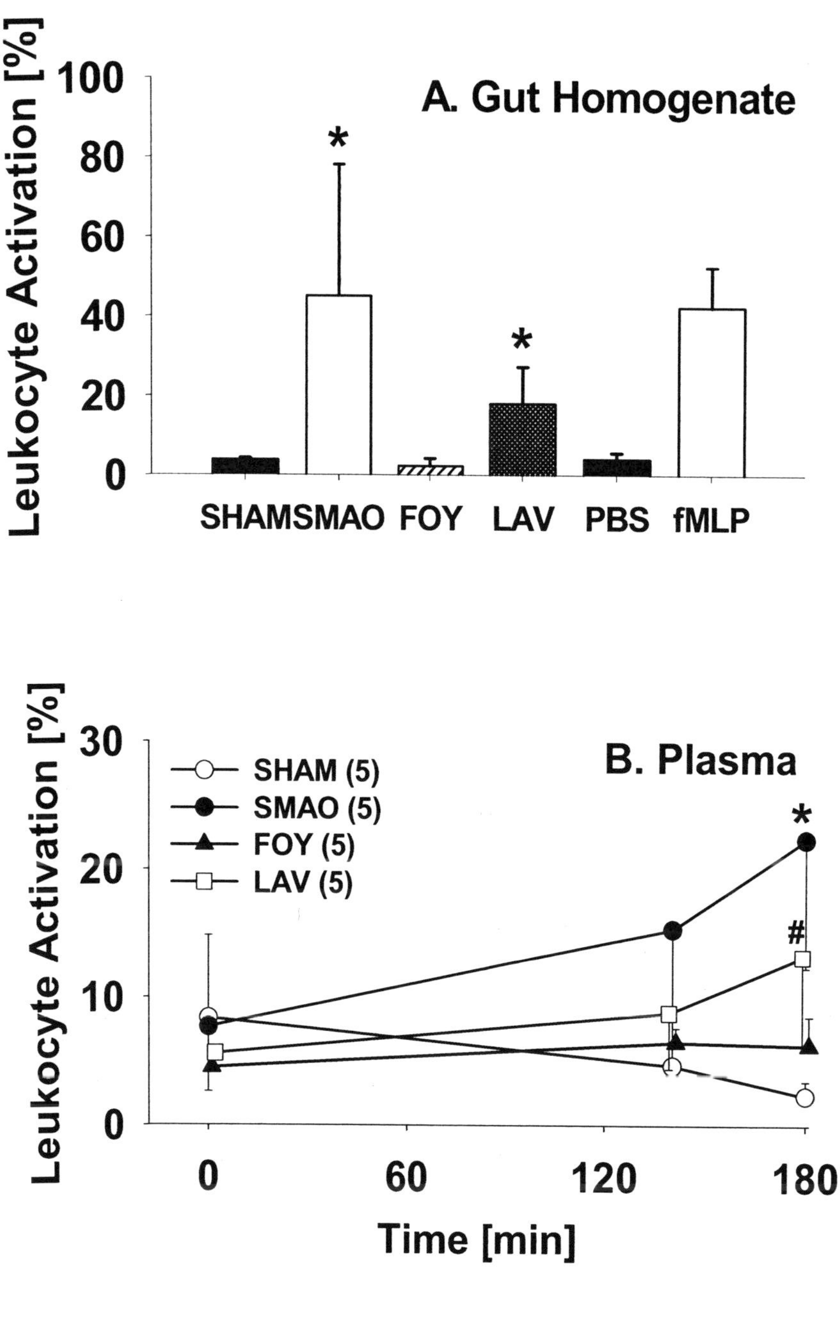

Figure 4.The number of naïve human leukocytes activated [as detected by pseudopods longer than 1μm] by A] intestinal homogenate or B] heparinized plasma collected before ischemia and 40 min as well as 80 min after reperfusion. Intestinal homogenates were made at the end of the experiment with 1g of small intestine in 10mM PBS. FOY attenuated the presence of leukocyte activating factors when compared with LAV and SMAO animals. * $P<0.05$ compared with baseline, SHAM and FOY. # $P<0.05$ compared with baseline and SHAM. PBS indicates negative control, fMLP [10^{-4}] indicates positive control. Reproduced by permission from Karger Publishers from the article: Intestinal pancreatic protease inhibition attenuates intestinal-ischemia-induced shock by reducing cell activation and gut injury J Vasc Res Vol.39 2002 [34].

IPI Decreases Systemic Inflammation

Peripheral leukocyte activation in the microcirculation in shock was shown to be abolished by IPI treatment [34] [Fig.5]. The number of rolling leukocytes as well as the leukocyte adhesion to postcapillary venules was found to be attenuated by IPI as well [34]. This result provides evidence for a reduction in SIRS; however, other parameters to investigate systemic inflammation would be helpful in evaluating our hypothesis. In this regard Mitsuoka, et al [30] demonstrated that intestinal enzyme inhibition reduced MPO levels in several organs after intestinal ischemia/reperfusion-induced shock. Moreover, plasma of animals after intestinal ischemia and reperfusion is capable of depressing myocardial function and this has been found to be attenuated by intestinal enzyme inhibition [29], giving evidence for a systemic inflammatory effect of protease induced cell inflammatory mediators. Intra-intestinal inhibition of digestive enzymes [but not intravenous blockade] also reduces the level of inflammatory mediators within the mesenteric lymph duct during hemorrhagic shock [39, 45].

IPI Attenuates Endotoxic Shock

Is it possible that blockade of pancreatic digestive enzymes may not only block formation of inflammatory mediators and symptoms of shock under conditions associated with ischemia of the intestine? For example in endotoxic shock is it possible that, in addition to endotoxin, inflammatory mediators derived from pancreatic digestive enzymes may also be present? Endotoxin may serve as initial inflammatory mediator and trigger an enhancement of the intestinal permeability, which then in turn permits entry of pancreatic digestive enzymes into the wall of the intestine. In septic patients the systemic inflammation, organ dysfunction and hemodynamic alterations continue even after a initial stimulus [a septic focus] has been eliminated and the patient is receiving antibiotic treatment. Clinical evidence suggests that patients may still develop systemic inflammation and multiple organ failure in the absence of bacteremia [46] or in spite of drainage of the infection site [47]. Thus, endotoxin and bacteria may trigger endogenous cell activating factors that maintain and enhance the inflammatory reaction and multiple organ dysfunction.

To further test this hypothesis we examined one particular aspect of this hypothesis. After endotoxin administration, we studied the effect of IPI on central cardiopulmonary dynamics, systemic inflammation, the level of inflammatory mediators that cause leukocyte activation, and peripheral muscle parenchymal cell death [48]. IPI did not interfere with hemodynamic parameters during the first 20 to 60 min, indicating that at the beginning of endotoxemia, intestinal enzymes are not the main factors that control the early hemodynamic events. Beyond 60 min, however, IPI reduced endotoxin-induced hypotension, tachycardia and hyperventilation leading to microvascular and hemodynamic improvement [Table 1 and 2]. There was attenuation of the delayed inflammatory process [Fig.6] after the initial endotoxin administration when IPI was used. Inflammation appears to be a major cause of shock and multiple organ failure during sepsis. It is accompanied by a powerful form of cellular activation which includes leukocytes, endothelial cells, and possibly other cell types

[49]. Leukocyte activation leads to pseudopod formation and capillary plugging with enhanced leukocyte migration across the endothelial wall, local tissue inflammation and cell death [11]. Inflammation is also accompanied by a series of patho-physiologic processes, which may lead to cardiopulmonary dysfunction, including hypotension, tachycardia and hyperventilation. Attenuation of inflammation by IPI may be one of the major reasons for the improvement of microvascular perfusion. The fact that IPI serves to reduce the formation of inflammatory mediators supports the hypothesis that such mediators may be predominantly produced within the wall of the intestine by pancreatic digestive enzymes. IPI also reduced endotoxin-induced microvascular leukocyte and endothelial cell activation, parenchymal cell death [Fig.7] as well as the production of IL-6 [Fig.8] [48].

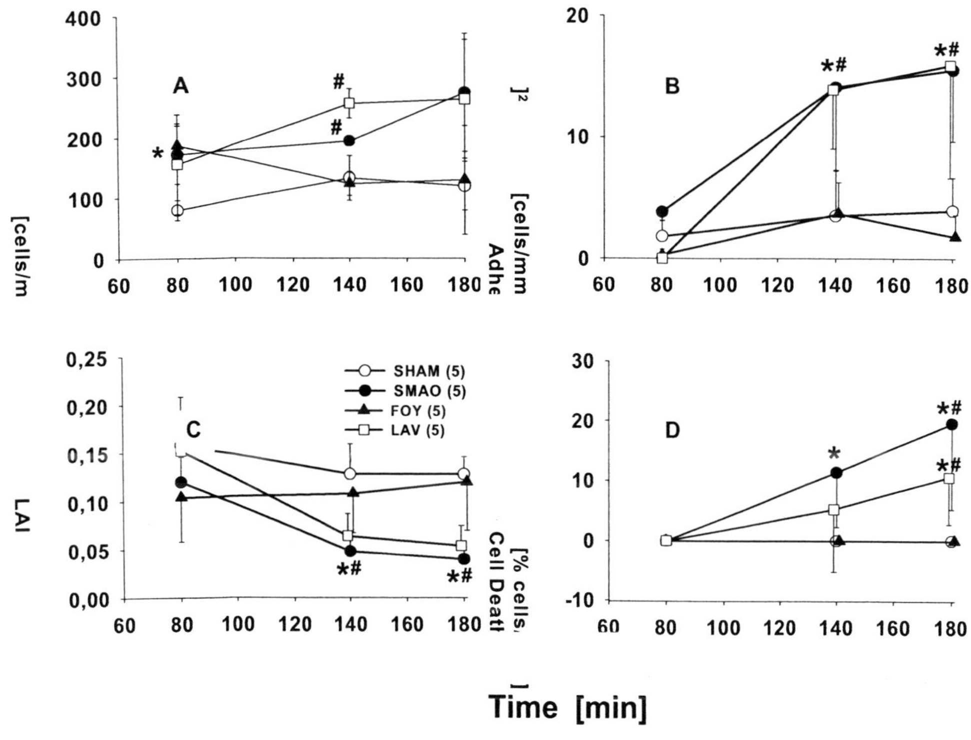

Figure 5. Microcirculatory measurements in post-capillary venules in the cremaster muscle starting at 80 min after ischemia with an intravital microscope [40x water objective]. Abscise starts at 60 min after the onset of ischemia.] The number of rolling leukocytes. * P<0.05 in all groups compared with SHAM group. # P<0.05 compared with the FOY group. B] The number of adherent leukocytes [cells sticking on the endothelial wall without moving for at least 30 sec]. * P<0.05 compared with baseline value in the SMAO and LAV group. # P<0.05 compared with the SHAM and FOY group. C] The leukocyte adhesion index [LAI = V_{WBC} / V_{RBC}]. * P<0.05 compared with baseline value in the SMAO and LAV group. # P<0.05 compared with the SHAM and FOY group.D] Cell death in the cremaster muscle as measured from the number of propidium iodide positive cells. SMAO and LAV animals showed a significant increase in cell death at 40 and 80 min after reperfusion when compared with their baseline [* P<0.05]. This was attenuated in FOY and SHAM animals [#P<0.05]. Reproduced by permission from Karger Publishers from the article: Intestinal pancreatic protease inhibition attenuates intestinal-ischemia-induced shock by reducing cell activation and gut injury J Vasc Res Vol.39 2002 [34].Clinical Impact of IPI

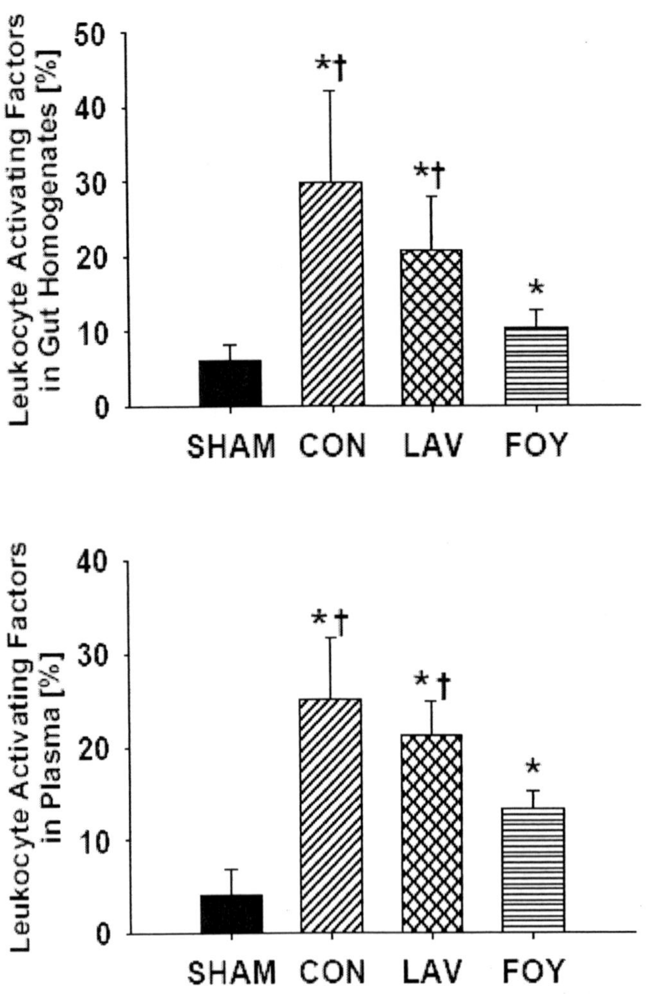

Figure 6. Neutrophil activation measured by pseudopod formation of naive human leukocytes mixed with [A] gut homogenates and [B] plasma before and after 300 min of i.v. endotoxin injection into rats. The increase in activating factors at 240 and 300 min after endotoxin injection was significantly reduced by intra-intestinal pancreatic protease inhibition with FOY. * $p<0.05$ compared with SHAM. † $p<0.05$ compared with FOY at the same time point. Reproduced by permission from Elsevier reprinted from Surgery Vol.134 2003 Pancreatic enzymes sustain systemic inflammation after an initial endotoxin challenge [48].

In all experiments described so far IPI was administered as pre-shock therapy. In practice, treatment is only possible after the onset of shock. Initial observations from our laboratory suggest that IPI, even administered at a delayed time point, serves to reduce shock induced hemodynamic alterations and cell activation [35]. Whether or not this intervention procedure is able to improve survival rates requires further investigation.

The experiments we have described so far have been carried out in rodents. Recently it was possible to demonstrate a similar level of protection using IPI in a porcine trauma model [50].

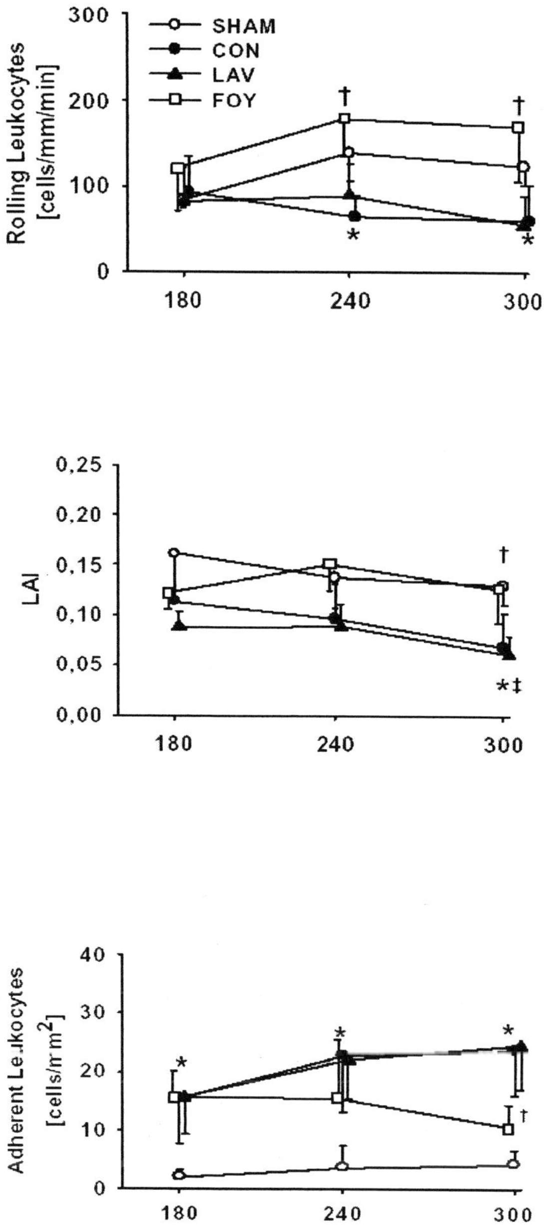

Figure 7. Systemic cell activation: Leukocyte and endothelial cell activation in the cremaster muscle in post-capillary venules measured by intravital microscopy at 180, 240 and 300 min after endotoxin injection. A] Number of rolling leukocytes B] Number of adherent leukocytes to endothelial cells C] Leukocyte adhesion index [LAI = VWBC /VRBC] as indicator for endothelial/leukocyte cell activation and interaction D] The number of propidium iodide [PI] positive parenchymal cremaster cells as marker for peripheral cell death. Data are presented as mean ± SD. *$p<0.05$ compared with SHAM at the same time point. † $p<0.05$ FOY compared with CON and LAV at the same time point. ‡ $p<0.05$ when compared with 180 min after endotoxemia. Reproduced by permission from Elsevier from Surgery Vol.134 2003 Pancreatic enzymes sustain systemic inflammation after an initial endotoxin challenge [48].

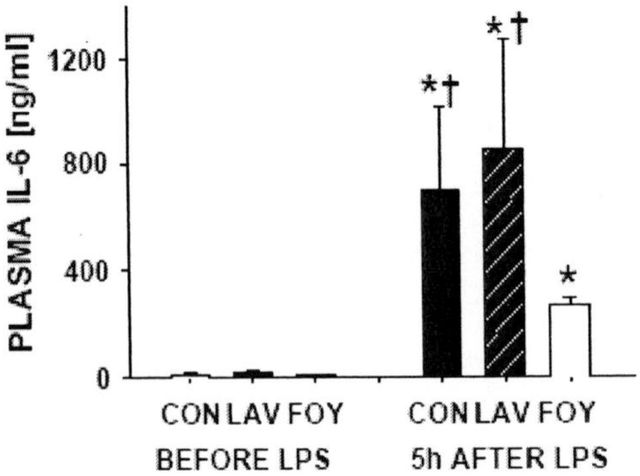

Figure 8. Plasma IL 6 levels in femoral arterial blood measured 300 min after intravenous endotoxin administration [4mg/kg]. * p<0.05 compared with baseline values before endotoxin application. † p<0.05 compared with FOY at the same time point. Reproduced by permission from Elsevier reprinted from Surgery Vol.134 2003 Pancreatic enzymes sustain systemic inflammation after an initial endotoxin challenge [48].

Table 1. Microvascular Parameters in Cremaster Muscle at Different Times After Endoxin Administration [4 mg/kg.i.v.] Functional Capillary Density

Cap/field	180min	240min	300min
SHAM	0.86 ± 0.05	0.65 ± 0.11	0.71 ± 0.16
CONTROL	0.69 ± 0.24	0.51 ± 0.33	0.31 ± 0.19†*
LAVAGE	0.45 ± 0.24	0.46 ± 0.28	0.25 ± 0.09*
FOY	0.47 ± 0.30	0.62 ± 0.31	0.62 ± 0.23

Rolling leukocytes in arterioles

Cells/min	180min	240min	300min
SHAM	0 ± 0	0 ± 0	0 ± 0
CONTROL	4 ± 9	13 ± 16	11 ± 12
LAVAGE	0 ± 0	9 ± 10	19 ± 26
FOY	0 ± 0	0 ± 0	0 ± 0

Adherent leukocytes in arterioles

Cells/mm^2	180min	240min	300min
SHAM	0 ± 0	0 ± 0	0 ± 0
CONTROL	4 ± 8	4 ± 6	7 ± 10
LAVAGE	0 ± 0	2 ± 2	4 ± 5
FOY	0 ± 0	0 ± 0	0 ± 0

Functional capillary density = the fraction of not-erfused capillaries in the cremaster muscle in three different tissue regions [area about 400μm x 400μm].

The number of rolling leukocytes in pre-capillary arterioles passing a given observation point and counted over 30 sec [cells/min].

The number of adherent leukocytes [without movement for at least 30 sec] per vessel area measured in a arteriolar vessel segment length of 100μm [cells/mm^2].

Mean ± SD are shown. † P<0.05 compared with value at 180min in the same group. *P<0.05 compared with SHAM and FOY at the same time point.

Characterization of Digestive Enzyme-Induced Cellular Activating Factors

The many inflammatory mediators generated during intestinal ischemia and shock have not yet been completely identified. They may arise early in shock because a significant increase in the level of activating factors has been observed within 40 min of reperfusion after intestinal ischemia [40]. This evidence suggests that activating factors are either preformed substances or produced by a rapid process such as enzymatic degradation [51].

Table 2. Cardiopulmonary Parameters Before [Baseline] and After I.V. Endotoxin Injection

	Mean Arterial Blood Pressure [mmHg]		
Experimental groups	Baseline	240min	300min
SHAM	110 ± 12	105 ± 9	105 ± 8
CON	114 ± 12	91 ± 11*	81 ± 12*†
FOYiv	107 ± 6	109 ± 4	99 ± 9
	Heart Rate [beats/min]		
SHAM	376 ± 12	396 ± 9	377 ± 16
CON	398 ± 11	491 ± 52*†	490 ± 69*†
FOYiv	391 ± 8	413 ± 12*†	413 ± 12*†
	Respiratory Rate [breaths/min]		
SHAM	73 ± 18	70 ± 10	66 ± 10
CON	76 ± 17	96 ± 15*†	101 ± 17*†
FOYiv	65 ± 5	103 ± 6*†	91 ± 6*†

Sham and CON are the same as in Fig. 1. FOYiv [n=5]: This group received endotoxin [4mg/kg over 5 min] and gabexate mesilate [FOY®] i.v during 5 hours every 30 min at a rate of 10mg/kg/h. This dosage has been shown to inhibit leukocyte activation and cytokine expression during ischemia and reperfusion and shock. In our experiment this dosage given intravenously had no significant improving effect on hemodynamics [except blood pressure] during endotoxemia while intraintestinal protease inhibition with FOY® significantly improved hemodynamics. Data are presented as mean ± SD. * significant different when compared with baseline value on the same group. † significantly different when compared with SHAM.

It is important to note that when pancreatic proteases are exposed to the various organs we have tested, they yield potent inflammatory mediators [10, 28]. Addition of platelet activating factor inhibitors to plasma in-vitro did not significantly reduce cellular activation [27]. Administration of a pancreatic enzyme inhibitor after the generation of the activating factors in-vitro did not reduce cell activation [27] suggesting that pancreatic enzymes are responsible for the formation of these factors but are not necessarily the activators themselves. Analysis of the inflammatory mediators derived from pancreatic homogenate indicated an interesting dichotomy. Both the hydrophobic [lipid] and the hydrophilic fractions caused rapid mortality when administered into the venous circulation, but only the lipid fraction caused leukocyte activation in-vitro [51]. Therefore, it appears there is a leukocyte dependent and a leukocyte independent pathway in shock.

Among other hypotheses, Hardaway postulated that aminophospholipids, strong complement activating proteins from the inner surface of cell membranes, might be released into the circulation after a proteolytic breakdown of cell membranes during shock [6]. Most recently, enzymatic fragments of extracellular matrix proteins have also been demonstrated to be important regulators in tissue responses to injury [37].

Conclusion

Pancreatic digestive enzymes in their fully activated state are one of the key requirements for normal digestion in the ileum. These enzymes are designed to break down a variety of biological molecules, proteins, lipids, carbohydrates and nucleotides. Self-digestion by these powerful enzymes is prevented to a large degree by the mucosal brush border barrier that prevents escape of pancreatic enzymes from the lumen of the intestine into the submucosal space and the wall of the intestine. Self-digestion is prevented by the barrier properties of this thin epithelial lining.

Under conditions when the intestinal permeability is compromised, pancreatic digestive enzymes can enter into the wall of the intestine where they may produce a variety inflammatory mediators that serve to activate cell and even cause direct cell death. These inflammatory mediators differ from cytokines and endotoxin and may be responsible for the systemic inflammatory response syndrome and multiple organ damage. Our current experimental results suggest that intra-intestinal enzyme inhibition may serve to block mediator generation and attenuate shock. Further studies are underway to elucidate the biochemical characteristics of these inflammatory mediators to help better understand the clinical impact of intra-intestinal enzyme inhibition.

Acknowledgement

The research summarised here has been supported by grant HL 67825 from the National Heart Lung and Blood Institute and by the MAX KADE foundation.

References

[1] D. J. J. Muckart, S. Bhagwanjee, *Crit Care Med* **25**, 1789-1795 [1997].

[2] F. Zeni, B. Freeman, C. Natanson, *Crit Care Med* **25**, 1095-1100 [1997].

[3] S. Bahrami, H. Redl, G. Schlag, *Wien Klin Wochenschr* **110 Suppl**, 2-10 [1998]; R. D. Berg, *J Med* **23**, 217-44. [1992]; G. Bounous, *Surgery* **107**, 118-9. [1990].

[4] J. C. Marshall, N. V. Christou, J. L. Meakins, *Ann Surg* **218**, 111-9. [1993]; E. A. Deitch, *Arch Surg* **125**, 403-4. [1990].
[5] H. S. Warren, *New Engl J Med* **336**, 952-953 [1997]; E. A. Deitch, D. Xu, L. Franko, A. Ayala, I. H. Chaudry, *Shock* **1**, 141-146 [1994].
[6] R. Hardaway, *Am Surg* **66**, 22-29 [2000].
[7] R. C. Bone, *JAMA* **276**, 565-566 [1996].
[8] M. C. Mazzoni, G. W. Schmid-Schönbein, *Cardiovasc Res* **32**, 709-719 [1996].
[9] J. Barroso-Aranda, G. W. Schmid-Schönbein, *Am J Physiol* **257**, H846-H852 [1989].
[10] E. B. Kistler, T. E. Hugli, G. W. Schmid-Schönbein, *Microcirc* **7**, 183-192 [2000].
[11] G. W. Schmid-Schönbein, T. E. Hugli, E. B. Kistler, A. Sofianos, H. Mitsuoka, *Microcirc* **8**, 5-14 [2001].
[12] S. Gelman, P. S. Mushlin, *Anesthesiology* **100**, 434-9. [2004].
[13] F. Tamion *et al.*, *Am J Physiol* **273**, G314-G321 [1997]; J. Fine, R. Minton, *Nature* **5031**, 97-98 [1966].
[14] W. E. Evans, R. T. Shore, L. C. Carey, J. C. Darin, *Arch Surg* **95**, 511-516 [1967]; W. E. Evans, R. T. Shore, J. C. Darin, *Arch Surg* **93**, 196-199 [1966].
[15] G. Bounous, D. Menard, D. E., *Gastroenterology* **73**, 102-108 [1977]; G. Bounous, *Can J Surg* **17**, 434 [1974]; G. Bounous, *Surgery* **99**, 92-94 [1985]; G. Bounous, *Gastroenterology* **82**, 1457-1467 [1982]; G. Bounous, *Surgery* **107**, 118-119 [1989];
[16] G. Bounous, J. Proulx, G. Konok, A. Wollin, *Int J Clin Pharma* **17**, 317-323 [1979]; G. Bounous, G. Konok, *Am J Surg* **133**, 304-306 [1977].
[17] E. B. De Koos, W. J. Gibson, G. Bounous, L. G. Hampson, *Can J Surg* **9**, 227-30. [1966]; L. R. Soma, G. R. Neufeld, D. C. Dodd, B. E. Marshall, *Ann Surg* **179**, 395-402. [1974].
[18] T. Manabe, T. Suzuki, I. Honjo, *Surg Gynecol Obstet* **146**, 577-82. [1978].
[19] A. Montgomery, A. Borgström, U. Haglund, *Gastronterology* **102**, 216-222 [1992].
[20] G. Bounous, L. G. Hampson, F. N. Gurd, *Ann Surg* **160**, 650-68. [1964].
[21] G. Bounous, R. A. Brown, D. S. Mulder, L. G. Hampson, F. N. Gurd, *Arch Surg* **91**, 371-5. [1965].
[22] A. M. Lefer, Y. Barenholz, *Am J Physiol* **223**, 1103-1109 [1972]; A. M. Lefer, *Klin Wochenzeitschr* **60**, 713-716 [1982].
[23] A. M. Lefer, T. M. Glenn, *Adv Exp Med Biol* **23**, 311-335 [1971].
[24] A. M. Lefer, J. A. Spath, *Ann Surg* **179**, 868-876 [1974].
[25] M. J. Galvin, A. M. Lefer, *Experientia* **35**, 55-56 [1979].
[26] T. M. Glenn, A. M. Lefer, *Circ Res* **29**, 338-49. [1971].
[27] J. T. Sambol, J. White, J. W. Horton, E. A. Deitch, *Shock* **18**, 272-6. [2002].
[28] E. B. Kistler, PhD Thesis, UCSD [1998].
[29] S. W. Waldo, H. S. Rosario, A. H. Penn, G. W. Schmid-Schonbein, *Shock* **20**, 138-43. [2003].
[30] E. B. Kistler, A. M. Lefer, T. E. Hugli, G. W. Schmid-Schönbein, *Shock* **14**, 30-34 [2000].
[31] H. Mitsuoka, E. B. Kistler, G. W. Schmid-Schönbein, *PNAS* **97**, 1772-1777 [2000].
[32] H. Mitsuoka, E. B. Kistler, G. W. Schmid-Schönbein, *Shock* **17**, 205-209 [2002].
[33] H. Mitsuoka, G. W. Schmid-Schönbein, *Shock* **14**, 522-527 [2000].

[34] H. S. Rosário, S. W. Waldo, S. A. Becker, G. W. Schmid-Schönbein, *Am J Pathol*, [2004].

[35] F. Fitzal, F. De Lano, C. Young, H. S. Rosario, G. W. Schmid-Schönbein, *J Vasc Res* **39**, 320-329 [2002].

[36] F. Fitzal, F. De Lano, C. Young, G. W. Schmid-Schonbein, *Arch Surg* **in press** [2004].

[37] C. J. Chiu, H. J. Scott, F. N. Gurd, *Arch Surg* **101**, 484-488 [1970].

[38] G. E. Davies, K. J. Bayless, M. J. Davies, G. A. Meininger, *Am J Pathol* **156**, 1489-1498 [2000].

[39] E. A. Deitch, C. Adams, Q. Lu, D. Z. Xu, *Surgery* **129**, 39-47 [2001].

[40] C. A. Adams, D. Z. Xu, L.Q., E. A. Deitch, *Surgery* **129**, 351-362 [2001].

[41] J. Barroso-Aranda, B. W. Zweifach, J. C. Mathison, G. W. Schmid-Schonbein, *J Cardiovasc Pharmacol* **25**, S23-9. [1995].

[42] N. Harada, K. Okajima, S. Mushimoto, *Crit Care Med* **27**, 1958-1064 [1999]; D. D. H. Koo, K. I. Welsh, J. A. Roake, P. J. Morris, S. V. Fuggle, *Am J Pathol* **153**, 557-566 [1998].

[43] E. Noack, in *Proteinasen Inhibitoren* K. H. Grötzinger, A. Schrey, R. W. Wabnitz, Eds. [Universitätsdruckerei und Verlag Dr C. Wolf und Sohn, München, 1981] pp. 44-56.

[44] K. M. Kerr *et al.*, *Am J Respir Crit Care Med* **162**, 14-20 [2000].

[45] K. Koike *et al.*, *Crit Care Med* **22**, 1438-1444 [1994].

[46] E. A. Deitch, H. P. Shi, Q. Lu, E. Feketeova, Z. Xu da, *Shock* **19**, 452-6. [2003].

[47] R. J. Goris, T. P. te Boekhorst, J. K. Nuytinck, J. S. Gimbrere, *Arch Surg* **120**, 1109-15. [1985].

[48] L. W. Norton, *Am J Surg* **149**, 347-50. [1985].

[49] F. Fitzal *et al.*, *Surgery* **134**, 1-11 [2003].

[50] G. A. P. Nieuwenhuijzen *et al.*, *Ann Surg* **218**, 791-799 [1993].

[51] J. J. Doucet *et al.*, *J Trauma*, [2004].

[52] W. J. Kramp *et al.*, *Shock* **20**, 356-62. [2003].

Index

A

B

C

D

H

I

J

K

L

M

N

O

P

R

S

T

U

V